Mosby's
Exam Review
for COMPUTED
TOMOGRAPHY

SECOND EDITION

Mosby's
Exam Review
for COMPUTED
TOMOGRAPHY

Daniel N. DeMaio, BS, RT(R)(CT)
Director
Radiologic Technology Program
University of Hartford
West Hartford, Connecticut

MOSBY

ELSEVIER

3251 Riverport Lane
St. Louis, Missouri 63043

MOSBY'S EXAM REVIEW FOR COMPUTED
TOMOGRAPHY, SECOND EDITION   ISBN: 978-0-323-06590-0
Copyright © 2011, 1996 by Mosby, Inc., an affiliate of Elsevier Inc.

Library of Congress Cataloging-in-Publication Data
DeMaio, Daniel N.
    Mosby's exam review for computed tomography / Daniel N. DeMaio. – 2nd ed.
      p. ; cm.
    Other title: Exam review for computed tomography
    Rev. ed. of: Registry review in computed tomography. c1996.
    Includes bibliographical references and index.
    ISBN 978-0-323-06590-0 (pbk. : alk. paper) 1. Tomography–Examinations, questions, etc.
    I. DeMaio, Daniel N. Registry review in computed tomography. II. Title. III. Title: Exam review
for computed tomography.
    [DNLM: 1. Tomography, X-Ray Computed–Examination Questions. WN 18.2 D369m 2011]
    RC78.7.T6D45 2011
    616.07'57076–dc22

                                                                      2010003503

Publisher: Jeanne Olson
Associate Developmental Editor: Amy Whittier
Publishing Services Manager: Pat Joiner-Myers, Radhika Pallamparthy
Senior Book Designer: Paula Catalano

Printed in the United States of America
Last digit is the print number: 9 8 7 6 5 4 3 2 1

For Thomas J. O'Rourke – a true inspiration.

CONTENT AND ORGANIZATION

Mosby's Exam Review for Computed Tomography is designed to prepare the radiologic technologist for successful completion of the American Registry of Radiologic Technologists (ARRT) Advanced Certification Examination for Computed Tomography. Since many general radiographers are now cross-training in computed tomography, and are performing computed tomography as part of their daily practice, this text will be a valuable resource for preparing for the Registry Exam.

This text first offers a thorough content review in an outline format of the three areas on the Computed Tomography Advanced Certification Exam: Patient Care, Imaging Procedures, and Physics and Instrumentation. The review is followed by, three 165-question mock examinations and answers keys.

FEATURES

Simulated Exams

The format of the questions is similar to the ARRT examination. Answers and rationales are provided for each question.

Evolve Resources

One of the most valuable features of this review resource is the accompanying Evolve site, http://evolve.elsevier.com/DeMaio/CT. The Evolve site contains 630 questions that can be randomly accessed to compile an unlimited number of variations of mock examinations. Exams on the Evolve site may be taken in quiz mode with immediate feedback or in a timed mode to simulate the actual exam experience.

Daniel N. DeMaio

ACKNOWLEDGMENTS

I wish to thank the professional staff of Elsevier for their support during the publication of this text. Ms. Jeanne Olson, Publisher, Health Professions, adeptly guided me through each step of the process from initial idea to finished product. Most important she is blessed with a dedicated and outstanding staff. I am extremely grateful to Ms. Amy Whittier, who served as the Developmental Editor for this book. Her relaxed style of gentle, yet purposeful encouragement always seemed to provide just the correct dose of prodding needed to move things along. My sincere thanks also to Mary Pohlman, Senior Project Manager, Radhika Pallamparthy, Project Manager, and Karen Baer, Editorial Assistant, for their assistance throughout this project.

Ms. Jennifer Gallagher graciously reviewed the sections on Cardiac CT and made many excellent suggestions for improvement. While I absolutely take full responsibility for any errors in content, I remain indebted to her for her efforts.

I have had the opportunity to work with and learn from many excellent educators, clinicians, technologists, and administrative support staff for more than 20 years and across three states. So to my friends and colleagues at the C.W. Post Campus of Long Island University, Great Neck Imaging, and Grappell & Walker Radiology in New York, Mercy Health System of Northwest Arkansas, and Milford Hospital in Connecticut, I offer my sincere gratitude.

To my colleagues at the University of Hartford, thank you for warmly welcoming me to campus and for your guidance, encouragement, and support. Thank you to all of my students from the past two decades. I continue to learn so much more from you than I could ever hope to teach.

To my wife Christine, you are the greatest friend and partner anyone could ever ask for. This book adds to the growing list of our joint accomplishments. As always, this one would not have been possible without you. To Ryan and Emily, you are the absolute joys of my life. I love you both more than words can describe. I can now answer that question you both asked me so, so many times, "Yes, Daddy is finally finished with that book!"

Daniel N. DeMaio

CONTENTS

Introduction

AMERICAN REGISTRY OF RADIOLOGIC TECHNOLOGISTS POST-PRIMARY CERTIFICATION IN COMPUTED TOMOGRAPHY

Technologists who wish to enter the post-primary pathway to certification in computed tomography (CT) must hold a registration in one of the following supporting categories:

- Radiography
- Nuclear Medicine Technology
- Radiation Therapy

In addition, candidates for CT certification are required to first document performance of core clinical procedures to establish eligibility. Specific clinical requirements and documentation procedures/forms may be obtained from the American Registry of Radiologic Technologists (ARRT).

The ARRT post-primary examination in CT was first offered in March of 1995. It was designed to give the technologist an opportunity to become certified in the specific modality of computed tomography. The CT registry is a 165-question, multiple-choice examination covering three major subject areas in the following manner:

Patient Care: 31 questions
Imaging Procedures: 76 questions
Physics and Instrumentation: 58 questions

The content specifications for the ARRT examination in CT are provided in the box at the end of this chapter. The approximate number of test questions for each major topic is provided in parentheses. The computer-based CT certification examination is currently given at specific test centers located throughout the United States. Please contact the ARRT (www.ARRT.org) for additional information regarding application procedures, deadlines, testing center locations, and so on.

USING THIS REVIEW BOOK

The first edition of this book, titled *Registry Review in Computed Tomography,* was developed shortly after I had successfully completed the CT registry examination in March of 1995. This second, expanded edition incorporates much of the information included in the first edition but has been vastly updated. It is designed for two different groups of examination applicants. For the established CT technologist, the review outline and examination questions help bridge the gap between clinical experience and cognitive knowledge. Those of you who are experienced in computed tomography will already be familiar with much of the subject matter covered. This review book allows you to answer questions concerning the principles and procedures that you put into practice each day. Used in conjunction with some additional reference materials, this book should adequately prepare you for the CT certification examination.

Keep in mind that the CT certification examination is an "advanced-level" examination. Some of the subject matter may go beyond the standard responsibilities of the staff CT technologist. Practical experience in computed tomography does not eliminate the need for study and preparation in order to achieve success on this examination.

Many examinees may be looking to use the advanced-level examination in CT as a vehicle towards developing a career in computed tomography. This second group of test applicants may have little experience in computed tomography beyond the ARRT clinical core requirements. If you are among this group, you have a significantly larger amount of work ahead of you. It would certainly be advisable to use several of the textbooks listed as references in the Bibliography during the initial stages of preparation. It is extremely important to review the physical principles of CT imaging along with the many clinical applications, such as patient care, scanning protocols, cross-sectional anatomy, and the identification of pathology on the CT image. *Mosby's Exam Review for Computed Tomography* will then serve as an invaluable tool to test your newly acquired knowledge and practice "registry-type" questions.

Please remember that the best way to reap benefits from review books such as this one is to concentrate on the material you are unfamiliar with: the questions that you *incorrectly* answer. It is not sufficient to simply grade each examination and calculate your score to determine whether or not you passed the examination. Take the time to carefully review each chapter. If you find that you are in need of further explanation, turn to the bibliography listed for additional study. Attempt the practice examinations with the mindset that they are "dry runs" for the real thing. After grading a practice examination, concentrate on the questions that you answered incorrectly. Look up each correct answer, read the brief explanation given, and then further review the topic in the review chapter and/or bibliography provided. You have much more to learn from the mistakes that you make, and when properly used, this book will give you the information you need.

TEXT FORMAT

Mosby's Exam Review for Computed Tomography contains a review, in outline form, of the three content areas covered on the ARRT certification examination in CT. The review chapters are followed by three full-length practice examinations. Each examination contains 165 multiple-choice questions. The topics for questions follow the content specifications of the ARRT advanced-level examination in computed tomography. Each practice examination is weighted concerning subject area in a similar manner to the certification examination.

Section III contains the correct answers to each examination. A brief explanation accompanies each correct answer and more detailed information about the question's subject may be found in the review chapters.

Many of the questions in each examination pertain to an included CT image. Be sure to use all of the information provided by the image when attempting to correctly answer these questions.

STUDY HABITS AND TEST-TAKING TECHNIQUES

Each of you preparing to take the ARRT examination in computed tomography is a registered and/or licensed medical imaging technologist. Most of you have already successfully completed an ARRT examination in an imaging discipline. You undoubtedly know how to take standardized examinations, and your previous results support this assumption. However, it may have been some time since you participated in a standardized examination, so here are some points to assist you in your preparation:

1. Do Not Wait Until the Last Minute to Prepare!

Although easier said than done, beginning to study early definitely improves your potential for success. The review chapters are just that—a review! They provide succinct outlines of the pertinent material and will serve as an excellent resource. But you may also find yourself in need of additional, more in-depth information. There is a multitude of excellent resources in both print and online forms. Start with a general text in the physical principles of computed tomography, and progress through the many clinical applications of CT. Also, a large proportion of the examination pertains to cross-sectional anatomy. Do not rely only on your practical experience in this area. Take care to review the CT images in this text. You may also want to refer to the cross-sectional anatomy books listed in the bibliography for additional review. For some people, this book may be sufficient as the sole preparatory tool for the CT examination. However, it is not a "quick fix" and will not make up for lack of adequate experience, research, and study.

2. Practice Your Time Management Skills

Time management is equally important during preparation and while you are taking the actual examination. You have 3.5 hours to complete 165 questions. This should be more than sufficient if you take care to keep track of your progress during the examination. Bring a watch with you to the testing center, and follow the standard rule of not spending too much time on any one question.

3. Zero In on the Correct Answer

Success on standardized examinations relies on your ability not only to choose the correct answer but also to identify the incorrect ones. The process of elimination is your most valued asset when you encounter a multiple-choice question. Carefully examine each answer, and eliminate those that are obviously incorrect. This step often narrows the possible choices and improves your chances when guessing becomes a necessity.

4. Have Confidence!

You are in the midst of a successful career in medical imaging. Your interest in the field and your dedication to continued learning has brought you here to this advanced-level examination. Have confidence in your ability, and put some faith in your preparation and experience: You know the material, so relax, and simply tap into this knowledge.

AMERICAN REGISTRY OF RADIOLOGIC TECHNOLOGISTS CT CERTIFICATION EXAMINATION: CONTENT SPECIFICATIONS

PATIENT CARE (31 QUESTIONS)

1. Patient Preparation (2 Questions)
 a. Consent
 b. Scheduling and Screening
 c. Patient Education
 d. Immobilization

2. Patient Assessment (4 Questions)
 a. History
 b. Monitoring
   • Vital signs
   • Heart rhythm and cardiac cycle
   • Oximetry
 c. Lab Values
   • Renal function (e.g., BUN, creatinine clearance, GFR, creatinine)
   • Blood coagulation (e.g., PT, PTT, platelet, INR)
   • Other (e.g., D dimer)
 d. Medications

3. IV Procedures (5 Questions)
 a. Venipuncture
   • Site selection
   • Aseptic and sterile technique
 b. Injection Techniques
   • Manual
   • Automatic
     ○ Single-phase
     ○ Multiphase
     ○ Flow rate

4. Contrast Agents (10 Questions)
 a. Types
   • Ionic, non-ionic
   • Hyper-osmolar, iso-osmolar
   • Barium sulfate
   • Water-soluble (iodinated)
   • Air
   • Water

 b. Administration Route and Dose Calculations
   • IV
   • Oral
   • Rectal
   • Intrathecal
   • Catheters
   • Intra-articular
 c. Special Considerations
   • Allergy preparation
   • Pathologic processes
   • Contraindications
   • Indications
 d. Adverse Reactions
   • Recognition and assessment of symptoms
   • Treatment (e.g., compresses, medications)
   • Documentation

5. Radiation Safety and Dosimetry (10 Questions)
 a. Technical Factors Affecting Patient Dose
   • kVp
   • mAs
   • Pitch
   • Collimation
   • mA modulation techniques
   • Multidetector configuration
   • Gating
 b. Radiation Protection
 c. Dose Measurement
   • CT Dose Index (CTDI)
   • Multiple Scan Average Dose (MSAD)
   • Dose Length Product (DLP)
 d. Patient Dose Reduction
   • Pediatric
   • Adult

IMAGING PROCEDURES (76 QUESTIONS)

Type of Study	Focus of Questions

1. Head (13 Questions)
  a. Cranial nerves
  b. Internal auditory canal
  c. Petrous pyramid
  d. Pituitary
  e. Orbit
  f. Paranasal sinuses
  g. Maxillofacial
  h. Temporomandibular joint
  i. Posterior fossa
  j. Brain
  k. Cranium
  l. Vascular

2. Neck (7 Questions)
  a. Larynx
  b. Soft tissue neck
  c. Vascular

3. Chest (14 Questions)
  a. Mediastinum
  b. Lung
  c. Heart
  d. Airway
  e. Vascular

4. Abdomen (23 Questions)
  a. Liver
  b. Biliary
  c. Spleen
  d. Pancreas
  e. Adrenals
  f. Kidneys/ureters
  g. Peritoneum
  h. Retroperitoneum
  i. GI tract
  j. Vascular

5. Pelvis (6 Questions)
  a. Bladder
  b. Colorectal
  c. Reproductive organs
  d. Vascular

6. Musculoskeletal (13 Questions)
  a. Upper extremity
  b. Lower extremity
  c. Spine
  d. Pelvis; hips
  e. Shoulder
  f. Sternum
  g. Vascular

Questions about each of the studies listed on the left may focus on any of the following relevant factors:

1. Sectional Anatomy
  • Sagittal plane
  • Transverse plane (axial)
  • Coronal plane
  • Off-axis (oblique)
  • Landmarks
  • Pathology recognition

2. Contrast Media
  • Types of agents
  • Indications
  • Contraindications
  • Dose calculation
  • Administration route
  • Scan/prep delay (e.g., bolus timing, test bolus)

3. Scanning Procedures
  • Positioning
  • Scout
  • Acquisition methods (e.g., volumetric, axial, sequential)
  • Parameter selection (e.g., slice thickness, mA, time, algorithm, pitch)
  • Protocol modification for pathology or trauma
  • CT angiography
  • Cardiac gating

4. Special Procedures
  • 3D studies
  • Biopsies
  • Radiation therapy planning
  • Drainage
  • Post myelography
  • CT arthrography
  • Hybrid imaging

Continued

PHYSICS AND INSTRUMENTATION (58 QUESTIONS)

1. CT System Principles, Operation and Components (17 Questions)
  a. Tube
    - kVp
    - mA
    - Warm-up procedures
  b. Generator and Transformers
  c. Detector Configuration
  d. Data Acquisition System (DAS)
  e. Collimation
  f. Computer and Array Processor
  g. Equipment Maintenance

2. Image Processing (10 Questions)
  a. Reconstruction
    - Filtered backprojection reconstruction
    - Reconstruction filters (algorithms)
    - Raw data vs. image data
    - Prospective/retrospective reconstruction
    - Effective slice thickness
    - Reconstruction interval
  b. Post-Processing
    - Multiplanar reformation
    - 3D rendering (MIP, SSD, VR)
    - Quantitative analysis (e.g., distance, diameter, calcium scoring, ejection fraction)

3. Image Display (10 Questions)
  a. Pixel, Voxel
  b. Matrix
  c. Image Magnification
  d. Field of View (scan, reconstruction and display)
  e. Attenuation Coefficient
  f. Window Level, Window Width
  g. Plane Specification (x, y, z coordinates)
  h. Cine
  i. ROI (single and multiple image)

4. Informatics (5 Questions)
  a. Hard/Soft Copy (e.g., DICOM file format)
  b. Storage/Archive
  c. PACS
  d. Security and Confidentiality
  e. Networking

5. Image Quality (10 Questions)
  a. Spatial Resolution
  b. Contrast Resolution
  c. Temporal Resolution
  d. Noise and Uniformity
  e. Quality Assurance
  f. CT Number
  g. Linearity

6. Artifact Recognition and Reduction (6 Questions)
  a. Beam Hardening
  b. Partial Volume Averaging
  c. Motion
  d. Metallic
  e. Edge Gradient
  f. Patient Positioning
  g. Equipment-Induced
    - Rings
    - Streaks
    - Tube arcing
    - Cone beam

Review of Patient Care in Computed Tomography

PATIENT PREPARATION

A. Consent

1. The patient is required to provide informed consent before the start of any invasive procedure.
2. Patient consent may be deemed "informed" only when the procedure, including its risks, benefits, and alternatives, are clearly explained in a language the patient fully comprehends.
3. Any patient questions must be adequately answered by qualified personnel before the procedure is begun.
4. The patient or a competent, legal representative must sign a form documenting informed consent for the procedure.
5. A parent or legal guardian must sign the informed consent form for a minor.
6. *Implied consent* occurs when a patient is in need of immediate medical services but is unconscious or is physically unable to consent to treatment. In this case, services are rendered with the assumption that the patient would consent if able.

B. Patient Screening/Education

1. Communication is the key to any successful patient interaction.
2. It should begin during the scheduling/screening process to identify concerns regarding exam tolerance, potential contrast agent contraindications, and so on.
3. Clear and thorough explanation by the technologist at the point-of-care helps make certain that the patient follows the instructions necessary for optimum exam quality.
4. Review breathing instructions when necessary, and include an opportunity for the patient to practice to ensure understanding and compliance.
5. Particularly during contrast studies, the patient should be instructed to empty the bladder before the start of the exam to reduce the possibility of discomfort or interruption.

6. Before contrast agent administration, discuss potential physical effects, such as warm sensation and metallic taste so that the patient is not surprised and upset during data acquisition.
7. High-density or metallic items, such as jewelry, hair fasteners, and electronic devices, should be removed when necessary and appropriate.
8. Care must be taken to ensure patient comfort on the CT table. This comfort will result in less patient motion and lead to higher-quality CT examinations.

C. Immobilization

1. As with any imaging procedure, patient motion during the CT exam can cause substantial image degradation.
2. CT scan manufacturers routinely include a variety of cushions, straps, and other safety devices that may be carefully used to help the patient hold still during data acquisition. These items are typically nonabrasive and can be utilized in place of medical tape.
3. The *breath-hold* is another form of patient immobilization required during many CT examinations. Carefully instruct the patient to suspend respiration at the end of inhalation or exhalation, providing a visual example when necessary. Cessation of breathing works to reduce motion and is particularly important during CT imaging of the chest and abdomen.

ASSESSMENT AND MONITORING

A. Patient History

1. Obtaining an accurate and pertinent patient history is one of the most important responsibilities of the CT technologist.
2. Proper documentation of the patient's recent procedures, surgeries, symptoms, possible trauma, and specific areas of pain or discomfort can greatly assist the radiologist in the diagnostic process.

3. General practices necessary to obtain a good patient history include the following:
   a. Non-leading or open-ended questions that allow the patient to provide the history in his or her own words.
   b. Keen listening and encouragement to maximize the information given.
   c. Focused questioning for additional information.
   d. Repeating and summarizing the information provided by the patient to check for accuracy.

B. Patient Monitoring

1. Vital sign assessment is the measurement of basic body functions to monitor critical information regarding the patient's physical condition.
2. Vital signs are temperature, pulse, blood pressure, and respirations:
   a. Normal body temperature is 97.7° to 99.5° F (36.5° to 37.5° C).
   b. Pulse rate for adults ranges from 60 to 100 beats per minute. Pulse rate for children ranges from 70 to 120 beats per minute.
   c. *Systolic blood pressure* indicates the pressure within arteries during cardiac contraction and should be less than 120 mm Hg. *Diastolic pressure* is measured during relaxation of the heart and should be less than 80 mm Hg.
   d. Normal respiration rate for an adult is 12 to 20 breaths per minute, and that for a child is 20 to 30 breaths per minute.
3. A *pulse oximeter* is an electronic device used to measure pulse and respiratory status. Placed on a patient's finger, toe, or ear lobe, the pulse oximeter measures blood oxygen levels, which are normally between 95% and 100%.
4. The *cardiac cycle* refers to the series of blood flow–related events that occur from the beginning of one heartbeat to that of the next.
5. It is the frequency of the cardiac cycle that determines the patient's heart rate.
6. As related to the cardiac cycle, *diastole* refers to relaxation of heart muscle, and *systole* refers to contraction of the heart muscle.
7. An electrocardiogram (ECG or EKG) is a graphic representation of the electrical activity of the heart. It is used particularly during cardiac CT procedures to evaluate the heart rhythm and cycle (Fig. 2-1).
8. The cardiac cycle can be divided into the following three distinct stages:
   a. Atrial systole:
      • Contraction of the left and right atria.
      • Corresponds to the onset of the P wave of the ECG.
   b. Ventricular systole:
      • Contraction of the left and right ventricles.
      • Beginning of the QRS complex on the ECG.

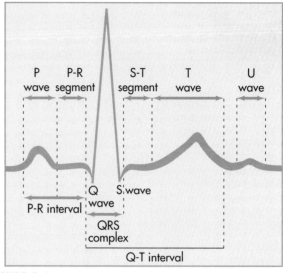

FIGURE 2-1 Normal ECG waveform. *(From Ehrlich RA, Daley JA: Patient Care in Radiography, 7th ed. St Louis, Mosby, 2009.)*

   c. Complete cardiac diastole:
      • Period of relaxation after heart contraction.
      • Consists of ventricular diastole and atrial diastole.
      • Corresponds to the T wave of the ECG.
9. Cardiac CT images are typically reconstructed from data acquired during the diastolic phase.
10. Patients with slower heart rates exhibit longer diastolic phases, which yield higher-quality cardiac CT exams.
11. β-Adrenergic receptor blocking agents (β-blockers) may be used to reduce a patient's heart rate. Sixty-five beats per minute (65 bpm) is the preferred rate for optimal imaging on most multislice CT (MSCT) systems.
12. Newer systems at the 64-slice level and beyond are capable of acquiring adequate cardiac CT images at higher heart rates. This capability may preclude the need for pharmaceutical intervention as clinically indicated.
13. If not contraindicated, sublingual nitroglycerine may be administered just before the cardiac MSCT study to cause dilation of the coronary vessels, improving their visualization.
14. Please consult the physician and/or department protocol for further information regarding administration of pharmaceuticals for cardiac CT procedures.

C. Laboratory Values

1. A number of laboratory values are important for the CT technologist to recognize and understand, particularly as they relate to the patient's capacity to undergo iodinated contrast agent administration (Table 2-1).

TABLE 2-1	Normal Assessment Signs and Laboratory Values in the Adult Patient
Temperature	97.7° to 99.5° F (36.5° to 37.5° C)
Pulse	60-100 beats per minute
Blood pressure	Systolic—less than 120 mm Hg Diastolic—less than 80 mm Hg
Respiration rate	12-20 breaths per minute
Pulse oximetry	95%-100%
Blood urea nitrogen (BUN)	7-25 mg/dL
Creatinine (Cr)	0.5-1.5mg/dL
BUN/Cr ratio	6-22:1
Glomerular filtration rate (GFR)	70 ± 14 mL/min/m² for men 60 ± 10 mL/min/m² for women
Prothrombin time (PT)	12-15 seconds
Partial thromboplastin time (PTT)	25-35 seconds
International Normalized Ratio (INR)	0.8-1.2
Platelet count	140,000-440,000 µL of blood

2. Blood urea nitrogen (BUN) and creatinine level are laboratory values used to indicate renal function. These values may be examined individually or in ratio form, as follows:
   a. Normal BUN values in adults range from 7 to 25 mg/dL. Range may vary depending on laboratory testing reference. By itself, BUN is not a sufficient indicator of renal insufficiency.
   b. Normal creatinine levels range from 0.5 to 1.5 mg/dL. Range may also vary with lab reference. An elevated creatinine value (>1.5 mg/dL) may not always indicate renal function compromise, because this value can vary widely with different populations. Recent changes in a patient's creatinine level are thought to be more informative as a renal function indicator.
   c. The BUN/creatinine ratio may also be used to evaluate renal function. Normal BUN/creatinine ratio is approximately 6:1 to 22:1, and this reference is laboratory-specific.
3. Glomerular filtration rate (GFR) is a more accurate measure of renal function. GFR is an approximation of creatinine clearance or the rate by which creatinine is filtered from the blood stream. GFR is calculated using the patient's measured serum creatinine level and takes into account the patient's age, sex, and race. The normal range of GFR is 70 ± 14 mL/min/m² for men and 60 ± 10 mL/min/m² for women.
4. Prothrombin time (PT) is a measure of blood coagulation. The normal range for PT is approximately 12 to 15 seconds.
5. Prothrombin time (PT) is measured in the lab after the addition of a protein called *tissue factor* to a patient's blood sample.

6. Owing to the inherent differences in manufactured batches of tissue factor, the International Normalized Ratio (INR) is calculated to standardize PT results. The INR compares a patient's PT with a control sample for a more accurate result.
7. The normal range for INR is 0.8 to 1.2.
8. Partial thromboplastin time (PTT) is an additional lab value used to detect abnormalities in blood clotting. Normal range for clotting time is generally 25 to 35 seconds.
9. Platelet count is also used to assess the patient's clotting ability. Normal platelet count is 140,000 to 440,000 per mm³ (or µL) of blood.
10. D-dimer testing is utilized for the diagnosis of deep vein thrombosis (DVT) and pulmonary embolism. Although nonspecific, the presence of elevated amounts of D-dimer in the bloodstream may indicate recently degraded blood clots. If the D-dimer value is elevated, additional testing such as CT angiography of the pulmonary arteries may be indicated.

D. Medications

1. Coumadin is a proprietary name for the generic drug warfarin, an anticoagulant. This drug is used to prevent the formation of blood clots in veins and arteries and may reduce the incidence of heart attack and stroke. Patients undergoing therapy with warfarin or any other anticoagulant are prone to excessive bleeding due to trauma, including intravenous (IV) access for contrast agent administration. The CT professional must take special precautions when providing care to the patient undergoing anticoagulant therapy. Adequate pressure must be applied to the site after IV removal to avoid excessive bleeding and bruising.
2. Metformin, also commonly referred to by the brand name Glucophage, is a drug used to treat type 2 diabetes. Patients are typically instructed not to take a metformin product for up to 2 days following a contrast-enhanced CT examination. There is a small risk of renal impairment from iodinated contrast agents, and reduced renal function can cause the potentially harmful retention of metformin within the body. The patient should consult the referring physician for instructions before resuming metformin treatment. A blood test to check renal function may be required.

INTRAVENOUS PROCEDURES

A. Venipuncture

1. The injection of a medication or contrast agent directly into the bloodstream is a type of parenteral administration.

2. Iodinated contrast agents are typically administered intravenously during CT examinations.
3. Sites commonly used for IV administration of radiopaque contrast agents include (Fig. 2-2):
   a. The anterior recess of the elbow, or antecubital space.
   b. The radial aspect of the wrist.
   c. The anterior surface of the forearm.
   d. The posterior portion of the hand.
4. IV administration requires strict adherence to standard precautions and aseptic technique.
5. *Aseptic technique* refers to the practices and procedures that a practitioner employs to reduce the risk of infection during the IV administration of contrast media.
6. Components of aseptic technique include:
   a. Thorough hand washing between patients.
   b. Wearing of disposable gloves.
   c. Cleaning of the site of venipuncture in a circular motion with an alcohol swab, moving from the center to the outside.

d. Application of gentle pressure with an alcohol swab to the venipuncture site after removal of the needle/catheter.
7. *Sterile technique* refers to the practices and procedures used to maintain a sterile, microorganism-free environment during invasive CT procedures such as biopsy, aspiration, and CT arthrogram.
8. Sterile technique involves establishing a field around the area of interest that is free of all microorganisms. The procedure is performed within this sterile field with the use of sterile equipment and supplies.

B. Injection Technique

1. There are generally two approaches to IV administration of iodinated contrast agents, as follows:
   a. *Drip infusion*, whereby the volume of contrast agent is administered at a slow rate over a long period. Because this method results in a slow rise in blood iodine concentration, it is no longer typically used in most CT procedures.

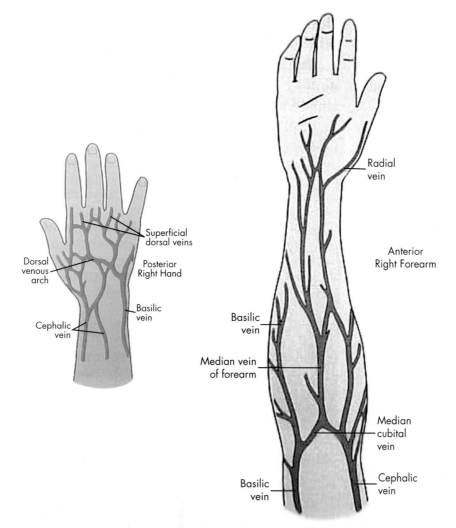

FIGURE 2-2 Upper extremity veins commonly used for venipuncture. *(From Jensen SC, Peppers MP: Pharmacology and Drug Administration for Imaging Technologists, 2nd ed. St Louis, Mosby, 2005.)*

b. *Bolus injection*, whereby the iodinated contrast agent is "pushed" into the bloodstream at a rapid rate over a short period. This results in a sharp peak of iodine concentration in the blood, yielding a more pronounced pattern of contrast enhancement.

2. Bolus administration may be accomplished by hand, meaning that the volume of contrast agent is manually injected into the bloodstream.

3. Automatic power injectors are commonly used for IV administration of contrast agents during CT examinations.

4. Power injectors are capable of consistently injecting large volumes of contrast agent at flow rates up to 5 to 6 mL/sec. Flow rate is determined by several factors, including clinical area of interest, contrast volume, venous access, patient condition, and pressure capacity of the IV materials utilized.

5. IV administration of contrast agent by power injector should be performed through flexible plastic angiocatheters rather than standard metal needles.

6. 22-gauge angiocatheters are sufficient for flow rates up to 3 mL/sec. 20-gauge or larger angiocatheters should be utilized whenever flow rates exceed 3 mL/sec.

7. Care must be taken to remove air from the injector syringe and connective tubing to eliminate the risk of air embolism.

8. Proper "bleeding" of the tubing eliminates air, and the injector syringe should remain in a downward position before administration of the contrast agent.

9. Once the total volume of contrast agent has been administered, scanning proceeds at set intervals based on the anatomic area of interest and the rate at which enhancement occurs.

10. Many CT systems have bolus tracking software to assist the technologist in acquiring CT images during periods of peak contrast enhancement.

11. During *single-phase imaging*, CT image acquisition occurs at a single specific time during or after the injection of the contrast agent. Images are acquired in this fashion during a single period of contrast enhancement.

12. *Multiphase imaging* involves the acquisition of multiple series of CT images over timed intervals. CT images may be acquired before, during, and after the administration of iodinated contrast agent. The periods of delay between subsequent acquisitions are determined by the clinical indication.

13. Automatic power injectors offer several advantages over manual injection of iodinated contrast during CT examination, including:
    a. Consistent, reproducible flow rates.
    b. Precise volume/dosage control.
    c. Higher injection rates for optimal contrast enhancement.
    d. Automatic delays for proper enhancement patterns and multiphase imaging.

14. The ability to administer normal saline as a flushing agent is an additional advantage of automatic power injectors in CT. Flushing the tubing with a volume of saline (30-50 mL) immediately after the contrast agent bolus allows for a reduction of contrast agent dose and helps eliminate the streaking artifact that often results from a high concentration of iodine in the mediastinal vasculature.

15. Dual-head power injectors can accommodate both the dose of iodinated contrast agent and the volume of saline flush in a convenient and accurate manner.

16. The major disadvantage of the use of a CT power injector is the increased risk of *extravasation*, or infiltration of the contrast agent outside the blood vessel. Extravasation of contrast agent into the surrounding tissue is extremely painful and a potentially serious consequence.

17. The technologist must take care to ensure the patency of the venous access before power injection. Before the injection is initialized, the technologist should check venous backflow by drawing back manually on the injector and observing blood flow into the connective tubing.

18. If venous backflow is not obtained, the catheter may need repositioning and should be checked with a test injection of saline before contrast administration.

19. The technologist must closely observe the contrast agent administration with initial palpation of the IV site. Power injection must be stopped immediately if extravasation occurs.

20. In the event of extravasation, the needle/catheter should be removed, and pressure applied with a warm, moist compress.

CONTRAST AGENTS

1. Contrast media are used during many CT procedures in an effort to increase the contrast between, and subsequent visibility of, the multitude of anatomic structures and pathologic conditions whose radiographic densities are too similar to be adequately separated.

2. The contrast agents utilized during CT procedures can be broken down into two basic types, positive and negative.

3. The positive contrast agents belong to a class of substances known as *radiopaque contrast media* (RCM).

4. The RCM typically used as for CT examinations are iodine and barium.

5. The degree of radiopacity exhibited by an iodinated contrast agent is directly proportional to the agent's concentration of iodine.

6. The degree of radiopacity exhibited by a barium contrast agent is directly proportional to the agent's concentration of barium.

7. Iodinated RCM are water-soluble compounds that may be administered:

a. Generally into the bloodstream intravenously.
b. Directly into a targeted vein or artery for localized enhancement.
c. Directly into the intrathecal space during CT myelography.
d. Into the joint space during CT arthrography.
e. Orally to opacify the gastrointestinal (GI) tract.

8. Suspensions of barium sulfate are commonly employed as positive contrast agents for opacification of the GI tract.

A. Types

1. Intravascular Radiopaque Contrast Media

a. Initial opacification of blood vessels allows for their anatomic visualization and differentiation from surrounding structures. Contrast enhancement of vasculature greatly aids in the diagnosis of many disorders, including aneurysm, thrombus, and stenosis.

b. Over time the contrast agent is distributed from the vasculature into the extravascular space. This interstitial redistribution of contrast agent can result in differentiation of normal from abnormal soft tissue on the basis of enhancement patterns.

c. As the kidneys excrete the contrast agent, opacification of the renal collecting system occurs. This process improves visualization of the renal pelvis, ureters, and bladder.

d. *Osmolality* is an important characteristic of an iodinated radiopaque contrast agent. It describes the agent's propensity to cause fluid from outside the blood vessel (extravascular space) to move into the bloodstream (intravascular space).

e. Iodinated RCM can be generally divided into the following categories:
   • *Ionic contrast media* are salts consisting of sodium and/or meglumine. Each molecule of ionic contrast agent consists of three iodine atoms. When injected into the bloodstream, each molecule dissociates into two charged particles, or ions. The production of osmotic ions is indicative of high-osmolar contrast media (HOCM). Examples of HOCM are iothalamate meglumine (Conray) and diatrizoate sodium (Hypaque).
   • *Non-ionic contrast media* are non-salt chemical compounds that also contain three atoms of iodine per molecule. They do not dissociate in solution. These substances are commonly referred to as low-osmolar contrast media (LOCM). Examples of LOCM are iohexol (Omnipaque), iopamidol (Isovue), and ioversol (Optiray).

f. The osmolality of an iodinated radiopaque contrast medium greatly affects its potential for adverse effects in the patient.

g. Non-ionic low-osmolar contrast agents are less likely to produce adverse side effects and/or reactions than ionic high-osmolar RCM.

h. Iso-osmolar contrast media (IOCM) have the same osmolality as blood and therefore may offer improved patient comfort and a reduced potential for untoward side effects.

i. Iodixanol (Visipaque) is an example of a non-ionic iso-osmolar contrast agent.

2. Enteral Radiopaque Contrast Media

a. Enteral RCM are administered orally and/or rectally to opacify the GI tract.

b. Generally an enteral agent is either a water-soluble iodinated solution or a suspension of barium sulfate.

c. Barium sulfate suspensions are readily used as oral and rectal contrast agents for opacification of the GI tract.

d. Barium sulfate is an inert compound with excellent attenuation properties.

e. Routine transit time for barium sulfate through the GI tract is typically between 30 and 90 minutes.

f. Water-soluble oral contrast media can also be either high-osmolar or low-osmolar iodinated solutions.

g. High-osmolar contrast agents, such as diatrizoate meglumine and diatrizoate sodium, have traditionally been used as oral/rectal CT contrast media.

h. Newer low-osmolar contrasts such as iohexol may also be used as oral/rectal contrast media for CT.

i. Routine transit time for water-soluble iodinated contrast agents through the GI tract is typically between 30 and 90 minutes.

j. The important considerations in the choice between a water-soluble iodine oral contrast agent and barium sulfate are as follows:
   • Barium sulfate may be not be utilized in cases of suspected perforation because it may be toxic to the peritoneum.
   • Barium sulfate is contraindicated in patients who are to undergo surgery or other invasive procedures of the abdomen and/or pelvis.
   • Barium sulfate can be potentially harmful if aspirated.
   • Water-soluble oral contrast agents, particularly of the low-osmolar type, are usually more palatable and result in less GI distress.
   • Water-soluble oral contrast agents may be contraindicated in patients with known iodine allergy.

k. The contrast agent used for rectal CT may be administered via enema to opacify the distal large colon and rectum.

3. Negative Contrast Agents

a. Air, gases, and water may be used as negative contrast agents during CT examination.

b. Water may be used as an oral contrast agent to fill the GI tract. Advantages include:
   • Increased palatability and improved patient comfort.

- Better demonstration of the enhancing bowel wall.
- Does not interfere with three-dimensional (3D) applications.

c. Effervescent granules used to treat gas and acid indigestion may also be administered as negative oral contrast agents. When swallowed, these granules add negative contrast in the form of gas to the stomach and proximal small bowel, allowing for better visualization of these structures.

d. Water-soluble iodinated solutions may be mixed with carbonated beverages to add negative contrast to the GI tract, improving the demonstration of subtle disease.

e. Air acts as a contrast agent during CT imaging of the chest much like it does on a chest radiograph. Image acquisition at the end of full inspiration improves image quality during a CT examination of the chest.

f. Air may also be administered via enema to insufflate the large bowel to improve image quality during CT colonography.

g. CT colonography may also involve insufflation of the large intestine with CO_2. Distention of the large intestine with room air or CO_2 is necessary for optimal visualization of the bowel wall.

4. Neutral Contrast Agents

a. Neutral oral contrast agents may be administered to opacify the small bowel during procedures such as CT enteroclysis and CT enterography.

b. Neutral contrast media distend the GI tract while still allowing for clear visualization of the bowel wall.

c. Very low-density (0.1%) barium sulfate solutions such as VoLumen may be administered for detailed CT examination of the small bowel.

B. Administration Route and Dose Calculations

1. The IV administration of a contrast agent typically consists of an intravenous bolus injection through an 18- to 23-gauge angiocatheter or butterfly needle.

2. An *angiocatheter* is an IV catheter placed within a vein and used to administer fluids, medication, and/or contrast media.

3. It consists of a small plastic catheter surrounding a solid needle that acts as a stylet to allow the catheter to be placed within a vein. Once the angiocatheter is inside the vessel, the needle is retracted and the catheter is advanced into the vein.

4. The angiocatheter may be connected to a contrast agent syringe or an automated contrast agent delivery system. Connective tubing may be attached to facilitate the administration of fluids and/or medications.

5. Most current angiocatheters contain a built-in safety shield or retraction mechanism that guards against accidental sharps exposure.

6. *Needleless* IV access systems feature a reusable port device that allows the blunt plastic cannulas of syringes and connective tubing to be attached without needles. Needleless systems improve occupational safety by reducing the risk of accidental needlesticks.

7. A *butterfly needle* consists of a hollow needle surrounded by plastic flaps or "wings." The wings are grasped and lightly pinched together to facilitate insertion of the needle into a vein. The needle is attached to a short length of connective tubing. Once the needle is inserted into a vein, the plastic wings are secured with tape, and the tubing is attached to a syringe or IV drip.

8. Intravascular RCM are generally administered in doses ranging from 50 to 150 mL. Specific dose depends on the patient's age, weight, and renal function and on the clinical indication for the CT procedure as directed by a radiologist.

9. The serum iodine concentration is a measure of the amount of iodine within the bloodstream. The range of serum iodine concentration for adequate opacification during CT examination is 2 to 8 mg/mL.

10. An IV contrast agent may also be administered through a central venous catheter if it is of adequate type, material, and diameter. The manufacturer of the venous catheter should be consulted for specific tolerances before contrast agent administration.

11. Common types of central venous catheters are subclavian lines, implanted access ports, and peripherally inserted central catheters (PICC lines).

12. Flow rates for injections through central venous catheters such as PICC lines are typically reduced to well below 2 mL/sec. Please refer to the manufacturer and the department's specific protocol before using a central venous catheter for contrast agent administration.

13. Patency of central venous catheters should be tested for venous backflow and may require a test injection of saline for complete assurance.

14. The total volume of oral contrast agent administered for a CT examination should be adjusted according to the extent of bowel opacification required clinically, that is, proximal small bowel, distal small bowel, proximal large bowel, and so on.

15. An example of oral contrast agent protocol for CT examinations limited to the abdomen is as follows:
   a. 300 mL of oral contrast agent 30 minutes before scan.
   b. 150 mL of oral contrast agent immediately before scan.

16. For CT examinations of the entire abdomen and pelvis, substantial opacification of the stomach, small bowel, and proximal large bowel is typically required. An example protocol is:
    a. 450 mL of oral contrast agent 60-90 minutes before scan.
    b. 300 mL of oral contrast agent 30 minutes before scan.
    c. 150 mL of oral contrast agent immediately before scan.
17. If complete distention of the stomach is clinically necessary, the last dose of oral contrast agent may be accompanied by a dose of effervescent granules.
18. For studies of the distal large bowel, including the sigmoid colon and/or rectum, an oral contrast agent may need to be administered 4 to 6 hours before scan time to ensure sufficient opacification.
19. When this delay is not clinically appropriate, an oral contrast agent may be administered rectally, through an enema.
20. A 150- to 300-mL CT contrast agent enema is usually sufficient to adequately opacify the rectum, sigmoid, and distal large bowel.
21. A small amount of air (negative contrast) may also be administered rectally to improve bowel distention when clinically indicated.
22. *Intrathecal* administration of an iodinated contrast agent is the injection of the agent directly into the space surrounding the spinal cord.
23. Intrathecal injections are performed during CT myelography for evaluation of the spinal cord and nerve roots.
24. *Intra-articular* administration of a contrast agent is the injection of the agent directly into a joint space.
25. Intra-articular injections are performed during CT arthrography of joints, including the shoulder, wrist, and knee.

C. Special Considerations

1. In general, for patients who are to undergo administration of iodinated contrast agent, attention should be paid to the four Hs as outlined by the American College of Radiology (ACR):
   a. *History:* The CT professional should obtain a thorough patient history. Details regarding the patient's allergic and contrast agent history must be reviewed.
   b. *Hydration:* Particularly with patients who may be renally compromised, adequate hydration must be ensured before, during, and after the examination.
   c. *Have equipment and expertise ready:* A detailed plan to treat contrast agent reactions should be in place and should be practiced regularly.
   d. *Heads up!* Constant assessment of the patient's condition is vital for early identification and proper treatment of an adverse reaction.

2. Patients with increased risk of adverse reaction to iodinated contrast agents may be required to undergo a premedication regimen.
3. Each CT department should have a specific regimen for pretreatment of patients who are at increased risk for adverse reaction to iodinated contrast agents. The regimen typically consists of a combination of an antihistamine such as diphenhydramine HCL (Benadryl) and a corticosteroid, taken at timed intervals beginning as early as 24 hours before contrast agent injection.
4. Please consult the radiologist, ordering physician, and/or department protocol for a specific contrast premedication protocol.
5. Physiologic and pathologic processes that may increase the risk of adverse reaction from iodinated contrast include:
   a. Asthma.
   b. Environmental and/or food allergies.
   c. Renal disease.
   d. Multiple myeloma.
   e. Diabetes mellitus.
   f. Pheochromocytoma.
   g. Sickle cell disease.
   h. Hyperthyroidism.
   i. Significant cardiac disease.
6. Contraindications to IV iodinated contrast agents include:
   a. Allergy to iodine.
   b. Prior severe allergic reaction to an iodinated contrast agent.
   c. Renal insufficiency/failure.
7. Patients who are in chronic renal failure and undergoing dialysis may be candidates for IV contrast agent administration at the discretion of the radiologist and referring physician.
8. Although iodinated contrast media are known to cross the placental barrier, pregnancy is not a direct contraindication to their administration. However, caution must be used in determining the potential benefit of contrast agent administration in the pregnant patient because the risk of adverse reaction in the fetus is unknown.
9. Nursing mothers may be injected with iodinated contrast agents as clinically warranted. Caution again must be exercised because many such agents are excreted in breast milk. Nursing mothers are typically instructed to pump and discard breast milk for 24 hours after administration of a contrast agent to effectively eliminate risk to the infant.

D. Adverse Reactions

1. The use of non-ionic or low-osmolar contrast media (LOCM) significantly reduces the incidence of adverse reaction in comparison with the of ionic or high-osmolar contrast media (HOCM).

2. Although the likelihood of severe adverse reaction to LOCM is low, the exact incidence is not known.
3. The majority of adverse reactions to iodinated contrast agents can be characterized as mild and non–life-threatening.
4. Mild reactions to iodinated contrast media include:
   a. Nausea/vomiting.
   b. Mild urticaria (hives).
   c. Pronounced sensation of warmth and/or flushing.
   d. Altered taste.
   e. Sweats/chills.
   f. Nasal stuffiness/sneezing.
   g. Anxiety.
5. Mild reactions to iodinated contrast agents typically require no treatment. The patient should be positively reassured and closely observed until the symptoms dissipate.
6. Moderate reactions are also usually non–life-threatening. However, they may progress rapidly, so treatment may be necessary.
7. Moderate reactions to iodinated contrast include:
   a. Mild bronchospasm.
   b. Moderate to severe urticaria.
   c. Vasovagal response.
   d. Tachycardia from hypotension.
8. Treatment for moderate adverse reactions to iodinated contrast include:
   a. Bronchodilator inhaler and/or oxygen therapy for bronchospasm (wheezing).
   b. Diphenhydramine (Benadryl) for urticaria.
   c. Elevation of legs and IV fluids for hypotension.
9. Severe reactions to iodinated contrast agents are those that are potentially life-threatening and require immediate treatment.
10. Severe adverse reactions are rare.
11. They may begin with mild symptoms, such as anxiety and respiratory distress, and then progress rapidly.
12. Severe reactions to iodinated contrast include:
    a. Profound hypotension.
    b. Laryngeal edema.
    c. Severe bronchospasm.
    d. Pulmonary edema.
    e. Cardiac arrhythmia.
    f. Seizure.
    g. Cardiopulmonary arrest.
    h. Death.
13. Table 2-2 outlines the ABCD approach to the management of adverse reactions to contrast media.
14. Fig. 2-3 summarizes the treatment for severe adverse reactions to iodinated contrast agents in adults, as recommended by the American College of Radiology.
15. Delayed reactions to contrast agent administration can occur in a small percentage of patients.
16. Common delayed reactions include:
    a. Urticaria (hives).
    b. Pruritus (itchiness).
    c. Nausea/vomiting.
    d. Drowsiness.
    e. Headache.
    f. Fever/chills.
17. Cutaneous reactions are the most common and can occur within 3 hours to 7 days after administration of a contrast agent.
18. Delayed reactions to a contrast agent must be well-documented, followed closely, and treated appropriately as needed.
19. Contrast-induced nephrotoxicity (CIN) is a potentially serious delayed effect of contrast agent administration.
20. It is a considerable decline in renal function that can occur after a patient receives an IV contrast agent.

TABLE 2-2	ABCD Guide for Management of Adverse Reactions to Contrast Agents		
A	**B**	**C**	**D**
Assessment: Categorize the type of reaction and assess its severity. May include BP and or ECG monitoring	Breathing: Begin cardiopulmonary resuscitation when necessary; use Ambu-bag or mouth mask	Common denominators: Assess cardiac output as it is related to decreased venous return, fluid third-spacing, pulmonary edema, and so on	Do assess and monitor patient Do use correct dose and administration route for drugs
Airway: Maintain an open airway and administer oxygen when necessary	Beware of atypical responses, such as prevention of a tachycardia response by beta-blocker therapy	Categorize type of reaction and current patient status	Don't delay! Don't use incorrect drugs and/or dose
Assistance: Immediately call for it		Call cardiopulmonary arrest team; perform CPR	
Access: Obtain and/or secure IV access		Circulatory assistance: Administer intravenous fluids	

Modified from the ACR Manual On Contrast Media, Version 6, 2008

MANAGEMENT OF ACUTE REACTIONS TO CONTRAST MEDIA IN ADULTS

Urticaria

1. Discontinue injection if not completed.
2. No treatment needed in most cases.
3. Give H_1-receptor blocker: diphenhydramine (Benadryl) PO/IM/IV 25 to 50 mg.

   If severe or widely disseminated: give α-agonist (arteriolar and venous constriction): epinephrine SC (1:1000) 0.1 to 0.3 mL (= 0.1 to 0.3 mg) (if no cardiac contraindications).

Facial or Laryngeal Edema

1. Give O_2 6 to 10 L/min (via mask).
2. Give α-agonist (arteriolar and venous constriction): epinephrine SC or IM (1:1000) 0.1 to 0.3 mL (= 0.1-0.3 mg) or, especially if hypotension evident, epinephrine (1:10,000) slowly IV 1-3 mL (= 0.1-0.3 mg).

   Repeat as needed up to a maximum of 1 mg. If edema is not responsive to therapy or if there is obvious acute laryngeal edema, seek appropriate assistance (e.g., cardiopulmonary arrest response team).

Bronchospasm

1. Give O_2 6 to 10 L/min (via mask). Monitor: electrocardiogram, O_2 saturation (pulse oximeter), and blood pressure.
2. Give β-agonist inhalers [bronchiolar dilators, such as metaproterenol (Alupent), terbutaline (Brethaire), or albuterol (Proventil or Ventolin)] 2 to 3 puffs; repeat as necessary. If bronchospasm is unresponsive to inhalers, use SC, IM, or IV epinephrine.
3. Give epinephrine SC or IM (1:1000) 0.1- to 0.3 mL (= 0.1-0.3 mg) or, especially if hypotension evident, epinephrine (1:10,000) slowly IV 1-3 mL (= 0.1-0.3 mg). Repeat as needed up to a maximum of 1 mg.

   Call for assistance (e.g., cardiopulmonary arrest response team) for severe bronchospasm or if O_2 saturation < 88% persists.

Hypotension with Tachycardia

1. Elevate legs 60 degrees or more (preferred) or use the Trendelenburg position.
2. Monitor: electrocardiogram, pulse oximeter, blood pressure.
3. Give O_2 6 to 10 L/min (via mask).
4. Rapid intravenous administration of large volumes of lactated Ringer's solution or normal saline.

   If there is poor response to these measures, give epinephrine (1:10,000) slowly IV 1 mL (= 0.1 mg). Repeat as needed up to a maximum of 1 mg. If response is still poor, seek appropriate assistance (e.g., cardiopulmonary arrest response team).

Hypotension with Bradycardia (Vagal Reaction)

1. Secure airway: give O_2 6 to 10 L/min (via mask).
2. Monitor vital signs.
3. Elevate legs 60 degrees or more (preferred) or use the Trendelenburg position.
4. Secur response to steps IV access: rapid administration of lactated Ringer's solution or normal saline.
5. Give atropine 0.6-1 mg IV slowly if patient does not show a quick response to steps 2 to 4.
6. Repeat atropine up to a total dose of 0.04 mg/kg (2 to 3 mg) in an adult.
7. Ensure complete resolution of hypotension and bradycardia before discharge.

Hypertension, Severe

1. Give O_2 6 to 10 L/min (via mask).
2. Monitor electrocardiogram, pulse oximeter, blood pressure.
3. Give nitroglycerine 0.4-mg tablet, sublingual (may repeat × 3); or, topical 2% ointment, apply 1-inch strip.
4. If no response, consider labetalol 20 mg IV, then 20 to 80 mg IV every 10 minutes up to 300 mg.
5. Transfer patient to intensive care unit or emergency department.
6. For pheochromocytoma: phentolamine 5 mg IV (labetalol may be used if phentolamine is not available).

Seizures or Convulsions

1. Give O_2 6 to 10 L/min (via mask).
2. Consider diazepam (Valium) 5 mg IV (or more, as appropriate) or midazolam (Versed) 0.5-1 mg IV.
3. If longer effect needed, obtain consultation; consider phenytoin (Dilantin) infusion 15 to 18 mg/kg at 50 mg/min.
4. Careful monitoring of vital signs required, particularly of pO_2, because of risk to respiratory depression with benzodiazepine administration.
5. Consider using cardiopulmonary arrest response team for intubation if needed.

Pulmonary Edema

1. Give O_2 6 to 10 L/min (via mask).
2. Elevate torso.
3. Give diuretics: furosemide (Lasix) 20-40 mg IV, slow push.
4. Consider giving morphine 1 to 3 mg IV.
5. Transfer patient to intensive care unit or emergency department.

IM, intramuscularly; IV, intravenously; PO, orally; SC, subcutaneously.

FIGURE 2-3 Treatment for severe adverse reactions to iodinated contrast agents in adults as recommended by the American College of Radiology. *(From American College of Radiology: Manual on Contrast Media, Version 6. Reston, VA, American College of Radiology, 2008.)*

21. CIN has varied definitions but is usually signified by a marked increase in serum creatinine level over a baseline measurement obtained before contrast agent administration.
22. The causative relationship between contrast agent administration and CIN is not completely understood but may be related to renal vasoconstriction and/or the toxicity of the contrast medium itself.
23. The overall risk of CIN is directly related to the patient's preexisting renal function and hydration level.
24. Other risk factors for contrast-induced nephrotoxicity include:
    a. Diabetes.
    b. Myeloma.
    c. Advanced age.
    d. Cardiovascular disease.

25. Adequate hydration of the patient is the best method of CIN prevention.
26. In the patient with normal renal function, the risk for development of CIN is extremely low.
27. A baseline serum creatinine measurement should be obtained in all patients who are determined to be at risk for CIN.
28. If the patient is deemed renally impaired, alternative imaging options that do not involve contrast agent administration may be indicated.
29. Patients with non–insulin-dependent diabetes who are taking an oral biguanide (metformin) drug may also have a higher risk of CIN-related effects.
30. Patients receiving metformin drug therapy are at increased risk for lactic acidosis, a condition that may be exacerbated by renal insufficiency.
31. If the patient's renal function is adversely affected by administration of a contrast agent, there is a potential increase in incidence of lactic acidosis in the metformin-treated patient.
32. Patients who have associated risk factors for renal insufficiency and are currently taking a metformin drug are typically instructed not to take the metformin following the contrast study.
33. A lab test of renal function may be necessary before the patient resumes metformin therapy.
34. Please refer to the department protocol and/or the appropriate physician guidelines when administering contrast agents to patients receiving metformin drugs.
35. All information regarding patient care, including the procedure(s) performed, contrast/medication administered, untoward event(s), and final outcomes must be documented by the practitioner.
36. Documentation within the patient's medical record must be clear, concise, and recorded in a timely manner.

RADIATION SAFETY AND DOSIMETRY

A. Technical Factors Affecting Patient Radiation Dose

1. The factors affecting CT patient radiation dose can be divided into the following categories:
   a. System configuration.
   b. User settings.
2. The individual technical configuration of a CT system determines several characteristics that may affect patient dose:
   a. Source–detector distance: As the distance from the x-ray tube to the detectors decreases, dose increases.
   b. Filtration within the CT x-ray tube varies between approximately 6 and 9 mm aluminum (Al) or equivalent material. Filtration acts to remove the unwanted, "low-quality" portion of the x-ray beam that adds to the patient radiation dose while failing to yield useful acquisition data. Beam-shaping or bow-tie filters are also added to the x-ray tube to compensate for the noncylindrical nature of most body shapes. Additional filtration material along the periphery of the x-ray beam absorbs radiation where it is not necessary, thereby reducing the overall patient dose.
   c. Detector efficiency plays an important role in patient radiation dose and can be described in several ways:
      • The *inherent absorption efficiency* of each detector element describes the ability of the detector to capture transmitted x-ray quanta and produce the appropriate response. Inefficiency here can result in the loss of data and a subsequent compensatory increase in patient dose.
      • The *geometric efficiency* of a detector array describes the spatial arrangement of detector elements, including the amount of interspace material required between adjacent elements. The interspace material absorbs transmitted radiation but yields no response. This results in a loss of acquisition data (signal) and requires an increase in radiation dose to compensate. This is of particular importance in MSCT, in which the complex arrangement of multiple rows of detectors requires increased interspace material, resulting in a reduction in geometric efficiency.
   d. In order to expose the widened detector array equally, MSCT utilizes a cone-shaped beam, instead of the fan-shaped beam traditionally used by single-slice CT (SSCT) systems. All detectors of the array must be exposed to x-radiation of equal intensity. The beam must be expanded even further to avoid exposing the detectors to undesirable "penumbra." This process is referred to as *overbeaming*. CT image data are acquired from only a portion of the exposed detector array. This results in a radiation dose to the patient that does not contribute to the formation of the CT image. Some CT manufacturers employ focal spot tracking systems to finely control the position of the x-ray beam on the detectors, reducing overbeaming and subsequent radiation exposure.
   e. *Overranging* occurs when radiation dose is applied before and after the acquisition volume to ensure sufficient data collection for the interpolation algorithms inherent in spiral CT. Up to a half-rotation both before and after the spiral scan are common and add to the patient radiation dose.

f. Noise reduction algorithms, or *adaptive filters*, are employed during the reconstruction process to reduce displayed noise within the CT image. Reduction of displayed noise allows for lower mAs (milliampere-seconds) settings during data acquisition.

3. Use of an MSCT rather than an SSCT system is associated with several technical pitfalls with the potential to increase the patient radiation dose. Dose can be considerably higher with MSCT because of:

   a. Decrease in the focal spot–detector distance.
   b. Use of a cone beam instead of a more z-axis–collimated fan beam.
   c. Increases in the number of phases of acquisition enabled by decreased scan times.
   d. Use of thinner section widths for improvement of three-dimensional and multiplanar reformation (MPR) images.

4. Scanning parameters should be routinely adjusted in an effort to minimize patient radiation dose. Adjustments should consider the exam indication, region(s) of interest, and patient's age and body habitus.

5. *Protocol optimization* is the process of adjusting parameters such as mA/kVp, slice thickness, and pitch for the purpose of reducing patient radiation dose while maintaining adequate image quality.

6. In certain applications, such as pediatric scanning and CT angiography, reduced kVp settings may be used without a loss in image quality, resulting in a dose reduction.

7. There is a directly proportional relationship between the milliampere (mA) setting, scan time, and patient radiation dose. For example, if the mAs value is doubled, the patient radiation dose is doubled.

8. During CT data acquisition, the section of the patient exposed to radiation may be referred to as the *dose profile*. As measured at the isocenter of the gantry, the longitudinal (z-axis) dimension of the dose profile is directly controlled by collimation of the x-ray beam.

9. When only a single slice is scanned, an increase in collimation (thinner section width) will result in a decrease in patient radiation dose. However, CT examinations rarely consist of a single slice.

10. Within the context of the standard CT examination, collimation may indirectly affect patient radiation dose. Increases in collimation (i.e., thinner slices) yield images with more noise. Although usually unnecessary, it is common practice for the user and/or system to compensate for the resultant noise generated by thin sections with an increase in mA, thereby increasing patient dose.

11. During multidetector CT (MDCT), wider collimation results in improved dose efficiency because less overbeaming occurs. Narrow beam widths, i.e., thin slices, increase overbeaming and reduce dose efficiency.

12. Although reconstruction algorithm (*kernel*) and window width and level settings are not primary controllers of patient radiation dose, they can play an indirect role. Noise levels in the CT image are a function of dose: Decreased dose typically yields an increase in image noise. Displayed noise can be reduced with the utilization of an appropriate reconstruction algorithm, or kernel. Also, displaying the reconstructed image with the correct window settings can help reduce the low image qualities inherent with noise. Both of these solutions are alternatives to increasing the patient dose.

13. Image noise is directly related to patient size. As a patient size decreases, noise decreases. Protocol optimization should include size-based dose (mAs) adjustments. For example, optimal scans in children can be acquired with a substantially lower radiation dose than scans in larger patients.

14. The clinical indication for a CT study should also be considered in the attempt to reduce patient radiation dose. For example, during renal stone survey scans of the abdomen and pelvis, more noise can be tolerated because of the high inherent contrast of the pathology in question.

15. Overall scan length and repeat scans, including multiple phases, should be kept to a minimum.

16. During SSCT, pitch values greater than 1 allow for the acquisition of a given scan volume in a shorter time, resulting in a reduction in patient radiation dose.

17. However, an increase in pitch during MSCT results in a marked increase in image noise. It is typically compensated for by an increase in mA, yielding little net improvement in patient radiation dose.

18. The modern CT scanner comes equipped with a form of automatic exposure control (AEC) to manage patient radiation dose on the basis of the size, density, and overall attenuation of the part being examined. Automatic tube current modulation (ATCM) can occur as either:

    a. Angular (x- and y-axis) tube current modulation, whereby the mA setting is adjusted according to the difference in thickness of the part as the tube rotates. For example, during imaging of the oval torso, mA can be reduced as the beam passes from anterior to posterior. Less attenuation occurs in the AP path than in the lateral path through the patient.
    b. Longitudinal (z-axis) tube current modulation, which allows for the adjustment of the mA

setting as the scan proceeds along the z-axis of the patient. Differences in attenuation as the body thickness and tissue density change from the chest to the abdomen, and so on, are met with appropriate adjustments in mA, resulting in an overall reduction in radiation dose.

19. Radiation dose reduction is maximized in CT scanners that employ both the angular and longitudinal current modulation techniques.

20. During MSCT cardiac studies, prospective gating can be used to reduce the patient radiation dose. ECG-triggered tube current modulation allows for pulses of x-ray energy rather than continuous exposure to be used.

21. Tube current is reduced during the cardiac phase not utilized for image reconstruction.

22. The potential radiation dose savings gained with ECG-triggered tube current modulation depend on the patient's heart rate. As heart rate increases, the radiation dose savings decrease.

B. Radiation Protection

1. Radiation protection in CT should follow the ALARA (*as* *low* *as* *reasonably* *achievable*) concept.

2. Radiation protection of the CT patient should also encompass three general principles:
    a. Strict clinical indication.
    b. Protocol optimization.
    c. Shielding.

3. Limiting CT examination to strict indications is the best way to reduce radiation exposure.

4. Scan lengths should be limited to the clinically indicated region(s).

5. Multiple phase acquisitions should be held at a minimum.

6. An optimized protocol is one that acquires CT images with acceptable levels of noise at the lowest possible dose.

7. Lead shielding should be utilized during CT whenever clinically possible.

8. Shielding of radiosensitive tissues, such as the eye lenses, breasts, and gonads, is critical.

9. Shielding must be applied both above and below the patient, to account for the rotational nature of the exposure in CT.

10. In-plane bismuth shielding of particularly radiosensitive areas, such as the orbits, thyroid, and breast tissue, can substantially reduce the effective radiation dose.

11. Scatter radiation does occur in the immediate area surrounding the CT scanner.

12. Room shielding requirements must be evaluated by a qualified radiologic health physicist.

13. Consideration for shielding requirements should account for exam workload, scanner position, and construction of doors, windows, and so on.

14. When it is clinically necessary to have the patient accompanied by a guardian or family member during a CT procedure, or when other health personnel remain in the room during scanning, the guardian/ family member or health personnel must wear appropriate lead shielding.

C. Dose Measurement

1. *Slice sensitivity profile* (SSP) may be used to describe the reconstructed CT section.

2. However, the section of tissue exposed to ionizing radiation, or *dose profile*, is greater in width than the SSP. The accurate calculation of CT patient radiation dose must take this fact into account.

3. *Exposure* is the term used to describe the ability of x-rays to ionize a volume of air. It is measured in roentgens (R).

4. *Absorbed dose* describes the amount of x-ray energy absorbed in a unit of mass. It is measured in grays (Gy).

5. *Kerma* may also be used to describe absorbed dose. *Air kerma* describes the amount of radiation absorbed in a quantity of air.

6. *Effective dose* accounts for the type of tissue that the radiation is deposited in. Different tissues are assigned weighting factors based on their individual radiosensitivity. Effective dose approximates the relative risk from exposure to ionizing radiation. It is measured in sieverts (Sv).

7. The CT dose index (CTDI) is an approximate measure of the dose received in a single CT section or slice.

8. CTDI is calculated for the central slice in a series that is surrounded by seven slices on each side.

9. CTDI is measured by performing scans of both head- and body-sized CT phantoms using specific technical parameters. A thermoluminescence dosimeter (TLD) is placed within each phantom during the scans.

10. The exposure measured by the TLD is used to calculate the CTDI for each acquisition.

11. Exposure from the scan is measured by the TLD, and the CTDI is calculated from those measurements.

12. $CTDI_{100}$ is a fixed measurement taken with a 100-mm-long pencil ionization chamber and makes no reference to a specific number of slices.

13. Because of absorption, dose varies within the CT image across the acquired field of view. $CTDI_w$ is an internationally accepted, weighted dose index. It is calculated by summing two-thirds of the exposure recorded at the periphery of the field with one-third of the centrally recorded dose. This weighting yields a more accurate dose approximation.

14. CTDI$_w$ is calculated from measurements made with TLDs positioned at the center and periphery of the phantom to account for the variance in dose distribution.
15. The CTDI$_w$ is measured utilizing a conventional step-and-shoot mode of axial CT scanning and does not account for the affects of helical scanning on patient radiation dose.
16. CTDI$_{vol}$ is used to approximate the radiation dose for each section obtained during a helical scan.
17. It corresponds to the axially acquired CTDI$_w$ divided by the helical pitch, as follows:

$$CTDI_{vol} = \frac{CTDI_w}{pitch}$$

18. As the pitch increases, the dose per section (CTDI$_{vol}$) decreases.
19. CTDI$_w$ approximates dose along the x- and y-axes of the acquired CT image. CTDI$_{vol}$ also includes the dose along the z-axis of the scan acquisition; it is given in units of milligrays (mGy).
20. CTDI$_{vol}$ is similar in principle to an older term used for conventional step-and-shoot scanning, *multiple scan average dose* (MSAD).
21. MSAD is a calculation of the average cumulative dose to each slice within the center of a scan consisting of multiple slices.
22. The MSAD is higher than the dose from an acquisition of a single slice, because of the contribution of scatter radiation.
23. The doses at the beginning and end slices in a series are slightly less, owing to the lack of dose from their outer sides.
24. MSAD may be calculated for axial scanning as follows:

$$MSAD = \frac{T}{I} \times CTDI$$

where T is slice thickness and I is increment or image spacing.
25. MSAD accounts for the affects of image spacing or *bed index* on the patient dose during axial scanning.
26. During axial scanning, overlapping scans increase the patient radiation dose, whereas gaps between slices decrease it.
27. MSAD increases when slice thickness is greater than image spacing—overlapping scans.
28. MSAD decreases when slice thickness is less than the bed index—noncontiguous scans.
29. When slice thickness equals the bed index, MSAD is equal to CTDI.
30. During spiral or helical scanning, MSAD is controlled by pitch, as follows:

$$MSAD = \frac{CTDI}{pitch}$$

where *pitch* is the amount of table travel per tube rotation divided by the collimation.

31. MSAD is most accurate at the center of a scan series. At either end of an acquisition, MSAD tends to overestimate patient radiation dose.
32. Both CTDI$_{vol}$ and MSAD are used to approximate average radiation dose within a scan volume. Total scan length along the z-axis is not considered. Therefore, neither provides an estimate of the total dose along a given scan volume.
33. *Dose length product* (DLP) is an internationally accepted measure of CT patient dose defined as:

DLP = MSAD × slice width (cm) × No. of slices in scan volume

where *slice* again equals the pre-patient collimator setting and *not* the reconstructed slice thickness.
34. The DLP can also be illustrated as the product of CTDI$_{vol}$ and scan length and is given in units of milligray-centimeters (mGy-cm), as follows:

DLP = CTDI$_{vol}$ × scan length

35. When evaluating patient radiation dose from a MDCT study, one must bear in mind that CTDI$_{vol}$ is still controlled by the pre-patient collimator setting, regardless of the number of reconstructed slices.
36. Because direct measurement of effective dose from CT is not possible, estimations must be made on the basis of exposure to a phantom. Once the air kerma or absorbed dose in a phantom is measured, an estimate of effective dose can be calculated.
37. CTDI$_{vol}$ and DLP are displayed on many CT scanners to help the technologist achieve protocol optimization.
38. It is important to remember that CTDI$_{vol}$ and DLP do not account for patient size and so overestimate the radiation dose to the larger patient and underestimate the dose to the smaller patient.
39. CTDI$_{vol}$ and DLP may also be expressed by the newer terms *computed tomography air kerma index* (C$_a$) and *air kerma length product* (P$_{kl}$), respectively.

D. Patient Radiation Dose Reduction

1. A dose gradient exists across the field of view (FOV) of the CT image.
2. Dose at the periphery can be markedly greater than that at the center of the image, along the x- and y-axes.
3. The magnitude of this gradient is size dependent. The difference in absorbed dose is greater in larger patients.
4. Smaller adults and pediatric patients exhibit little to no radial dose gradient.
5. For smaller patients, the entrance radiation and exit radiation are equal in intensity, resulting in a more uniform distribution of dose.

6. When all other technical factors remain constant, absorbed dose is greater in the smaller patient.

7. This difference in dose distribution illustrates the importance of dose reduction for the smaller, i.e., pediatric, patient.

8. Recommendations for the reduction of pediatric dose include:
   a. Eliminate CT scans for inappropriate indication.
   b. Reduce multiphase scanning (pre-contrast, delays, and so on).
   c. Reduce mA.
   d. Increase pitch.

9. Regardless of age, the CT protocol should be optimized on the basis of the individual patient's size and/or weight.

10. Patient size–based protocols should be developed for each specific CT system to include adjustments in mA, kVp, and pitch.

11. The *Image Gently* campaign was developed by the Alliance for Radiation Safety in Pediatric Imaging and sponsored by the Society for Pediatric Radiology (SPR). The widely recognized campaign offers guidelines to help reduce pediatric radiation exposure from CT imaging. Like the dose reduction techniques listed here, the *Image Gently* guidelines suggest that:
    a. mA and kVp should be "child-sized."
    b. One single-acquisition phase is often enough.
    c. Only the indicated area should be scanned.

Review of Imaging Procedures in Computed Tomography

HEAD

Technical Considerations

A. Brain

1. Axial plane computed tomography (CT) images are acquired parallel to the infraorbital-meatal line (IOML) on the sagittal localizer (scout, topogram) image. Acquisition may be performed at an angle 15 degrees above the IOML, parallel to the skull base, to reduce orbital dose and minimize beam-hardening artifact (Figs. 3-1 to 3-5).

2. The axial (sequential) mode of data acquisition is used for improved z-axis resolution. Thin sections (2-5 mm) are acquired from the skull base through the posterior fossa, then 5- to 10-mm sections through the vertex. Thinner sections through the posterior fossa reduce beam-hardening artifact caused by the petrous pyramids.

3. The excellent z-axis resolution of thin-section volumetric multidetector CT (MDCT) studies allows for high-quality helical examinations of the brain. Helical (volumetric) acquisition may also be preferred whenever multiplanar reformation (MPR) or three-dimensional (3D) imaging is anticipated or when exam speed is a critical issue.

4. A standard or soft tissue reconstruction algorithm (filter, kernel) is used.

5. Additional image reconstruction with a high spatial frequency (bone) algorithm may be used to maximize bony detail for suspected fractures or other skeletal anomalies.

6. Sample window level (WL) and width (WW) settings for optimal image display of various structures or irregularities are as follows:
   a. Gray/white matter: WL 35, WW 100.

FIGURE 3-1 Brain—axial image.

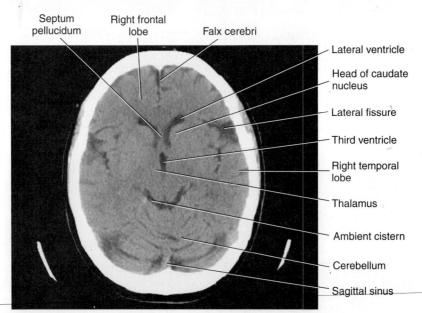

Septum pellucidum · Right frontal lobe · Falx cerebri · Lateral ventricle · Head of caudate nucleus · Lateral fissure · Third ventricle · Right temporal lobe · Thalamus · Ambient cistern · Cerebellum · Sagittal sinus

FIGURE 3-2 Brain—axial image.

Left frontal lobe · Corpus callosum · Left parietal lobe · Septum pellucidum · Partially calcified choroid plexus · Corpus callosum · Lateral ventricle · Occipital lobe

FIGURE 3-3 Brain—axial image.

b. Bone: WL 400, WW 3000.
c. Hemorrhage/hematoma: WL 75, WW 150.
d. Acute ischemia: WL 35, WW 25 (variable, high-contrast windowing improves the CT visualization of acute stroke).

7. Non-contrast CT examinations of the brain are routinely indicated for trauma to diagnose intracranial hemorrhage or hematoma. Administration of contrast media in the trauma patient is initially contraindicated because contrast enhancement may mask subtle signs of hemorrhage.

8. Unenhanced CT of the brain is also typically the first component of a comprehensive protocol for the evaluation of acute stroke. Hemorrhage must be first excluded on the non-contrast images obtained before thrombolytic therapy.

9. Other indications include:
a. Congenital abnormalities.
b. Hydrocephalus (abnormal accumulation of cerebrospinal fluid [CSF] on the ventricles).
c. Mass or tumor.
d. Primary neoplasms of the brain, including meningioma, schwannoma, and gliomas such as astrocytoma.
e. Metastatic lesions, which are commonly from lung, breast, renal, or gastrointestinal (GI) cancer.

FIGURE 3-4 Brain—axial image.

FIGURE 3-5 Brain—axial image.

f. Infectious fluid collections or abscess.

g. Bony abnormalities.

h. Endocrine pathology.

10. Unless contraindicated, IV administration of an iodinated contrast agent is essential in cases of arteriovenous malformation, suspected neoplasm, or attention to the pituitary gland.

11. Coronal plane, thin-section (1-3 mm) helical imaging may be performed through the pituitary gland.

12. CT studies of the temporal bones and internal auditory canal require a high-resolution imaging technique, which consists of the following:

a. Thin slices.

b. Small targeted display field of view (DFOV).

c. High-resolution reconstruction algorithm.

13. Thin sections (1-2 mm) are obtained in both the axial and coronal planes (Figs. 3-6 to 3-9). Multislice CT (MSCT) axial acquisitions allow for isotropic MPR, which can eliminate the added patient radiation dose from direct coronal acquisition.

14. Targeted thin-section (1-2 mm) reconstructions should be performed bilaterally utilizing a small DFOV or increased zoom factor to maximize resolution of the small bony components of the inner ear.

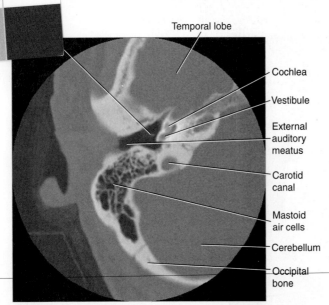

FIGURE 3-6 Internal auditory canal (IAC)—axial image.

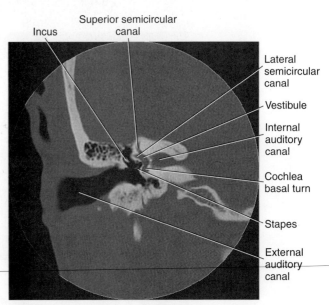

FIGURE 3-8 Internal auditory canal (IAC)—coronal image.

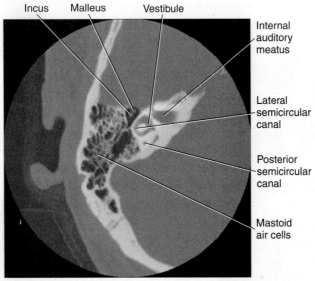

FIGURE 3-7 Internal auditory canal (IAC)—axial image.

FIGURE 3-9 Internal auditory canal (IAC)—coronal image.

15. CT images of the temporal bones are reconstructed with a high spatial frequency (bone) algorithm.
16. The patient must be instructed to hold completely still, because even the slightest motion may cause severe image degradation.
17. CT examinations of the temporal bones are typically performed without contrast enhancement, although IV contrast media may be indicated in cases of suspected soft tissue neoplasm, vascular anomalies, and so on.

B. Orbits

1. For imaging of the orbits, axial plane, thin-section (1-3 mm) images are acquired parallel to the IOML (Fig. 3-10).

2. Direct thin-section (1-3 mm) coronal images may be acquired perpendicular to the axial plane (Fig. 3-11). The acquisition angle may be adjusted slightly to avoid streaking from metal dental apparatus.
3. MSCT axial acquisitions allow for isotropic MPR, which can eliminate the added patient radiation dose from direct coronal acquisition.
4. Oblique sagittal and/or oblique coronal MPR images through the optic nerve may be included (Fig. 3-12).
5. A standard or soft tissue reconstruction algorithm is used.
6. Additional image reconstruction with a high spatial frequency (bone) algorithm may be used for trauma indications.

FIGURE 3-10 Orbits—axial image.

Anterior chamber
Medial rectus muscle
Lens
Posterior chamber
Lateral rectus muscle
Optic nerve
Ethmoid cells
Sphenoid sinus
Optic canal

FIGURE 3-11 Orbits—coronal image.

Superior rectus muscle
Medial rectus muscle
Superior oblique muscle
Superior opthalmic vein
Lateral rectus muscle
Ethmoid sinus
Inferior rectus muscle
Optic nerve
Maxillary sinus

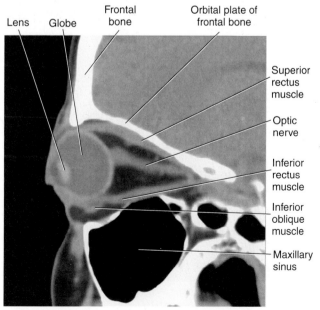

FIGURE 3-12 Orbit—multiplanar reformation (MPR) image in the sagittal plane.

Lens
Globe
Frontal bone
Orbital plate of frontal bone
Superior rectus muscle
Optic nerve
Inferior rectus muscle
Inferior oblique muscle
Maxillary sinus

7. Sample WL and WW settings for optimal image display are:
   a. Soft tissue: WL 40, WW 400.
   b. Bone: WL 400, WW 3000.
8. Protocol optimization is vital to limit unnecessary exposure of the highly radiosensitive eye lenses.
9. IV administration of an iodinated contrast agent is indicated for evaluation of vascular abnormalities, inflammation, suspected neoplasm, and so on.

C. Sinuses and Facial Bones

1. CT examinations of the sinuses should include axial images parallel to the hard palate (Figs. 3-13 and 3-14).
2. Acquisition should extend inferiorly and anteriorly to include the maxillary and ethmoid sinuses, superiorly to include the frontal sinus, and posteriorly to include the sphenoid sinus.
3. Direct coronal imaging perpendicular to the axial plane may be obtained with the patient in the prone position. The supine position with the head dropped back may also be used.
4. MSCT axial acquisitions allow for isotropic MPR, which can eliminate the added patient radiation dose from direct coronal acquisition. However, the additional coronal position may be valuable in demonstrating changing air-fluid levels and other sinus-related disease.
5. Coronal plane imaging best visualizes the osteomeatal complex, a common site for sinus inflammation (Figs. 3-15 and 3-16). Sagittal MPR images are also useful for demonstrating the osteomeatal complex.
6. Low-dose survey CT scans consisting of limited coronal acquisition through the sinuses are common.

7. Examination of the facial bones should also include axial and coronal images. Scan coverage should be adjusted to the area(s) of interest.
8. Both standard algorithm and bone algorithm reconstructions are necessary to optimally display soft tissue and bony structures.
9. Sample WL and WW settings for optimal image display are:
   a. Soft tissue: WL 40, WW 400.
   b. Bone: WL 400, WW 3000.
10. CT examinations of the temporomandibular joints (TMJ) also include axial and coronal thin sections (1-3 mm).
11. Images may be acquired in both the open-mouth and closed-mouth positions, as clinically indicated.
12. Examinations of the sinuses and facial bones are usually performed without IV contrast media, except in cases of suspected neoplasm.

Contrast Media

1. The administration of IV iodinated contrast media during CT examinations of the head has multiple indications, including:
   a. Neoplasm.
   b. Inflammatory processes.
   c. Vascular abnormalities.
2. Administration of an iodinated contrast agent raises the attenuation values of normal brain gray matter, thereby increasing contrast and CT visualization.
3. A contrast agent enhances an intracranial neoplasm that has disrupted the normal blood-brain barrier.

FIGURE 3-13 Sinus—axial image.

FIGURE 3-14 Sinus—axial image.

FIGURE 3-15 Sinus—coronal image.

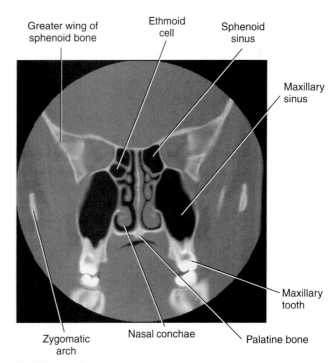

FIGURE 3-16 Sinus—coronal image.

4. Total volumes of non-ionic contrast agents typically range between 75 and 150 mL, according to study type, patient weight, renal function, and so on.
5. Injection rates vary from less than 1 mL/sec during general examinations of the brain to upwards of 4 mL/sec during angiographic or perfusion studies.
6. Scan timing for general contrast-enhanced studies of the brain is not as critical as in other applications. In fact, delays of up to 5 minutes may be utilized to maximize sensitivity of the CT scan to detect neoplasm.
7. Contrast-enhanced CT studies of the temporal bones, pituitary, and facial bones, follow department-specific protocols with regard to volumes, flow rates, and scan delays.
8. An example general protocol is as follows: 100 mL of a non-ionic contrast agent, 1 to 3 mL/sec injection rate, 60-second scan delay.

Special Procedures

A. Brain CT Angiography

1. Brain CT angiography (CTA) consists of advanced multidimensional CT imaging of the cranial blood vessels (circle of Willis), which have been opacified

by an intravenously administered iodinated contrast agent.

2. The vascular components of the circle of Willis are as follows:
   a. Right and left anterior cerebral arteries.
   b. Anterior communicating artery.
   c. Right and left internal carotid arteries.
   d. Right and left posterior cerebral arteries.
   e. Right and left posterior communicating arteries.

3. Although they do not form part of the circle of Willis, the basilar artery and middle cerebral arteries are also of importance during CTA imaging of the brain and its blood supply.

4. CTA of the brain is used to identify and evaluate cerebral aneurysm, intracranial thrombosis, traumatic cerebrovascular injury, arteriovenous malformation, and stenosis.

5. Thin-section (0.5-1.5 mm) helical acquisition is performed in the caudocranial direction from the level of the second cervical vertebra (C2) to at least 1 cm above the dorsum sella. CT systems with sufficient technical capabilities (16-slice or greater) may extend the acquisition through the vertex.

6. Before contrast agent administration, a survey scan of the brain is performed to evaluate anatomy and to identify underlying pathology.

7. The CTA spiral acquisition is then made during a rapid bolus infusion of iodinated contrast agent at a rate of 3 to 4 mL/sec.

8. Proper timing of the acquisition with regard to the contrast agent bolus is critical and may be accomplished by:
   a. Use of an empiric delay of 12 to 20 seconds.
   b. Performing a bolus-timing sequence, whereby multiple scans through the cranial vessels are acquired during a test bolus. The proper delay can be determined by visually identifying the time at which peak vessel enhancement occurs.
   c. Use of automated triggering, or bolus-tracking software that monitors vessel opacification during contrast agent administration. The scan automatically begins once a predetermined Hounsfield unit (HU) value of attenuation within the target vessel(s) is reached.

9. Thin sections are reconstructed with a minimum 50% overlap to maximize the quality of MPR and 3D images.

10. The axial "source" images are reformatted into various coronal, sagittal and oblique planes.

11. 3D techniques such as maximum intensity projection (MIP), surface rendering, and volume rendering are employed (Fig. 3-17).

12. Protocols for brain CTA depend strictly on the technical capabilities of the CT system employed. Example technical parameters for a CTA of the brain (circle of Willis) using a 64-slice system are:
   a. Performance of a standard non-contrast axial brain sequence first.

FIGURE 3-17 Volume-rendered three-dimensional reformation of the Circle of Willis (COW). This coronal perspective is produced from a CT angiographic acquisition through the brain. *PICA* - Posterior Inferior Cerebellar, *PCA* - Posterior Cerebral Artery, *ICA* - Internal Carotid Artery, *MCA* - Middle Cerebral Artery, *SCA* - Superior Cerebellar Artery. *(From Kelley L, Peterson C: Sectional Anatomy for Image Professionals, 2nd ed. St Louis, Mosby, 2007.)*

   b. 50 to 75 mL of a non-ionic contrast agent at 4 mL/sec (15- to 20-second scan delay).
   c. Helical CTA acquisition with 0.625-mm collimation.
   d. 120 kVp/300 mA/0.4 sec.
   e. Overlapping 0.75-mm source images reformatted into coronal and sagittal MPR, MIP, and volume-rendered 3D images.

13. CT angiography in the emergency setting is often deployed as part of a comprehensive acute stroke imaging protocol.

14. For evaluation of acute stroke, both the intracranial and extracranial vessels are included in the CTA acquisition, which extends from the aortic arch through the circle of Willis.

15. CT angiography source images (CTA SIs) can be utilized to produce subtraction maps, which may provide valuable information about acute brain infarct. The maps are obtained by subtracting the unenhanced CT brain images from the contrast-enhanced CTA source images.

16. CT venography (CTV) of the brain is a variation of the CTA technique. The CTA protocols can be modified with respect to bolus timing in order to evaluate venous structures.

B. CT Perfusion of the Brain

1. The comprehensive MSCT management of acute stroke consists of:
   a. Pre-contrast head CT.
   b. CTA of the brain and carotid arteries.
   c. CT perfusion (CTP) imaging.

2. *Cerebral perfusion* refers to the level of blood flow throughout brain tissue.
3. CT perfusion evaluates cerebral perfusion by monitoring the initial passing of iodinated contrast media through the vasculature of the brain.
4. The factors used to describe cerebral perfusion are as follows:
   a. *Cerebral blood volume (CBV)*: The quantity of blood (in mL) contained within a 100-g volume of brain tissue. Normal range is 4 to 5 mL/100 g.
   b. *Cerebral blood flow (CBF)*: The quantity of blood (mL) that moves through 100 g of brain tissue each minute. Normal range in gray matter is 50 to 60 mL/100 g/min.
   c. *Mean transit time (MTT)*: The average transit time, in seconds, for blood to pass through a given region of brain tissue. MTT varies according to the distance traveled between arterial inflow and venous outflow for a particular area.
5. The *central volume principle* illustrates the relationship between these factors as follows:

$$CBF = \frac{CBV}{MTT}$$

6. The primary indication for CTP is for the evaluation of acute stroke.
7. The primary goal of CTP is to identify and differentiate the infarct core and the penumbra.
8. Brain tissue within the *infarct core* is beyond repair by thrombolytic therapy.
9. The *penumbra* is the ischemic yet still viable tissue immediately surrounding the infarct core.
10. Ischemic tissue demonstrates a greater than 34% decrease in blood flow in comparison with normal brain tissue.
11. The penumbra can be described as the region of ischemic brain parenchyma where CBV is still greater than 2.5 mL/100 g.
12. Brain parenchyma with a CBV less than 2.5 mL/100 g is identified as the infarct core.
13. CTP imaging of the brain generates quantitative maps of CBF, CBV, and MTT. These maps can help distinguish regions of ischemic penumbra from an infarct core.
14. The technical procedure for CTP brain acquisition and quantitative display includes:
    a. Bolus administration of 50 mL of a contrast agent at a rate of 4 to 7 mL/sec.
    b. Cine acquisition of at least 2 cm of applicable brain region over a period of 45 to 60 seconds to allow for complete tracking of the first pass of the contrast agent through the intracranial vasculature. Careful attention must be paid to ensure that patient dose is kept to a minimum during the extended cine-acquisition required for a perfusion-CT examination.
    c. The acquisition may be broken down into multiple slabs for greater coverage. Each slab must

contain a major intracranial artery for accurate CTP map reconstruction.
    d. The slice thickness and subsequent coverage area depend on the detector configuration and technical capabilities of the individual CT system.
    e. Region of interest (ROI) measurements are placed over a well-opacified artery and an area of venous outflow, for example, the anterior cerebral artery and superior sagittal sinus, respectively.
    f. Computer software utilizes the ROI information to generate color-coded CBF, CBV, and MTT maps.
    g. The mathematical technique utilized for generation of perfusion maps is referred to as *deconvolution*.
15. Xenon CT perfusion (Xe-CT) is performed with the inhalation administration of a nonradioactive isotope of xenon (Xe) gas. The xenon enters the bloodstream and can be used to calculate a brain perfusion map on the basis of cerebral blood flow.

NECK

Technical Considerations

A. Soft Tissue of the Neck
1. Helical axial plane images of the soft tissue of the neck are acquired from the superior orbital rim inferiorly through the lung apex (Figs. 3-18 to 3-20)
2. The gantry should be angled to avoid streak artifact from dental hardware, as follows:

FIGURE 3-18 Neck—axial image.

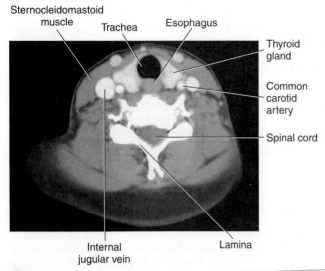

Sternocleidomastoid muscle

Trachea

Esophagus

Thyroid gland

Common carotid artery

Spinal cord

Internal jugular vein

Lamina

FIGURE 3-19 Neck—axial image.

a. From the superior orbital rim to the hard palate, the gantry may be angled superiorly, parallel to the hard palate.
   b. The remainder of the acquisition is acquired with the gantry angled parallel to the mandibular body.
   c. The two scan groups should overlap slightly to ensure complete coverage of the posterior skull base and neck.
3. The patient is supine with the arms relaxed caudally to reduce artifact from the thicker area of the shoulders.
4. An increase in mAs may be required to adequately demonstrate the lower neck and thoracic inlet as the patient dimension increases through the shoulders.
5. Slice thickness of 3 to 5 mm is adequate for most CT studies of the soft tissue neck. Thinner sections

(0.5-2 mm) may be employed for detailed examinations of the larynx or CT angiographic studies of the neck vasculature.
6. A medium to large scan field of view (SFOV) is required to accommodate the variation in part size as the scan progresses from the skull base through the thoracic inlet.
7. The DFOV typically ranges between 18 and 25 cm and should be tailored to individual patient size.
8. Sample WL and WW settings for optimal image display are:
   a. Soft tissue: WL 50, WW 400.
   b. Bone: WL 300, WW 2000.
9. Image quality degradation due to motion is a primary concern during CT examinations of the soft tissue of the neck.
10. The patient should be instructed to breathe quietly and to suspend swallowing during data acquisition.
11. Clinical indications for CT examination of the soft tissues of the neck include:
    a. Inflammation or swollen glands.
    b. Infection or abscess.
    c. Malignant neoplasms, such as carcinoma, sarcoma, and parotid gland tumor.
    d. Benign masses such as cysts and lipomas.
    e. Lymphadenopathy.
    f. Trauma.
    g. Endocrine pathology involving the thyroid and parathyroid glands.

B. Larynx
1. The patient is positioned supine with the head extended to place the plane of the larynx perpendicular to the CT image. In this position, the gantry angle

Internal jugular vein

Trachea

Esophagus

Thoracic vertebral body

Clavicle

Ribs

Spinal cord

Rt. lung apex

Subclavian artery

FIGURE 3-20 Neck—axial image.

FIGURE 3-21 Thin-section CT image of the larynx during quiet breathing and phonation. Wide "lung" windows may be used to demonstrate the vocal cords.

is adjusted so that images are acquired parallel to the plane of the true vocal cords.

2. Thin-section (0.5-2.0 mm) helical acquisition extends from just above the hyoid bone inferiorly through the cricoid cartilage (Fig. 3-21).

3. Detailed examinations of the larynx may be obtained during suspended respiration (breath-hold) in an effort to improve visualization of the true vocal cords.

4. Phonation may be used to demonstrate abnormal mobility of the vocal cord(s).

5. After an initial acquisition through the larynx during quiet respiration, an additional sequence is obtained during which the patient is instructed to phonate a low, steady "EEE" sound during the entire scan length.

6. A wide window setting (WL −300, WW 1000) may be used to visually separate the small soft tissue vocal structures from the surrounding air-filled endolarynx.

7. MPR images in the coronal and sagittal planes may also be employed during MDCT examinations of the larynx, or any other applicable area of the neck.

8. Virtual endoscopic CT examinations of the nasopharynx and larynx may also be performed for evaluation of inflammatory processes, vocal cord lesions, and so on.

Contrast Media

1. Pre-contrast imaging of the soft tissues of the neck may be indicated to evaluate the enhancement pattern of a suspicious mass or to identify salivary gland calculi.

2. Contrast media (CM) should be employed for most other CT examinations of the soft tissues of the neck unless contraindicated. Contrast enhancement vastly improves differentiation of soft tissue structures such as lymph nodes, tumors, and vasculature.

3. Total volume of contrast media depends on clinical indication, CT system capabilities, and patient physiologic factors. It ranges from 50 to 150 mL.

4. Automated injection of a contrast agent is performed at 1 to 3 mL/sec with appropriate scan delays of 30 to 60 seconds.

5. Scan delay should be sufficient to prevent data acquisition through the thoracic inlet during active bolus administration. This delay avoids image degradation from dense contrast agent in the subclavian vein.

6. The bolus may be divided to accommodate any change in gantry angle necessary to reduce metal artifact.

7. The thyroid gland is hyperdense on CT owing to its inherent iodine content. This density increases further with administration of iodinated contrast media.

Special Procedures

Carotid CT Angiography

1. Similar to the CTA of the brain, CT angiographic examinations of the neck involve imaging of the major neck vasculature, which has been opacified by IV administration of an iodinated contrast agent.

2. CTA of the neck is used primarily to evaluate the carotid arteries.

3. Indications for CTA of the carotids include:
   a. Stenosis.
   b. Occlusion.
   c. Aneurysm.
   d. Trauma.

4. Thin-section (0.5-1.5 mm) helical acquisition is performed in the caudocranial direction.

5. The MDCT carotid angiogram typically includes from the aortic arch to the skull base. If the intracranial vessels (circle of Willis) are to be evaluated, the acquisition proceeds to at least 1 cm above the dorsum sella. The scan extent may be limited as required by the clinical indication and the CT system capabilities.

6. The mA value is system dependent but should be kept at the minimal allowed to reduce patient radiation dose. The typical range is 300 to 400 mA for sub-second scan rotation.

7. Utilizing a reduced kVp setting of 120 (rather than 140) can improve the visualization of vessel opacification by an IV contrast agent.

8. When possible, the gantry should be angled to avoid artifact from dental hardware.

9. The CTA spiral acquisition occurs during a rapid bolus infusion of iodinated contrast agent at a rate of 3 to 4 mL/sec.

10. Proper timing of the acquisition with regard to the contrast agent bolus is critical and may be accomplished by:
    a. Use of an empiric delay of 15 to 18 seconds.
    b. Performing a bolus-timing sequence, whereby multiple scans through a level of the carotid arteries are acquired during a test bolus. The proper delay can be determined by visually identifying the time at which peak vessel enhancement occurs.
    c. Use of automated triggering, or bolus-tracking software that monitors vessel opacification during contrast agent administration. The scan automatically begins once a predetermined HU value of attenuation within the target vessel(s) is reached.

11. Thin sections are reconstructed with a minimum 50% overlap to maximize the quality of MPR and 3D images.

12. The axial "source" images are reformatted into various coronal, sagittal and oblique planes.

13. MIP, surface-rendered, and volume-rendered 3D techniques are employed.

14. Protocols for CTA of the neck depend on the technical capabilities of the CT system employed. Example technical parameters for a CTA of the neck (carotid arteries) using a 64-slice system are:
    a. Non-contrast helical axial neck images may first be acquired.
    b. Administration of 50 to 75 mL of a non-ionic contrast agent at 4 mL/sec (12- to 15-second scan delay).
    c. Helical CTA acquisition with 0.625-mm collimation.
    d. 120 kVp/350 mA/0.8 sec.
    e. 0.75 mm × 0.5 mm (overlapping) source images are reformatted into coronal and sagittal MPR, MIP, and volume-rendered 3D images.

CHEST

Technical Considerations

1. MDCT of the chest encompasses a variety of clinical areas, including:
   a. Interstitial lung disease.
   b. Evaluation of the mediastinum.
   c. Detection and differentiation of pulmonary nodules/masses.
   d. Oncologic staging
   e. CT angiography of the major vessels.
   f. Cardiac CT.
   g. Assessment of the airways.

2. Speed is one of the key attributes of helical MDCT. The acquisition of volumetric data for the entire lungs within a single breath-hold is now routine.

3. Some MDCT systems possess sufficient scanning speeds to allow for motion-free image acquisition without the need for suspended respiration by the patient.

4. Reduction of respiratory motion has all but eliminated the misregistration artifacts historically encountered during single-slice CT (SSCT) of the chest. This development has dramatically improved the quality of CT chest imaging.

5. The ability to retrospectively reconstruct thin-section images is another distinct advantage of MDCT. Better visualization and differentiation of small pulmonary nodules, high-quality MPR and 3D techniques, and simultaneous high-resolution CT (HRCT) imaging are just a few of the technical improvements made possible by MDCT.

A. Lungs and Mediastinum

1. The patient is positioned supine with the arms brought above the head to reduce artifact from the shoulder area.

2. Axial plane helical images are acquired from above the lung apices through at least the costophrenic angles.

3. Oncologic CT surveys of the chest to evaluate for disease progression should extend through the adrenal glands, which are a common site for metastatic deposit.

4. Data acquisition is typically performed at the end of a patient's full inspiration.

5. Scanners with detector configurations of 64 rows or more typically acquire CT data through the chest with very narrow detector width, on the order of 0.5 to 2 mm. These data are then reconstructed into thicker sections (3-5 mm) for easy review, with the potential for thin sections to be used in MPR or 3D applications.

6. Settings are 120 kVp with automatically modulated exposure in the range of 40 to 300 mA at rotational scan times of 0.33 to 1.0 seconds.

7. Low-dose CT of the chest should be considered for all patients when clinically possible, particularly in the pediatric or potentially-pregnant patient. Reduced kVp settings and very low mA (down to 1/4 of the routine setting) may still produce images of sufficient quality for interpretation.

8. Pitch varies greatly according to the configuration of the SSCT or MDCT helical system. Overall pitch selection should strike a balance between the requirement for high-quality images and the lowest patient radiation dose possible. Pitch must also be set in accordance with the patient's ability to hold the breath for the length of the scan.

9. A standard reconstruction algorithm (kernel) is used for evaluation of the mediastinum and soft tissues (Figs. 3-22 to 3-26). A given CT system may also have specific algorithms available for review of the lung parenchyma.

FIGURE 3-22 Chest—axial image displayed with a soft tissue window.

FIGURE 3-23 Chest—axial image displayed with a soft tissue window.

Superior vena cava   Ascending aorta   Pulmonary trunk

Left atrium

Pulmonary vein

Descending aorta

Pulmonary vessels

FIGURE 3-24 Chest—axial image displayed with a soft tissue window.

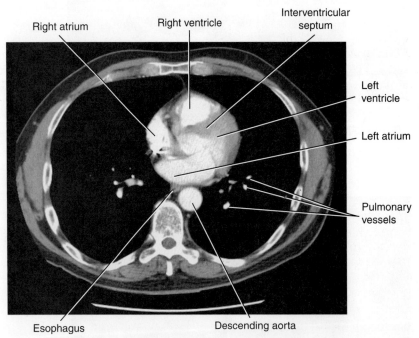

Right atrium   Right ventricle   Interventricular septum

Left ventricle

Left atrium

Pulmonary vessels

Esophagus   Descending aorta

FIGURE 3-25 Chest—axial image displayed with a soft tissue window.

10. Additional retrospective reconstructions utilizing a high spatial frequency algorithm (bone, edge) may be used for indications such as small airways disease, bone metastases, and fractures of the thorax.

11. High spatial frequency algorithms should not be utilized for the evaluation of small pulmonary nodules because of the risk of a false-positive demonstration of nodule calcification.

12. The chest consists of a wide range of anatomic structures and, subsequently, of CT densities: lung, mediastinum, bone, and so on. Images must be viewed in multiple window settings for proper evaluation.

13. Sample WL and WW settings for optimal display are:
    a. Lung parenchyma: WL −450, WW 1400.
    b. Mediastinum: WL 40, WW 350.
    c. Bone: WL 300, WW 2000.

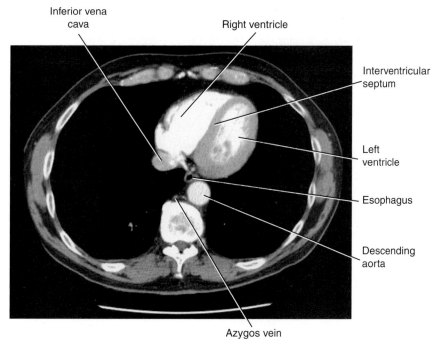

FIGURE 3-26 Chest—axial image displayed with a soft tissue window.

14. MPR and 3D techniques are often valuable tools for diagnosis during CT imaging of the thorax. For example, pulmonary vessels displayed in cross section can be mistaken for pulmonary nodules. MIP reconstructions assist in differentiating surrounding pulmonary vasculature from true nodules.
15. Thin sections are reconstructed with a minimum 50% overlap to maximize the quality of MPR and 3D images.

Contrast Media

1. Because of the inherent high contrast of the anatomic structures of the thorax, use of IV iodinated contrast media is often not necessary.
2. However, there are several indications for contrast agent administration, including:
   a. Evaluation of the mediastinum and/or major vessels.
   b. Hilar or pleural abnormalities.
   c. Assessment of lymphadenopathy.
   d. CTA of the chest.
3. Contrast enhancement of a lung mass or nodule can indicate tumor vascularity and malignancy.
4. Sufficient opacification of vascular structures can be typically obtained with injection rates of 2.5 to 4.0 mL/sec.
5. The delay utilized before scanning is specific to the vessel(s) of interest and must be coordinated with the injection rate.

6. Contrast agent dose ranges from approximately 50 to 150 mL. The total dose depends on the patient's condition and the clinical indication for the study. The rapid acquisition of MDCT makes it possible to greatly reduce contrast media volume during CT of the chest.
7. There is often significant artifact within the mediastinum from high concentrations of iodine in the superior vena cava. It may be alleviated by administering a bolus of contrast agent with reduced iodine concentration, which is achieved by diluting the full-strength contrast agent with saline. Another option is to scan in the inferior-to-superior direction so that acquisition of the superior mediastinum occurs after the period of peak contrast density within the superior vena cava.
8. An oral contrast agent such as barium sulfate paste may be administered to improve visualization of the esophagus when necessary.

A. High-Resolution CT of the Lungs
1. HRCT is used in the chest to demonstrate diffuse lung disease (Figs. 3-27 to 3-29).
2. Indications for HRCT of the lungs include:
   a. Emphysema.
   b. Bronchiectasis.
   c. Sarcoidosis.
   d. Cystic fibrosis.
   e. Chronic obstructive pulmonary disease (COPD).
   f. Asbestosis.
   g. Asthma.

FIGURE 3-27 High-resolution CT of the chest—axial image displayed with a lung window.

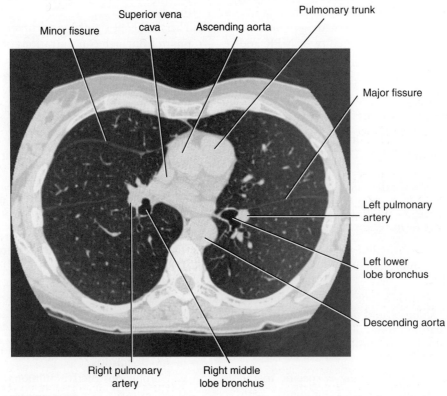

FIGURE 3-28 High-resolution CT of the chest—axial image displayed with a lung window.

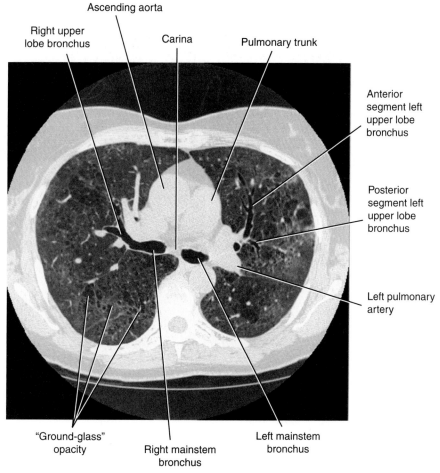

FIGURE 3-29 High-resolution CT of the chest—axial image displayed with a lung window.

3. HRCT of the lung incorporates the following technical parameters to maximize resolution:
   a. Axially acquired thin slices (1-2 mm).
   b. Reconstruction with a high spatial frequency algorithm.
   c. Reduced (targeted) DFOV to include only the lung parenchyma.
4. Although the slices acquired are narrow to improve resolution, image spacing can be considerably wider (10-15 mm), accounting for the diffuse nature of interstitial disease.
5. HRCT imaging of the lung is a sampling technique that is often performed as an adjunct to a general helical CT exam of the lungs.
6. The patient is typically scanned in the supine position. Data acquisition occurs with suspension of respiration at full inspiration.
7. HRCT images with the patient in the prone position can be acquired to differentiate the dependent edematous changes often seen in the lung bases.

8. Suspension of breathing at the end of forced expiration (static expiratory HRCT) may be utilized to demonstrate air trapping in patients with suspected small airways disease.
9. MDCT scanners allow for retrospective reconstruction of helically acquired data utilizing high-resolution parameters. Additional images with a targeted DFOV or zoom factor, a high-resolution algorithm or kernel, and a width down to 0.6 mm can be reconstructed. This may be an alternative to direct HRCT imaging in some applications, thus eliminating the need for additional scanning.
10. MDCT volumetric HRCT of the lungs also offers the added benefit of high-quality MPR and 3D techniques using the acquired isotropic data.
11. In the min-IP (minimum intensity projection) technique, displayed pixels represent the minimum attenuation value encountered along each sampled ray. This type of multiplanar volume reconstruction (MPVR) can be applied to a volume of the thorax to demonstrate air trapping within the trachea and bronchial tree.

Special Procedures

A. CT Pulmonary Angiography

1. A pulmonary embolism occurs when a thrombus (blood clot) breaks free from elsewhere in the venous system (usually the lower extremities) and migrates into a pulmonary artery. The pulmonary artery becomes blocked, causing reduced blood flow to the lung tissue.
2. The main tenets of chest CTA for evaluation of the pulmonary arteries (CTPA) are:
   a. Helical scan through the thorax with thin-slice reconstruction ranging from 0.5 to 1.25 mm.
   b. Short scan acquisition time performed within a single patient breath-hold.
   c. Acquisition during the period of peak contrast enhancement of the pulmonary arteries.
3. The scan progresses from the diaphragm superiorly to the lung apex.
4. Scanning is best performed in the caudocephalad direction, for two reasons:
   a. If the patient is unable to hold the breath for the entire scan, motion artifacts are reduced higher in the chest.
   b. There is less streaking artifact from dense contrast agent in the superior vena cava as the scan progresses.
5. Iodinated contrast agent is administered as a bolus injection at a rate of 4 to 5 mL/sec through an 18- or 20-gauge catheter.
6. Low-osmolarity or iso-osmolar non-ionic contrast agents are preferred to increase patient comfort and cooperation.
7. Contrast agent volume ranges from 80 to 150 mL, on the basis of patient physiologic factors and CT system capabilities.
8. Care must be taken to ensure that scan acquisition occurs during peak contrast enhancement of the pulmonary arteries. The previously mentioned test bolus and automated bolus-tracking methods are available for study optimization.
9. An injection of saline immediately after administration of the contrast agent bolus can increase enhancement within the pulmonary vessels. The saline flush makes use of any contrast agent remaining in the injector tubing and peripheral veins. This maneuver improves contrast agent utilization efficiency and may allow for an overall reduction in contrast agent dose for the patient.
10. The use of a saline flush also reduces artifact from dense contrast agent in the superior vena cava. It may also work to decrease the incidence of nephrotoxicity from administration of contrast media.
11. Protocols for pulmonary CTA strictly depend on the technical capabilities of the CT system employed. Example technical parameters for CTPA with a 64-slice MDCT system are:

FIGURE 3-30 A coronal multiplanar reformation (MPR) image from a CT angiographic acquisition through the chest and abdomen.

   a. 100 mL of non-ionic contrast agent at 4 mL/sec (20- to 25-second empiric scan delay or use of automated bolus tracking).
   b. Helical CTA acquisition with 0.625-mm detector collimation.
   c. 120 kVp/400 mA/0.8 sec.
   d. Overlapping 0.75-mm source images are reformatted into coronal and sagittal MPR, MIP, and volume-rendered 3D images (Fig. 3-30).
12. MPR and MIP images in the coronal, sagittal, and para-axial planes may aid in the identification of pulmonary embolism or other pathology.
13. Electrocardiogram (ECG) gating can be utilized to eliminate pulsation artifacts due to cardiac motion during the study.
14. *Prospective gating* or *triggering* is the synchronization of the data acquisition process with the cardiac cycle. Data are acquired only during the periods when the heart is at rest (diastole).
15. *Retrospective gating* involves scanning throughout the entire cardiac cycle. Only data from specific user-determined portions of the ECG waveform are reconstructed into images.
16. During a CTPA study, CTV of the lower extremities for the identification of deep vein thrombosis may also be performed.
17. After the CTPA acquisition, a delay of 2 to 3 minutes is employed. An additional acquisition is made from the iliac crest to the ankles using a 5.0- to 7.5-mm slice thickness.

B. Cardiac CT

1. *Cardiac CT* is a general term that covers several clinical applications:
   a. Coronary artery calcium (CAC) quantitation.

b. Coronary CTA.

c. Noncoronary cardiac imaging.

2. The primary clinical indication for MDCT CAC quantitation is the assessment of atherosclerotic disease.

3. The presence of CAC is a specific indicator of atherosclerotic disease.

4. CAC quantitation by MDCT provides a measurement of calcified atherosclerotic plaque burden, a possible predictor of future cardiovascular events.

5. A limitation of this evaluation is the inability to measure and characterize noncalcified atherosclerotic plaque.

6. CAC quantification is often employed as the precontrast component of a more comprehensive cardiac CTA procedure.

7. MDCT for CAC quantitation typically employs a prospective gating approach for data acquisition:

   a. With simultaneous ECG monitoring, scanning occurs only during diastole, when the heart demonstrates the least motion.

   b. A user-defined percentage of the R-R interval is set as the trigger for data acquisition to occur during the T wave of the ECG.

8. Prospective gating reduces patient radiation dose and scan variability.

9. The Agatston scoring system quantifies the volume and density of calcium within the coronary arteries.

10. Areas of calcium are identified as those greater than 1 mm^2 in area with HU values above 130.

11. The scores are characterized and compared on the basis of the patient's age and sex.

12. CAC scores can be graded as follows:

    a. 1-10: minimal.

    b. 11-100: mild.

    c. 101-400: moderate.

    d. >400: extensive.

13. MDCT for CAC quantitation is performed as a low-dose (120 kVp, <200 effective mAs) cine-axial exam.

14. Contiguous 2.5- to 3.0-mm axial sections are sequentially acquired from the aortic arch through the cardiac base.

15. The prospectively gated scans are obtained in a cine mode during diastole with fast gantry revolution times (0.35 second) to maintain excellent temporal resolution and provide motion-free images.

16. CAC studies of patients with elevated heart rates are subject to motion artifact because such patients are typically imaged without the administration of β-blockers for heart rate control.

17. In an effort to reduce motion, some CT systems may have the ability to obtain multiple images at each axial location at set time intervals. For example, three images are obtained at each axial position, separated by 50-msec intervals. The user then chooses the image with the least motion artifact.

18. System software yields measurements of calcium volume, mass, and Agatston score.

19. Newly developed dual-energy MDCT technology allows voltage switching within the same scan from 80 kVp to 140 kVp. The system is then able to differentiate calcified plaque from iodinated contrast agent during CTA of the coronary arteries. This capability may eliminate the need for a separate CAC quantitation scan, thereby saving time and patient radiation dose.

20. Dual-energy scanning is also available on dual-source MDCT systems, which consist of two separate x-ray tubes and detector arrays mounted 90 degrees from each other on the rotating gantry.

21. The development of MDCT, particularly 64-slice and beyond, has enabled CT to assume a primary role in the noninvasive evaluation of the arterial blood supply to the heart known as *coronary CTA* (CCTA).

22. The coronary arteries consist of a right coronary artery (RCA) and a left coronary artery (LCA), both arising from the aorta (Fig. 3-31).

23. The main branches of the RCA, in proximal-to-distal order, are:

    a. Conus artery.

    b. Sinus node artery.

    c. Right atrial branches.

    d. Right ventricular branches.

    e. Posterior descending artery (PDA).

    f. Posterior left ventricular branches (PLBs).

24. The LCA typically has two main branches:

    a. Left anterior descending (LAD) artery.

    b. Left circumflex artery (LCX).

25. A normal variant may produce a third LCA branch, or trifurcation, known as the *ramus intermedius*. Such a variant is commonly called a *diagonal branch*.

26. The LAD divides further into left ventricular, right ventricular, and interventricular diagonal branches.

27. The LCX divides into obtuse marginal arteries to the left ventricle and left posterolateral branches (in codominant or left-dominant patients).

28. *Dominance* refers to the source of the PDA in a particular patient. It is an important consideration in the evaluation of the coronary artery anatomy during CCTA.

29. 85% of the population is said to be right dominant—the PDA branches from the RCA.

30. 8% is said to be left dominant—the PDA branches from the LCX.

31. In patients who have *codominant anatomy* (7%), the PDA is supplied by the RCA, and the left posterior ventricular branches arise from the LCX.

32. Indications for coronary CTA include:

    a. Coronary artery stenosis.

    b. Evaluation of coronary stents and bypass grafts.

    c. Coronary anatomic anomalies.

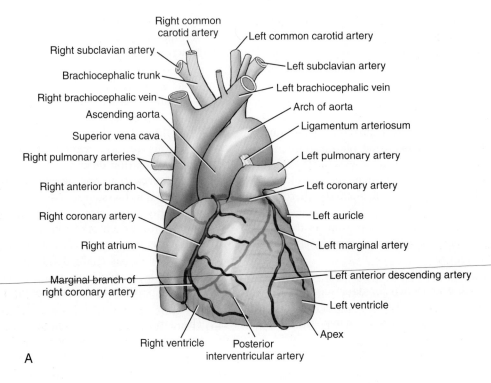

Right common
carotid artery
Left common carotid artery
Right subclavian artery
Left subclavian artery
Brachiocephalic trunk
Left brachiocephalic vein
Right brachiocephalic vein
Arch of aorta
Ascending aorta
Ligamentum arteriosum
Superior vena cava
Left pulmonary artery
Right pulmonary arteries
Left coronary artery
Right anterior branch
Right coronary artery
Left auricle
Right atrium
Left marginal artery
Marginal branch of
right coronary artery
Left anterior descending artery
Left ventricle
Apex
Right ventricle   Posterior
interventricular artery

A

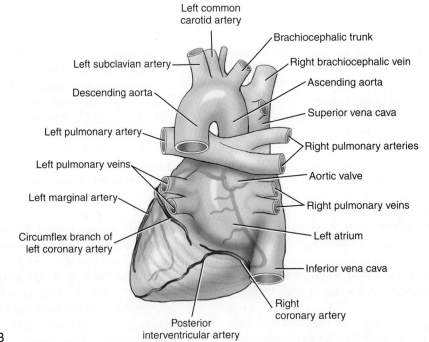

Left common
carotid artery
Brachiocephalic trunk
Left subclavian artery
Right brachiocephalic vein
Descending aorta
Ascending aorta
Superior vena cava
Left pulmonary artery
Right pulmonary arteries
Left pulmonary veins
Aortic valve
Left marginal artery
Right pulmonary veins
Circumflex branch of
left coronary artery
Left atrium
Inferior vena cava
Right
coronary artery
Posterior
interventricular artery

B

FIGURE 3-31 Heart with coronary vessels. **A,** Anterior view; **B,** posterior view. *(From Kelley L, Peterson C: Sectional Anatomy for Image Pro-fessionals, 2nd ed. St Louis, Mosby, 2007.)*

33. Contraindication to use of iodinated contrast agents is the only absolute contraindication to coronary CT.
34. Other relative contraindications are:
    a. Severe arrhythmia.
    b. Very densely calcified coronary artery plaque.
    c. Severe tachycardia that is not pharmaceutically controllable.
    d. Contraindication to β-blockers.

35. The major controlling factor of coronary CTA is the patient's heart rate. Stable, steady heart rates below 65 to 70 beats per minute (bpm) yield the best results.
36. Heart rate may be controlled pharmaceutically with the administration of oral or IV β-blockers before the study.
37. As MDCT technology improves (i.e., allows faster scanning), the need for low heart rates and pharmaceutical intervention is reduced.

38. The following technical attributes of MDCT allow for coronary artery CTA:
    a. High temporal resolution.
    b. High spatial resolution.
    c. ECG waveform synchronization.
39. The ability of an MDCT system to scan the heart quickly relies on its gantry revolution speed. Current CT systems have shorter gantry rotation times, as low as 0.33 sec (330 msec).
40. The *temporal resolution* of an MDCT system describes its ability to freeze the motion of the heart as well as the arterial motion velocity within the coronary vasculature.
41. The *gantry rotation time* is the technical parameter controlling a CT system's temporal resolution. For example, a gantry of rotation time of 400 msec results in a temporal resolution of 400 msec.
42. With gantry revolution times below 0.5 second, current, state-of-the art MDCT systems employ additional modifications to achieve temporal resolution below 100 msec, as follows:
    a. *Half-scan reconstruction*: Single-segment reconstruction in which data from only half a gantry rotation are used, thereby halving the scan time. As a result, the temporal resolution equals one-half the gantry rotation time. Image reconstruction can be further reduced into two-segment and four-segment techniques for improved temporal resolution. For example, a CT system's minimum gantry rotation time is 400 msec. Single-segment reconstruction results in 200-msec temporal resolution (half-scan). Two-segment and four-segment reconstruction may also be available, providing temporal resolution of 100 msec and 50 msec, respectively.
    b. The *multisegment reconstruction* method combines data from multiple heartbeats to form an image equaling 180 degrees of acquisition. The number of segments, and therefore the number of successive heartbeats scanned, is set by the user and determined by the patient's heart rate.
    c. For a *two-segment reconstruction*, two heartbeats are used for a single axial image. With this method, temporal resolution is reduced by one half, allowing for a freezing of the heart motion even with heart rates up to 100 bpm.
    d. In *four-segment reconstruction*, data from four heartbeats is used (45 degrees of data per cycle), reducing the temporal resolution by a factor of 4. Four-segment reconstruction yields high-quality, motion-free coronary CTA images in patients with heart rates exceeding 100 bpm.
    e. Multisegment reconstruction requires a stable cardiac cycle, with the heart maintaining an equal size and shape during successive beats. Severe arrhythmia, premature contractions, and so on, may be contraindications to coronary CTA.
    f. Dual-source CT systems utilize two separate sources of x-ray and two detector arrays. With each half-rotation of the system, temporal resolution may be reduced up to one quarter.
43. The *spatial resolution* of a CT system describes its ability to image small objects. During CTA of the coronary arteries, the MDCT system must be capable of adequately demonstrating very small blood vessels with diameters averaging 2 to 5 mm in size.
44. Spatial resolution has two main components:
    a. *In-plane resolution*, which is controlled by factors related to the x- and y-axes of the CT image. A large (512 × 512) image matrix, small DFOV (18-22 cm), and smooth reconstruction algorithm (kernel) are preferred.
    b. *Z-axis resolution* is controlled by the minimum detector width. 64-slice MDCT systems utilize detectors between 0.5 and 0.625 mm wide.
45. If not contraindicated, administration of sublingual nitroglycerine immediately before the CTA procedure can improve spatial resolution by dilating the coronary vessels. Please consult the referring physician and/or department protocol for guidelines regarding medication administration.
46. Ventricular diastole is the portion of the cardiac cycle in which coronary artery motion velocity is slowest and cardiac motion is at its lowest.
47. Data used for reconstruction of coronary CTA images are synchronized with the ventricular diastolic portion of the cardiac cycle to eliminate motion artifact.
48. The R-R interval on ECG waveform corresponds to the entire cardiac cycle.
49. *Diastole* is the portion of the R-R interval (cardiac cycle) when the heart is at rest. During *systole*, the heart is in motion.
50. During retrospective ECG-gated MDCT, data acquisition and simultaneous ECG monitoring occur throughout the entire cardiac cycle for a predetermined number of heartbeats.
51. For evaluation of the coronary arteries, the MDCT system then includes only the portion of the acquisition attained during diastole in the reconstruction process.
52. The user selects the phase percentage of the R-R interval to reduce motion artifact and optimize image quality on a case-by-case basis, as it relates to the patient's heart rate.
53. The least heart motion occurs from approximately 55% to 75% of the R-R interval, typically corresponding to the point of mid-diastole.
54. CTA acquisition is performed during suspension of respiration to reduce image degradation due to breathing.
55. During prospective ECG-gated cardiac CTA, data are acquired in an axial *step-and-shoot* mode.

The x-ray and data acquisition systems are activated only during the diastolic portion of the R-R interval.

56. Prospective ECG gating requires a steady heartbeat to limit motion artifact.

57. Evaluation of cardiac function is not possible because data are acquired only during diastole.

58. The main benefit of prospective ECG gating is the potential for up to a 70% reduction in patient radiation dose.

59. Administration of an iodinated contrast agent is a necessary component of coronary CTA. Proper timing of the contrast agent bolus is crucial to maximizing coronary artery opacification.

60. A test bolus technique can be used to determine timing delay, but the preferred method is to utilize system bolus tracking with the trigger ROI set in the ascending aorta.

61. 100 mL of a non-ionic or iso-osmolar contrast agent is injected into an antecubital vein at a rate of 4 to 6 mL/sec.

62. Additional saline flush may also be employed to improve the efficiency of contrast agent utilization.

63. Protocols for coronary CTA depend strictly on the technical capabilities of the CT system employed. Example technical parameters for a coronary CTA using a 64-slice system are:
    a. Initial non-contrast CAC scoring scan or low-dose chest CT.
    b. Administration of 75 to 100 mL non-ionic contrast agent at 4 to 6 mL/sec (automated bolus tracking).
    c. Helical CTA acquisition with 0.625-mm detector width.
    d. Scan extending from the carina through the base of the heart.
    e. 120 kVp/700-900 effective mAs (automatic mA modulation techniques may be employed).
    f. Pitch at 0.2 or less.
    g. Table feed/rotation of 3.8 mm.
    h. Reconstructed slice thickness of 0.75 mm; spacing at 0.5 mm.
    i. Small DFOV or zoom factor (18-22 cm).
    j. Sequences reconstructed at 10% intervals of R-R interval from 0 to 90%.

64. MPR, curved reformatted, and MIP images are used to evaluate the coronary arteries for stenoses. Volume-rendered and shaded-surface displays may also be of diagnostic value.

65. Acquisition data from multiple phases may be demonstrated in a cine loop for four-dimensional (4D) evaluation (x-, y-, and z-axes + time = 4D)

66. In addition to the evaluation of the coronary arteries, retrospectively gated cardiac CT can be used to assess:
    a. Morphology of the heart chambers and valves.
    b. Myocardial perfusion.
    c. Ventricular volume and ejection fraction.
    d. Wall thickness and motion abnormalities.

67. Noncoronary cardiac imaging can also be performed for the identification and evaluation of pericardial disease and differentiation of cardiac masses.

68. Cardiac function can be assessed by collecting CT data throughout the entire cardiac cycle in what is termed a *multiphase data set*. A cine-loop is then used to view the heart in motion from systole to diastole.

69. MPR images along the heart's long and short axes are also used to evaluate cardiac function, morphology, and pathology.

C. CT Angiography of the Aorta

1. MDCT angiography is a primary diagnostic tool in the evaluation of aortic aneurysm.

2. Aortic dissection occurs when an inner layer of the aorta tears and a false lumen is created. These lesions may be classified as follows:
   a. Stanford type A, involving the ascending aorta.
   b. Stanford type B, involving the descending aorta.

3. CTA acquisition should extend from the base of the neck inferiorly to include the celiac trunk.

4. When indicated, scan coverage may extend superiorly to include the carotid arteries or inferiorly through the bifurcation and iliac arteries.

5. Protocols are system-specific, with detector collimation, gantry rotation time, and pitch adjusted to ensure that the entire acquisition is attained within a single breath-hold.

6. The guiding principle of contrast agent administration is that the bolus should last throughout the entire scan but not beyond it.

7. Total volumes of contrast agent range from 75 to 125 mL, determined by the flow rate and the scan duration.

8. Good venous access is required because flow rates in the range of 4 to 5 mL/sec are recommended.

9. An antecubital IV catheter should be placed in the right arm whenever possible. This practice helps avoid the streaking artifact that may obscure the main branches off the aortic arch when contrast agent is administered in the arm and enters through the left brachiocephalic vein.

10. Scan delay is determined by test bolus or automated bolus tracking.

11. Thin-section images (0.5 to 1.5 mm) as well as thicker images (3 to 5 mm) may be reconstructed for MPR applications and general chest evaluation, respectively.

12. Pulsation artifacts, particularly in the ascending aorta, can be avoided with the use of retrospective ECG gating.

13. Protocols for CTA of the aorta depend strictly on the technical capabilities of the CT system employed. Example technical parameters using a 64-slice system are:
    a. Initial non-contrast, low-dose, thick-slice (3-5 mm) acquisition through the chest to evaluate for calcium, intramural hematoma (IMH), and so on.
    b. Administration of 75 to 125 mL of a non-ionic contrast agent at 4 mL/sec (automated bolus tracking).
    c. Helical CTA acquisition with 0.625-mm detector width.
    d. Scan extending from the base of the neck through the celiac trunk.
    e. 120 kVp/automatic mA modulation.
    f. 0.33 to 0.35 second gantry rotation time.
    g. Pitch <1.
    h. Reconstructed slice thickness of 0.75 mm; spacing at 0.5 mm.
    i. Small DFOV or zoom factor (18-22 cm).
    j. Additional reconstruction at 5 × 5 mm with sufficient DFOV to evaluate entire thorax field.
    k. MPR, MIP, and volume-rendering imaging techniques.
14. The "triple rule-out" MDCT procedure consists of a comprehensive evaluation of the chest for cardiac and noncardiac pain. Multiple clinical considerations are possible with a single MDCT procedure:
    a. Coronary CTA for coronary artery disease.
    b. CTA of the aorta for aneurysm.
    c. CTA of the pulmonary arteries for embolism.
15. In order to assess the thorax in its entirety, a full field of view is utilized to identify additional sources of chest pain, such as focal masses, pleural abnormalities, and pulmonary infiltrate.

D. CT Bronchography
1. *CT bronchography* is 3D CT visualization of the tracheobronchial tree.
2. It consists of MPR and volume-rendered 3D images reconstructed from thin, overlapping MDCT axial images acquired through the airways.
3. CT bronchography may also include "fly-through" endobrachial views, commonly known as *virtual bronchoscopy.*
4. Indications for CT bronchography and virtual bronchoscopy include:
    a. Airway stenosis.
    b. Foreign body aspiration.
    c. Trauma.
    d. Anatomic variants.
    e. Stent planning and evaluation.
    f. Bronchogenic carcinoma.
    g. Interventional guidance.

ABDOMEN AND PELVIS

1. The ability of MDCT to rapidly acquire large volumes (greater anatomic coverage) of extremely thin (isotropic) images has revolutionized the CT evaluation of the abdomen and pelvis.
2. Protocol selection and adaptation for MDCT of the abdomen and/or pelvis are vital to ensure that the scan produced meets the needs of the patient, referring physician, and radiologist.
3. Proper MDCT evaluation of the abdomen and pelvis is highly individualized. Great attention must be paid to the patient's history and the clinical indication.
4. There are many vital considerations that need to be tailored to any given examination, including:
    a. Extent of the area to be scanned.
    b. Necessity of IV and/or oral contrast media, and the administration details.
    c. Phases of contrast enhancement required.
    d. Technical parameters, such as slice thickness, imaging planes, and 3D applications.
5. The CT examination of the abdomen begins just above the diaphragm and extends through the aortic bifurcation at the general area of the iliac crest. An exam that includes the pelvis extends through at least the pubic symphysis.
6. The anatomic area scanned is based on the physician order and clinical concern—abdomen only, abdomen and pelvis, chest, abdomen, and pelvis, and so on.
7. The contents of the abdominal-pelvic cavity may be further divided as follows:
    a. The peritoneum forms a membranous sac called the *peritoneal cavity* that contains the following organs:
       • Stomach.
       • Small bowel, a small portion of the duodenum, and all of the jejunum and ileum.
       • Transverse colon.
       • Liver and gallbladder.
       • Spleen.
       • Ovaries.
    b. The peritoneal cavity is a closed sac in males but opens to the exterior in females through the fallopian tubes, uterus, and vagina.
    c. The peritoneum contains double layers and folds that surround and support the abdominal organs:
       • *Mesentery:* A thickened portion of the peritoneum that attaches portions of the intestines to the abdominal wall.
       • *Omentum:* A mesentery that is divided into lesser and greater components, each responsible for attaching portions of the stomach and intestines.
    d. *Retroperitoneum:* The space located between the peritoneum and the posterior abdominal wall. It includes the following organs and structures:
       • Duodenum.

- Pancreas.
- Adrenal glands.
- Kidneys, ureters, and bladder.
- Aorta and inferior vena cava (IVC).
- Prostate.
- Uterus.

Technical Considerations

General guidelines regarding the technical parameters for MDCT examinations of the abdomen and/or pelvis are outlined here. This section is followed by more specific technical details for the major organ systems of the abdomen and pelvis.

A. Exam Preparation

1. When possible, patients fast for 2 to 6 hours before the examination. Fasting results in an empty proximal GI tract, facilitating its evaluation and also limiting the potential hazard of aspiration of stomach contents in the event of GI upset due to IV administration of a contrast agent.
2. In most cases, an oral contrast agent is administered to distend the GI tract and clearly demonstrate the intestinal lumen. The agent used may be a dilute solution of an iodinated contrast medium, barium sulfate, or water. For general studies of the abdomen and pelvis, 750 to 1500 mL of oral contrast agent is administered 30 to 120 minutes before the exam.
3. Example protocol for oral contrast agent administration is:
   a. 450 mL given 90 to 120 minutes before the exam for opacification of the distal intestines.
   b. 300 to 450 mL given 30 minutes before the exam for opacification of the proximal intestines.
   c. An additional volume of 150 to 250 mL given just before scanning for opacification of the stomach and duodenum.

B. Patient Position and Instructions

1. The patient is positioned supine with the arms placed overhead to eliminate scatter artifact.
2. Additional positions (prone, decubitus) may be employed to improve the demonstration of normal anatomy and the differentiation of pathologic processes.
3. Whenever possible, the patient is instructed to suspend respiration (hold the breath) during scan acquisition.

C. Scan Parameters

1. Detector configuration and section width: 64–detector row (or larger) MDCT systems allow for detector collimation as thin as 0.5 to 0.625 mm, with images reconstructed at widths based on the anatomy or pathology in question. For general survey studies, section widths of 3 to 5 mm are sufficient. Section widths of 1 to 2 mm or less may be preferable during multiphasic studies and in anticipation of 3D and multiplanar reconstructions.
2. Table travel speed and pitch: The relationship among detector collimation, table travel speed, and pitch is important in determining the amount of data acquired per gantry rotation and the overall scan time. A state-of-the-art MDCT system is capable of long z-axis acquisitions in a short time, often within a single, comfortable breath-hold.
3. The detector configuration, table speed, and pitch should be optimized according to the clinical indications of the exam while keeping scan time and patient radiation dose to a minimum.
4. The mA and kVp settings should be based on patient size, yielding to the noise requirements of the particular exam.
5. Patient radiation dose may also be reduced with the utilization of automatic tube current modulation (ATCM) techniques, which are available on most CT systems.
6. DFOV is patient specific, being set as small as possible while still including the abdomen and pelvis in their entirety.
7. A standard soft tissue algorithm is used for reconstruction. When indicated, additional reconstruction with a high-resolution algorithm may be used to demonstrate bony detail.
8. Sample WL and WW settings for optimal display are:
   a. Soft tissue of the abdomen: WL 40, WW 350.
   b. Lung bases: WL −450, WW 1400.
   c. Bone: WL 300, WW 2000.

D. Administration of Intravenous Contrast Agents

1. When not contraindicated, the administration of an iodinated IV contrast agent improves the quality of abdominal and pelvic CT imaging by:
   a. Enhancing, or increasing the CT density of, abdominal organ parenchyma.
   b. Increasing the detectability of lesions from normal structures.
   c. Opacifying vascular structures.
   d. Providing assessment of organ perfusion and function.
2. There are also clinical indications for non-contrast or pre- and post-contrast imaging, including:
   a. Characterizing the enhancement pattern of a lesion.
   b. Evaluation of calcifications within organ parenchyma.
   c. Assessment of unenhanced parenchymal attenuation values.
   d. Identification of calculi within the bile ducts, gallbladder, urinary tract, and appendix.

3. Contrast agent dose ranges from approximately 50 to 150 mL. The total dose depends on the patient's condition and the clinical indication for the study.
4. Injection rates vary between 2.0 and 5.0 mL/sec. The rate selected depends on the enhancement phase(s) to be acquired and the capacity of the venous access.
5. The delay between the initiation of contrast agent administration and scanning is tailored to the required phase of enhancement and coordinated with the injection rate.
6. Specific contrast agent injection rates, acquisition delays, and a description of the pertinent phases of contrast agent enhancement are described here for each anatomic region.

HEPATOBILIARY SYSTEM

1. The primary role of MDCT in evaluation of the liver is the identification and characterization of hepatic lesions.
2. When not contraindicated, most CT examinations of the liver involve the IV administration of an iodinated contrast agent to improve the differentiation between lesions and normal hepatic parenchyma.
3. However, non-contrast imaging may be indicated in cases of suspected hepatic calcifications, fatty infiltration, and visualization of hemorrhage or to characterize the enhancement pattern of hepatic lesions.
4. Normal unenhanced hepatic parenchyma is homogeneous in appearance, with CT densities in the range of 45 to 65 HU. The CT density of the unenhanced liver is normally slightly greater than densities of blood vessels and the splenic parenchyma.
5. Soft tissue masses may appear less dense (*hypodense*) or more dense (*hyperdense*) than the structures that surround them.
6. Upon enhancement with an IV contrast agent, a tumor may be described as *hypovascular* if it is lower in density than the surrounding organ parenchyma or *hypervascular* if it is higher in density.
7. The most common malignant hepatic neoplasms are metastases, which usually appear as hypodense.
8. Examples of hypervascular tumors are hemangiomas, hepatocellular carcinomas (HCCs), focal nodular hyperplasia (FNH), and hypervascular metastases.
9. Tumors with densities equal to those of surrounding tissue or structures are said to be *isodense*. These structures may not be well-defined on the CT image. HCC is an example of a neoplasm that may appear isodense on routine contrast-enhanced CT. Scanning during multiple phases of contrast enhancement may improve the visualization of HCC and other tumors like it.

10. Benign neoplasms of the liver include:
    a. *Hemangioma:* Often an incidental finding, this commonly occurring vascular lesion is characterized by peripheral globular enhancement during initial post-contrast imaging. Progressive fill-in of enhancement occurs over time, until the mass becomes isodense with surrounding hepatic parenchyma
    b. *Focal nodular hyperplasia:* Another common vascular lesion often identified along the surface of the liver, FNH is characterized by intense homogeneous enhancement with contrast agent administration. There is usually a central scar that remains hypodense until delayed imaging, during which it may also enhance.
    c. *Hepatic cysts:* They appear as well-defined, thin-walled, round or oval masses, with attenuation close or equal to that of water (0-20 HU). The hallmark feature is lack of enhancement with IV contrast agent administration.
11. Malignant neoplasms of the liver include:
    a. *Hepatocellular carcinoma:* The most common primary malignant neoplasm of the liver. HCC typically appears hypodense on non-contrast scans and hyperdense or hypervascular on arterial phase imaging.
    b. *Metastases:* The liver is a common site for the metastatic spread of cancer. Primary neoplasms that commonly metastasize to the liver include those of the colon, lung, breast, pancreas, and stomach. The CT appearance of hepatic metastases varies greatly and is nonspecific. They may appear as solitary or multiple, hypodense or hyperdense, necrotic or calcified, and so on.
12. Additional indications for MDCT of the liver include:
    a. Diffuse liver disease:
       • *Fatty liver (steatosis):* Normal liver parenchyma exhibits a CT density approximately 10 HU greater than that of the spleen. A liver with fatty infiltration demonstrates an overall density that is at least 10 HU less than that of the spleen. Areas of focal sparing of fatty infiltration appear hyperdense to surrounding tissue and may mimic hepatic neoplasm.
       • *Cirrhosis:* Chronic destructive disease characterized by a variety of features, including hepatomegaly, fatty infiltration, irregular nodular contour, enlargement of the left and caudate lobes of the liver, and portal hypertension. Common causes of cirrhosis are hepatitis and chronic alcoholism.
    b. Trauma: The liver is the second most commonly injured abdominal organ (after the spleen). Hematoma, hemorrhage, and laceration are typical signs of traumatic liver injury.

c. Infection or abscess.

d. Pre- and post-operative assessments of the patient who may undergo hepatic transplantation.

13. The liver has a dual blood supply, receiving 75% of its supply from the portal vein and the remaining 25% via the hepatic artery. The dual nature of this blood supply has important ramifications with regard to IV contrast agent administration and scan timing.

14. There are three distinct phases of hepatic contrast enhancement:

   a. *Arterial phase:* The period of peak arterial enhancement typically occurs at 25 to 35 seconds after the initiation of contrast agent administration. During this phase, hypervascular tumors, or tumors supplied by the hepatic artery, undergo maximal enhancement. The lesions are made conspicuous by the relatively unenhanced hepatic parenchyma surrounding them.

   b. *Portal (or hepatic) venous phase:* The period of peak hepatic parenchymal enhancement during which contrast material redistributes from the blood into the extravascular spaces. Typically occurring at 60 to 70 seconds after the initiation of contrast agent administration, this is the phase during which hypovascular lesions are most conspicuous owing to their density difference from the enhancing hepatic parenchyma.

   c. *Equilibrium phase:* Usually occurs at 2 to 3 minutes after the initiation of contrast agent administration. During this phase, hepatic parenchymal enhancement dissipates, and there is minimal difference in contrast enhancement between the intravascular and extravascular spaces. Many hepatic lesions become indistinguishable from their surroundings. The rapid acquisition made possible by MDCT helps avoid scanning during this phase.

15. An *early arterial phase*, occurring at 15 to 20 seconds after the initiation of contrast agent administration, has also been identified. During this phase the hepatic arterial supply is well opacified with little or no parenchymal enhancement. This is the optimal phase for angiographic applications of liver CT.

16. The *delayed phase* of hepatic data acquisition occurs approximately 5 to 20 minutes after contrast agent administration. This phase is used primarily to demonstrate the complete "fill-in" of a hemangioma as it becomes isodense with surrounding parenchyma.

17. The timing of each of these phases depends on a number of factors:

   a. Cardiac output: As it is reduced, peak arterial and parenchymal enhancement is delayed.

   b. Injection duration: A function of the total contrast agent volume and the injection rate. A short duration, via smaller volume, faster injection rate, or a combination thereof, results in a faster delivery of the iodine load and earlier peak arterial and parenchymal enhancement. Rapid injection rates also provide a greater temporal separation between the arterial and venous enhancement phases.

   c. Iodine concentration of contrast agent: The use of media with higher iodine concentrations (at or above 350 mgI/mL) results in a higher administered iodine load, which helps widen the window of peak arterial and parenchymal enhancement.

18. The degree of hepatic parenchymal enhancement depends on the overall dose of iodine delivered. Iodine dose may be increased directly, with the use of contrast agents with a higher concentration, or indirectly, through using a higher injection rate.

19. Lesion detectability improves as parenchymal enhancement improves. Care must be taken to ensure that CT scanning of the liver is performed during the highest level of enhancement possible.

20. Automated bolus-tracking software can be utilized to improve the timing accuracy of multiphasic acquisitions of the liver.

21. Current MDCT technology allows for scanning of the liver during multiple phases of contrast enhancement. This improves characterization of both hypovascular and hypervascular lesions.

22. Protocol considerations for a multiphasic MDCT scan of the liver are department-specific but may include any or all of the following:

   a. Non-contrast survey of the liver to evaluate baseline lesion density, fatty infiltration, calcifications, and so on.

   b. Early arterial phase (15-20 seconds) for assessment of the hepatic arterial supply. Important in cases of preoperative planning for resection, transplantation, or placement of a chemotherapy infusion pump.

   c. Arterial phase (25-35 seconds) for optimal visualization of hypervascular hepatic lesions such as hemangioma and HCC.

   d. Portal venous phase (60-70 seconds) for evaluation of the maximally enhanced hepatic parenchyma and demonstration of hypovascular lesions such as hepatic metastases.

   e. Delayed phase (5-20 minutes) for demonstration of hemangioma fill-in, FNH central scar, and so on.

   f. Reconstructed images 3 to 5 mm thick from data obtained with detector collimation as low as possible. Section width may range from 2.5 mm in a 4-slice MDCT system to 0.6 mm in a 64-slice system.

g. Thinner (0.5-2.5 mm), overlapping reconstructions may be used for angiographic, MPR, and 3D applications.

23. The gallbladder is demonstrated as a bile-filled (near water density) oval sac positioned within a fossa along the inferior surface of the liver.

24. CT is not usually the modality of choice for evaluation of the gallbladder. However, MDCT is capable of adequately demonstrating many pathologic etiologies of gallbladder symptoms in the patient who is undergoing CT evaluation of the abdomen and pelvis:

a. *Cholelithiasis* (gallstones): The ability of CT to demonstrate gallstones depends primarily on the stone composition. Cholesterol stones may exhibit a CT density less than that of the surrounding bile. Calcified gallstones are easier to identify. Mixed-composition stones may be obscured on CT.

b. *Cholecystitis:* Inflammation of the gallbladder is nonspecific but may be characterized on CT by a thickened and contrast-enhancing wall, distention, gallstones, and/or pericholecystic fluid.

c. Neoplasms of the gallbladder such as benign adenoma and malignant carcinoma.

25. Components of the biliary tract commonly demonstrated on CT examination include:

a. Common hepatic duct (CHD).

b. Common bile duct (CBD).

c. Intrahepatic bile ducts (IHBDs).

26. Common clinical indications for CT examination of the biliary tree include:

a. Biliary dilatation or obstruction.

b. *Choledocholithiasis* (bile duct stones).

c. *Cholangitis* (inflammation of the bile ducts).

d. Biliary duct neoplasms.

27. Optimal CT demonstration of the gallbladder and biliary tree requires thin-section (0.5 to 2.0 mm), dual-phase (arterial and portal venous) acquisition.

28. Water is used as an oral contrast material to eliminate the streak artifact that may occur from the positive contrast agent within the duodenum.

29. Pre-contrast imaging may be performed initially to look for stones.

SPLEEN

1. The spleen is evaluated concurrently with the remaining organs and structures of the abdomen on CT examination (Fig. 3-32).

2. The CT density of the unenhanced spleen is between +40 and +60 HU, which is approximately 10 HU less than that of the unenhanced liver.

3. The spleen is optimally imaged after administration of a contrast agent.

4. On arterial phase imaging, the spleen demonstrates a heterogeneous enhancement pattern. The preferred timing for CT acquisition of the spleen is the portal venous phase (60-70 seconds), when a more homogeneous pattern of enhancement is demonstrated.

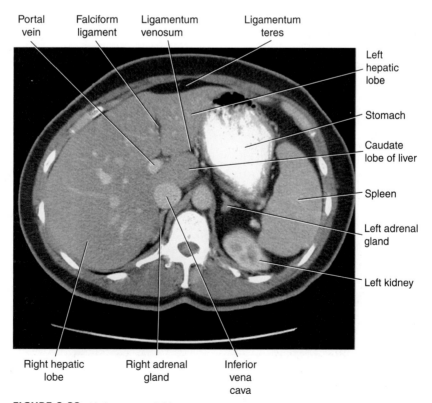

FIGURE 3-32 Abdomen—axial image.

5. Common indications for CT evaluation of the spleen include:
   a. Trauma: The spleen is the most common site of organ injury due to blunt abdominal trauma. Hematoma, hemorrhage, and laceration are typical signs of traumatic splenic injury.
   b. Focal lesions: Benign masses such as cysts and hemangiomas, and malignant lesions, including those from lymphoma and metastatic disease.
   c. *Splenomegaly:* An enlargement of the spleen with numerous etiologies, including lymphoma, cirrhotic portal hypertension, and infection.
6. Accessory spleens (*splenules*) are common incidental findings on CT examinations of the abdomen. They appear as small nodules of splenic tissue just adjacent to the main spleen. They usually have little clinical significance but may be mistaken for other types of abdominal masses.

PANCREAS

1. MDCT is capable of thin-section acquisition through the entire pancreas, in a single breath-hold, during multiple phases of contrast enhancement (Fig. 3-33).
2. The isotropic nature of current MDCT acquisition also allows for high-quality reformation of the pancreas in multiple planes and volume-rendered techniques, further improving its diagnostic capabilities.
3. Indications for CT of the pancreas include:
   a. Evaluation of pancreatitis: The role of CT is to assess pancreatic and peripancreatic inflammatory changes and to identify the presence of pancreatic necrosis.
   b. Identification of pancreatic neoplasms, including:
      • Adenocarcinoma, the most common pancreatic neoplasm.
      • Cysts or pseudocysts.
      • Endocrine masses, such as islet cell tumors.
   c. Trauma.
   d. Complications of cystic fibrosis.
4. Most pancreatic tumors appear hypodense in comparison with surrounding contrast-enhanced pancreatic parenchyma.
5. Imaging the pancreas during the phase of peak parenchymal enhancement vastly increases the conspicuity of most pancreatic neoplasms.
6. The pancreatic phase of contrast enhancement is a delayed arterial phase occurring approximately 35 to 45 seconds after the start of contrast agent administration, assuming that an adequate volume is injected at a rate of 3 mL/sec or higher.
7. Protocol considerations for a multiphasic MDCT scan of the pancreas are department-specific but may include any or all of the following:
   a. Water as an oral contrast agent to distend the proximal GI tract without the streaking artifact possible when positive contrast media are used.
   b. Injection of 100 to 150 mL of iodinated contrast agent at 3 to 5 mL/sec.

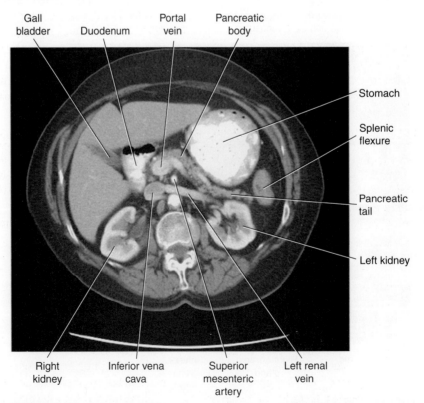

FIGURE 3-33 Abdomen—axial image.

c. Pre-contrast imaging for localization of the pancreas and identification of calcifications.

d. Arterial phase acquisition through the pancreas after a 20- to 25-second delay from the start of the injection. During this period there is maximum opacification of the surrounding vasculature, including the aorta and superior mesenteric artery. An important goal of pancreatic CT is to evaluate the involvement of surrounding vessels by pancreatic neoplasm.

e. Pancreatic (delayed arterial) phase acquisition after a 35- to 45-second delay from the start of injection. This is the phase of optimal pancreatic parenchymal enhancement.

f. Venous phase acquisition through the entire abdomen after a 60- to 70-second delay from the start of injection. This phase provides imaging during portal opacification and optimal hepatic enhancement.

g. Images 1 to 3 mm thick are reconstructed from data obtained with detector collimation as low as possible. The detector collimation may range from 1.25 mm in a 4-slice MDCT system to 0.5 mm in a 64-slice system.

h. Thinner (0.5-1.25 mm), overlapping reconstructions may be used for angiographic, MPR, and 3D applications.

8. The primary goal of multiphasic CT evaluation of a pancreatic mass is the determination of tumor resectability. There are several factors that determine the potential for surgical removal of a pancreatic tumor, including:

a. Vascular involvement of the mass.

b. Local tumor spread.

c. Metastases.

9. Patients who have been determined to be candidates for surgical intervention typically undergo a resection of the pancreas and duodenum known as a Whipple procedure.

ADRENAL GLANDS

1. CT is the primary imaging modality for the evaluation of the adrenal glands.

2. The *adrenal glands* are small, soft tissue structures with a CT density similar to that of muscle (25-40 HU).

3. They lie in the space just superior to each kidney and are surrounded by fat, a feature that improves their inherent contrast and subsequent visualization by CT.

4. During routine abdominal CT imaging, the adrenal glands are usually adequately imaged with slice thicknesses in the 3 to 5 mm range.

5. Specific CT assessment of the adrenal glands benefits from thinner slice widths, in the range of 0.5 to 2.0 mm, depending on the CT system's capabilities.

6. When not contraindicated, both pre- and post-contrast imaging is usually necessary to fully characterize adrenal pathology.

7. Acquisition is made routinely during the portal venous phase of contrast enhancement. Delayed imaging (10-15 minutes) may also be employed for tumor characterization.

8. Beyond assessment during routine scanning of the abdomen, there are several indications for specific CT evaluation of the adrenal glands, including:

a. Endocrine abnormality, to rule out an adrenal mass.

b. Oncologic staging; the adrenal gland is a common location for metastatic disease from lung carcinoma.

c. Characterization of an adrenal lesion identified on another study/modality (adrenal "incidentaloma").

9. Adrenal hyperplasia is an enlargement of the adrenal gland(s), usually associated with a disorder of endocrine function.

10. The majority of focal adrenal masses are benign adenomas.

11. Differentiation between a metastatic lesion and a benign adenoma is an important goal of the CT evaluation of an adrenal mass:

a. On pre-contrast imaging, ROI measurements of a mass that are less than 10 HU indicate a benign process.

b. On delayed post-contrast imaging, metastatic lesions of the adrenal gland remain enhanced longer than adrenal adenomas.

c. The extent of the dissipation of enhancement, or "washout" can be calculated during delayed (10-15 minutes) imaging of the adrenal glands.

12. The pancreatic tail, tortuous vasculature, splenules, bowel loops, and so on, may appear as pseudotumors on axial CT images. The utilization of MPR (coronal, sagittal) images improves differentiation of pseudotumors from true adrenal masses.

GENITOURINARY SYSTEM

1. CT is the primary imaging modality for the evaluation of the *urinary tract*, which consists of the kidneys, ureters, and bladder.

2. The kidneys are enveloped and supported by a sheath of connective tissue called *Gerota fascia*.

3. The renal parenchyma consists of the internal medulla surrounded by the renal cortex.

4. The renal pelvis contains the minor and major calyces, which lead inferiorly into the ureters.

5. The epithelial lining of the urinary tract is called the *urothelium*.

6. General indications for CT assessment of the urinary tract include:

a. Identification of urinary calculi.

b. Evaluation of the kidney, ureters, and/or bladder for tumor, infection (pyelonephritis), and trauma.

c. Assessment of renal vasculature.

7. Unenhanced helical CT of the urinary tract has become the standard for the investigation of urinary tract lithiasis (stones).

8. Thin-section (3-5 mm) acquisition is made from above the kidneys through the base of the bladder.

9. Per specific department protocol, the scan may begin above the diaphragm to include the entire abdomen. CT holds a distinct advantage over other imaging modalities in its ability to identify non-genitourinary pathology—pancreatitis, cholelithiasis, appendicitis, diverticulitis—in patients with abdominal pain.

10. No patient preparation is typically required because this is a non-contrast study. However, better patient hydration through the ingestion of water before the study can help eliminate small hyperdensities of the renal pyramids that can mimic stones.

11. When there is a question of stones within the bladder or at the uterovesical junction (UVJ), additional imaging with the patient in the prone position may be indicated.

12. Patient radiation dose should be kept at a minimum through either weight-based manual or automated modulation techniques.

13. In a further effort to reduce overall patient radiation dose, all non-contrast renal stone survey studies may be performed in the prone position. This alternative may help reduce the need for additional sequences by initially differentiating UVJ stones and pelvic *phleboliths* (calcifications within pelvic veins).

14. The diagnosis of distal ureteral stones may be complicated by the presence of phleboliths, regardless of patient position. An IV contrast agent may be administered to better distinguish the ureter from adjacent phleboliths.

15. Administration of an iodinated contrast agent also aids in demonstrating the inflammation of the renal fascia and obstruction of the collecting system that are often associated with urinary lithiasis.

16. The characterization of most renal masses also requires the IV administration of an iodinated contrast agent.

17. Cystic renal masses are common, are usually benign, and may be identified before the administration of contrast agent, as follows:
    a. *Simple cysts:* Smooth, round, thin-walled masses with homogeneous near-water CT density (<20 HU).
    b. *Hyperdense cysts:* Complicated cystic masses with CT densities in the range of 25 to 90 HU on unenhanced scans. Because of infection or hemorrhage, these masses have CT densities greater than the density of surrounding normal renal parenchyma and therefore appear "hyperdense."
    c. *Polycystic kidney disease (PKD):* A genetic disorder characterized by the formation of numerous renal cysts.
    d. *Parapelvic cysts:* Instead of arising from the renal cortex as most simple cysts do, parapelvic cysts occur within the renal pelvis. They can sometimes appear as hydronephrosis, or distention of the pelvis and calyces, which would be secondary to renal obstruction. Delayed imaging after IV administration of a contrast agent opacifies the renal pelvis, clearly differentiating hydronephrosis from parapelvic cysts.

18. After administration of a contrast agent, a renal cyst should not "enhance" or exhibit a significant increase in CT density.

19. *Pseudoenhancement* describes the minimal "enhancement" of a renal cyst following contrast agent administration. This apparent increase in attenuation, of 15 to 20 HU, likely results from volume averaging primarily due to dense cortical enhancement of the kidneys. The occurrence of pseudoenhancement has increased with the advent of MDCT.

20. An *angiomyolipoma* of the kidney is a benign mass of blood vessels (angio-), muscle tissue (myo-), and fat (lipoma). An ROI measurement of less than −10 HU characterizes a renal mass as an angiomyolipoma.

21. Malignant masses of the kidney include:
    a. Renal cell carcinoma (RCC): The most common primary renal malignancy. RCC is typically characterized by marked contrast enhancement (>20-25 HU).
    b. *Transitional cell carcinoma* (TCC): A tumor originating in the urothelium. Most TCCs arise in the bladder, with the possibility of additional masses in the ureters, renal pelvis, or both. On pre-contrast imaging, TCC usually appears as a hypodense lesion within the renal collecting system that has a CT density greater than that of urine but less than that of renal parenchyma (<40 HU). TCC significantly enhances after administration of a contrast agent.
    c. Metastases: Lung, colon, and breast cancers are primary malignancies that commonly result in renal metastases.

22. Like other abdominal organs, the kidneys undergo distinct phases of contrast enhancement. The described phases are transient in nature, and their reported times assume a contrast agent bolus of adequate volume administered at a rate of 2 mL/sec or higher:
    a. *Corticomedullary phase:* A late arterial phase beginning 30 to 40 seconds after the initiation of contrast agent administration. Optimal enhancement of the renal cortex and renal veins occurs during this period. The renal medulla is minimally enhanced, allowing for its maximum differentiation from the renal cortex.

b. *Nephrographic phase:* Time between 70 and 90 seconds after the start of injection. Enhancement differences between renal cortex and medulla reach equilibrium, providing optimal sensitivity for parenchymal lesions. Imaging during the nephrographic phase also allows for portal opacification and optimal hepatic enhancement, which are important for the assessment of disease spread (Fig. 3-34).

c. *Excretory phase:* A delayed imaging phase that begins approximately 3 minutes after the initiation of contrast agent administration. During this phase, the contrast agent has been excreted into the renal calyces, opacifying the renal pelvis and the remainder of the urinary collecting system (ureters, bladder). The excretory phase best demonstrates the filling defects and the potential lesions involving the urothelium.

23. A *CT urogram* (CT intravenous pyelogram [IVP]) is a comprehensive, multiphasic evaluation of the urinary tract. Although variation in specific protocols exists, the key components to a CT urogram are:
   a. Non-contrast image acquisition of the urinary tract.
   b. Post-contrast image acquisition of the abdomen and pelvis.
   c. Thin-section delayed (excretory phase) imaging of the urinary tract.
   d. Coronal MIP and volume-rendered images for CT urographic display.

24. Opacification of the urinary tract may be improved by the IV drip administration of approximately 250 mL of normal (0.9%) saline during the delay before the excretory acquisition.

25. Another approach combines axial CT with 2D excretory urography. Post-contrast CT sequences are followed by an appropriate delay (5-15 minutes). Conventional radiographs are then obtained with or without compression to form a combination CT-radiography urogram.

26. Protocol considerations for a multiphasic MDCT scan of the kidneys and urinary tract are department-specific but may include any or all of the following:
   a. Use of water as oral contrast agent to distend the proximal GI tract while avoiding interference from positive contrast media during MPR and 3D techniques. A positive oral contrast agent (iodine or barium) may be utilized to simultaneously evaluate the GI tract for alternative etiologies, assess lymphadenopathy, and so on.
   b. Pre-contrast imaging through the kidneys, ureters, and bladder for identification of calculi.
   c. Injection of 100 to 150 mL of iodinated contrast agent at 3 to 5 mL/sec.
   d. Arterial phase image acquisition through the kidneys and renal vasculature following a 20- to 25-second delay after the start of injection. During this period there is maximum opacification of the aorta and renal arteries.
   e. Corticomedullary (late arterial) phase acquisition through the kidneys following a 30- to 40-second delay after the start of injection. This phase best demonstrates the interface between renal cortex and medulla as well as the potential vascular involvement of a renal mass.
   f. Nephrographic (parenchymal) phase acquisition through the entire abdomen following a 70- to

FIGURE 3-34 Abdomen—axial image.

FIGURE 3-35 Abdomen—coronal multiplanar reformation (MPR) image.

90-second delay after the start of injection. The nephrographic phase best demonstrates parenchymal renal masses.

g. Excretory (delayed) acquisition through the kidneys, ureters, and bladder following a 3- to 15-minute (or longer) delay. This phase allows for optimal opacification of the renal collecting system. The excretory acquisition is utilized in MPR, VR, and MIP techniques for the production of a CT urogram. This is also the phase that best demonstrates TCC of the urothelium.

h. Images 1 to 3 mm thick reconstructed from data obtained with detector collimation as low as possible. Detector collimation may range from 1.25 mm in a 4-slice MDCT system to 0.6 mm in a 64-slice system.

i. Thinner (0.5-1.25 mm), overlapping reconstructions may be used for angiographic, MPR, and 3D applications.

j. Selection of acquired phases of enhancement should balance the clinical needs of the exam while reducing patient radiation dose to a minimum. (Figs. 3-35 and 3-36)

27. The most common abnormality of the ureters is a dual collecting system, or ureteral duplication. This condition is often an incidental finding characterized by the appearance of a second ureter descending from an individual kidney.

28. Ureteral duplication is more symptomatic in the pediatric patient and may present as urine reflux or obstruction.

29. TCC and obstruction from stones are two additional pathologic conditions of the ureters demonstrated on CT examination.

30. The bladder varies in size and appearance according to the amount of urine held. The unenhanced CT density of urine is similar to that of water.

31. Nephrographic (70-90 seconds) imaging provides an enhanced bladder wall used to evaluate the extent of tumor infiltration.

FIGURE 3-36 Coronal maximum intensity projection (MIP) image of the abdomen and pelvis. This image was produced from a delayed (excretory) phase acquisition during a CT urogram.

32. The additional delayed phase (>5 minutes) imaging of CT urography can be helpful in displaying the filling defects associated with bladder cancer.

33. Additional sequences with the patient in a prone and/or decubitus position may improve visualization of bladder wall tumors.

GASTROINTESTINAL SYSTEM

1. The *gastrointestinal tract* consists of the esophagus, stomach, small intestine, and large intestine.

2. Anatomic structures of the GI system are evaluated on all CT studies of the abdomen and/or pelvis (Figs. 3-37 and 3-38).

FIGURE 3-37 Abdomen—axial image.

FIGURE 3-38 Pelvis—axial image.

3. Although its findings are often nonspecific, CT plays an important role in the identification of disease within the GI tract.
4. General indications for CT evaluation of the GI system include:
   a. Inflammatory disease.
   b. Identification, evaluation, and staging of GI neoplasm.
   c. Trauma.
   d. Vascular disease.
5. CT imaging is also extremely valuable in the evaluation of various complications of GI disease processes, such as:
   a. *Perforation:* Puncture in the wall of the GI tract. Contents within the stomach or intestine may then spill into the abdominal cavity, with

the potential to cause infection known as *peritonitis*.

   b. *Fistula:* An abnormal connection between the intestine and an adjacent structure. Fistulas are commonly associated with inflammatory bowel disease.

   c. *Abscess:* A collection of pus caused by an infectious or inflammatory process within the GI tract.

6. The most important identifying sign of GI pathology on CT examination is wall thickening. The ability to evaluate the gastric and bowel walls is a crucial component of successful CT evaluation of the GI system.

7. Historically, CT evaluation of the bowel wall has been hampered by the muscular digestive motion of peristalsis. The acquisition speed of MDCT effectively eliminates peristaltic motion artifact and greatly improves the CT evaluation of intestinal wall pathology.

8. Distention and opacification with oral media, coupled with contrast enhancement through IV administration, offer the best level of GI wall demonstration.

9. The factors governing optimal bowel opacification and distention from oral contrast agents are:

   a. Contrast agent type: Dilute barium and water-soluble iodine oral contrast media are available as positive contrast agents. Water may serve as a negative oral contrast agent, providing bowel distention without the artifact possible with denser material. Air and gas are negative contrast agents used for stomach or bowel distention.

   b. Contrast agent volume: 750 to 1500 mL of oral contrast agent is typical for general studies of the abdomen and pelvis.

   c. Timing: Delay of scanning after the administration of oral contrast agent is based on the area of clinical concern. Opacification of the stomach and proximal small bowel may take only 30 minutes, whereas proper evaluation of the large intestine requires a delay of at least 90 minutes. Delays of up to 24 hours are not uncommon for complete opacification of the distal large intestine. Transit time varies with the patient's physiologic condition.

   d. Route of administration: Direct and immediate opacification of the distal large colon is possible with an enema of 150 to 250 mL of a positive contrast agent.

   e. Patient position: CT of the abdomen and/or pelvis is performed predominantly with the patient in the supine position. Additional positions may be used to improve opacification and distention of a particular portion of the GI tract.

10. Bowel wall enhances with the IV administration of an iodinated contrast agent. Enhancement improves demonstration of bowel wall thickening, mass lesions, inflammatory processes, and vascular perfusion abnormalities such as bowel ischemia.

11. Injection techniques for studies of the GI system are similar to those for general abdominal indications. 100 to 150 mL of non-ionic contrast agent administered at a rate of 2 to 4 mL/sec provides adequate wall enhancement.

12. Acquisition is typically obtained during the portal venous phase for optimal gastric and intestinal wall enhancement.

13. Contiguous 3- to 5-mm sections through the abdomen and pelvis, from above the diaphragm to the pubic symphysis, are acquired for complete evaluation of the GI system.

14. MDCT systems may utilize a narrow detector collimation (0.5-1.25 mm) for optimal MPR quality when clinically indicated (Fig. 3-39).

15. For evaluation of potential esophageal pathology, the acquisition may begin more superiorly as dictated by the area(s) of clinical concern.

16. The esophagus appears as an air- or contrast-filled cylindrical structure on axial CT imaging.

17. In addition to oral and IV contrast agents, a thick barium paste may be given immediately before scanning to further outline the esophagus.

18. CT of the esophagus is performed predominantly for evaluation of a neoplasm and staging of esophageal malignancy.

19. Inflammation of the esophagus, or *esophagitis*, is characterized on CT by uniform cylindrical thickening of the esophageal wall. Esophagitis is often secondary to gastroesophageal reflux disease (GERD).

20. Other abnormalities demonstrated during CT of the esophagus include:

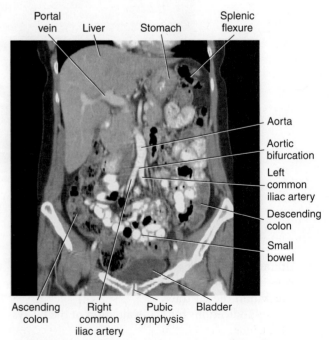

FIGURE 3-39 Coronal multiplanar reformation (MPR) image of the abdomen and pelvis.

a. Foreign bodies.

b. *Esophageal varices*, which are dilated veins of the esophagus that result from portal hypertension. They are often seen in patients with cirrhosis of the liver.

c. *Hiatal hernia*, defined as a protrusion of the gastroesophageal junction through the diaphragm into the thorax.

21. The stomach must be distended with a positive or negative oral contrast agent, or both, for CT evaluation.

22. 150 to 250 mL of dilute barium or iodine contrast agent is administered immediately before scanning. Alternatively, use of water as an oral contrast agent improves visualization of the enhancing gastric mucosa when an IV contrast agent is administered.

23. The stomach may be further distended with the administration of effervescent granules.

24. Placing the patient in the prone or decubitus position may also improve the demonstration of gastric pathology. A positive oral contrast agent distends the dependent portion of the stomach, whereas gas-forming crystals provide distention of the side facing upward.

25. Patients should have fasted for 4 to 6 hours before the study to ensure that the stomach is empty of food, which otherwise may mimic abnormality.

26. Common indications for specific CT evaluation of the stomach include benign and malignant gastric neoplasms, lymphoma, hiatal hernia, and assessment of complications due to bariatric (weight loss) surgery.

27. The *small intestine* is divided proximally to distally as the duodenum, jejunum, and ilium.

28. The duodenal bulb connects to the stomach's pyloric sphincter. The ilium leads to the large intestine at the ileocecal valve.

29. The duodenum is suspended from the diaphragm by the ligament of Treitz.

30. Opacification with an oral contrast agent is typically necessary for CT evaluation of the small intestine.

31. An oral contrast agent should be administered in sufficient volume (>750 mL) and at least 30 minutes before scanning for the duodenum and jejunum. Opacification of the ilium and proximal large intestine may take an hour or more, depending on the individual patient.

32. Water as an oral contrast agent improves visualization of the enhancing enteral wall when an IV contrast agent is administered.

33. MPR and 3D techniques may aid in visualization of the small bowel in its entirety.

34. External hernia of the small intestine is a common occurrence. There are many types of external hernias, including:

a. *Inguinal:* lower anterior abdominal wall in the region of the groin.

b. *Umbilical:* near the umbilicus; umbilical hernia is most common in pregnant women and obese patients.

c. *Incisional:* a complication of surgery.

35. *Small bowel obstruction* (SBO) is a serious and potentially fatal pathologic condition amenable to CT assessment.

36. SBO is typically characterized by loops of dilated proximal small bowel terminating abruptly at an area of collapsed bowel. Oral contrast agent does not pass beyond the obstruction.

37. Causes of small bowel obstruction include adhesions, hernia, and tumor.

38. *Intussusception* describes the condition whereby a portion of the small intestine collapses or telescopes into itself. It is a rare occurrence that may result in obstruction.

39. *Ileus* is an area of intestine that has lost normal contractile motion, resulting in obstruction.

40. *Crohn's disease* is an inflammatory condition that often affects the small intestine. It is usually characterized on CT by wall thickening, edema, and haziness of the fat surrounding the affected bowel. Also referred to as *stranding*, this increase in density of fat usually indicates inflammation. Crohn's disease may also affect the large colon and the remainder of the GI tract.

41. Other conditions of the small intestine that are evaluated by CT are benign and malignant neoplasm, lymphoma, edema, and trauma.

42. The *large intestine* begins with the cecum at the ileocecal valve and progresses to the ascending, transverse, and descending portions, the sigmoid colon and rectum.

43. The appendix appears in most patients as a tubular structure extending from the cecum, near the ileocecal valve.

44. Anatomic location, haustral markings, and the presence of fecal matter help identify the large intestine on CT cross section.

45. Opacification with an oral contrast agent is typically a necessity for CT evaluation of the large intestine.

46. Oral contrast agents should be administered in sufficient volume (>750 mL) and at least 90 minutes before scanning. Opacification of the distal large intestine may take as much as 24 hours, depending on the individual patient.

47. Direct and immediate opacification of the distal large intestine is possible with an enema of 150 to 250 mL of a positive contrast agent.

48. Insufflation with air or gas distends the rectum and distal colon, allowing for improved visualization of wall pathology.

49. Clinical indications for CT evaluation of the large intestine include:

a. Neoplasm:

• Polyps (adenoma): precancerous growths of the colon.

• Colorectal carcinoma: CT is used primarily for staging of the disease and assessment for reoccurrence.

b. Inflammation:
- *Diverticulitis* refers to the inflammation of *diverticula*, which are pouches that develop outward from the colon wall. It is most common in the sigmoid and is characterized on CT by wall thickening and stranding of the surrounding fat.
- *Inflammatory bowel disease* (IBD) is a general term used to describe conditions of inflammation of the colon, or colitis:
  - *Crohn's colitis* is similar to Crohn's disease, which affects the small intestine.
  - *Ulcerative colitis* (UC) is characterized on CT by wall thickening and narrowing of the intestinal lumen.
- *Appendicitis*, inflammation of the appendix, is characterized on CT by distention, a thickened contrast-enhancing wall, and periappendiceal fat stranding. CT examinations to diagnose appendicitis should be optimized with thin-section (<5 mm) imaging through the entire abdomen and pelvis to identify potential causes of abdominal pain that are unrelated to the appendix. IV administration of a contrast agent may improve visualization of the appendix in the patient with limited intra-abdominal fat. Oral or rectal administration of a contrast agent can also improve identification of the appendicitis and its associated inflammatory changes.

50. Focused CT for appendicitis reduces patient radiation dose by limiting the acquisition to the area of the cecum and appendix only. Although the radiation dose is significantly reduced with this technique, the chances of detection of alternative diagnoses are also lower. Focused CT for appendicitis is usually employed in pediatric patients.

51. An *appendicolith*, a calcification within the appendix, is often associated with appendicitis.

52. An *enterovesical fistula* is an abnormal communication between the bowel and the bladder. It typically results from inflammatory processes of the colon such as diverticulitis. The role of CT in suspected fistula is to identify the entry of oral or rectal contrast agent into the bladder through the fistula. It is important that the bladder not be opacified. Therefore, acquisition of sections before the administration of an IV contrast agent is crucial.

PELVIS AND REPRODUCTIVE SYSTEM

1. Clinical indications for CT evaluation of the pelvis include:
   a. Identification of primary pelvic cancers, including those of the colon, bladder, and reproductive organs.
   b. Oncologic staging, which includes evaluation of pelvic adenopathy for metastatic spread of primary cancer to the pelvic lymph nodes and assessment of local tumor recurrence.
   c. Assessment of soft tissue and bony trauma.

2. The male reproductive organs are not commonly imaged by CT. However, the internal location of the prostate gland and seminal vesicles allows for their visualization during a routine examination of the male pelvis (Fig. 3-40).

Contrast-filled bladder

Rectus abdominus muscle

Sigmoid colon

External iliac artery

External iliac vein

Seminal vesicles

Right ureterovesical junction (UVJ)

Rectum

FIGURE 3-40 Male pelvis—axial image.

3. The external penis and testicles are not routinely evaluated by CT but may be included on scans that proceed inferiorly beyond the pelvic floor.

4. Ectopic or undescended testes appear internally within the pelvis. They are usually atrophic in appearance and have a greater propensity for malignancy.

5. A *hydrocele* of the testes is an abnormal accumulation of fluid around a testicle.

6. On axial CT, the prostate gland is positioned between the pubic symphysis anteriorly and the rectum posteriorly. It lies just inferior to the base of the bladder.

7. *Benign prostate hyperplasia* (BPH) is an increase in prostate volume, which can result in constriction of the urethra and interference with urination. It typically occurs in middle-aged to elderly men and is similar in CT appearance to prostate carcinoma.

8. CT findings in prostate carcinoma include prostatic enlargement and pelvic adenopathy. The primary role of CT in the diagnosis and treatment of prostate cancer is one of staging.

9. The pair of seminal vesicles forms a "bow-tie" shape between the prostate and the base of the bladder.

10. The *female reproductive organs* are routinely demonstrated on CT because of their internal location. They are the uterus, cervix, ovaries, and fallopian tubes (Figs. 3-41 and 3-42).

11. The uterus is typically demonstrated as an oval, homogeneous soft tissue mass positioned between the bladder and rectum.

12. The uterine wall is divided as follows:
    a. *Perimetrium:* Outer layer.
    b. *Myometrium:* Middle layer.
    c. *Endometrium:* Inner layer.

13. The myometrium enhances brightly after IV administration of a contrast agent, owing to its highly vascular composition.

14. The cervix extends inferiorly from the uterus and may also enhance after IV administration of a contrast agent.

15. *Adnexa* is used to describe an appendage of an organ; the ovaries and fallopian tubes constitute the uterine adnexa.

16. The ovaries may demonstrate a soft tissue or cystic CT density and are located in close proximity to the uterus. The ovaries are often not visualized in postmenopausal women.

17. The primary clinical indications for CT of the female pelvis and reproductive organs are the evaluation of pelvic pain and the identification or staging of gynecologic masses.

18. Benign masses of the uterus and adnexa include:
    a. *Leiomyoma,* or fibroid uterus.
    b. Ovarian cysts.
    c. *Cystic teratoma,* a dermoid mass consisting of various CT densities including those of soft tissue, fat, teeth, and bone.

19. Malignant masses of the uterus and adnexa include:
    a. Cervical cancer.
    b. Uterine cancer; endometrial carcinoma is the most prevalent gynecologic malignancy.

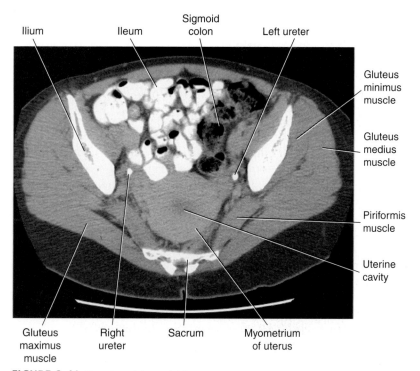

FIGURE 3-41 Female pelvis—axial image.

FIGURE 3-42 Female pelvis—axial image.

c. Ovarian cancer, the CT appearance of which may be uniformly solid or cystic, or a combination of the two.

20. For the evaluation of a gynecologic mass, the insertion of a tampon assists in identifying the vaginal canal.

Special Procedures

A. Body CT Angiography

1. MDCT systems with detector configurations of 16-slice and above are readily capable of scanning the entire abdomen with sub-millimeter collimation in less than 20 seconds. With careful bolus timing, the abdominal vasculature may be imaged during a single breath-hold and at peak arterial enhancement.

2. Isotropic data acquisition allows for high-quality vascular imaging in any plane, including volumetric 3D display.

3. Body CTA includes the CT angiographic evaluation of the following structures:
   a. Aorta.
   b. Renal arteries.
   c. Mesenteric arteries.
   d. Hepatic arteries.

4. The technical considerations for body CTA are similar to those outlined in previous sections on CT angiography. Additional information specific to each anatomic area are summarized in this section.

5. Protocols are CT system–specific, being adjusted according to the clinical area of concern. Detector collimation, gantry rotation time, and pitch are adjusted to ensure that the entire acquisition is attained during a single breath-hold.

6. The guiding principle of contrast agent administration for CTA is that the bolus should last throughout the entire scan, but not beyond it.

7. Total volumes of contrast agents used range from 75 to 125 mL, being determined by the flow rate and the scan duration.

8. Good venous access is required because flow rates in the range of 4 to 5 mL/sec are recommended.

9. Scan delay is determined by a test bolus or automated bolus tracking.

10. Arterial phase imaging is performed for arterial vascular mapping, and portal venous phase imaging for venous vascular mapping.

11. A positive oral contrast agent is not given because of its interference with MPR and 3D imaging techniques.

12. The primary indications for CTA of the aorta are aneurysm and dissection.

13. MDCT technology allows for scanning of the entire aorta in a single breath-hold from above the arch through the common iliac arteries. The extent of acquisition is determined by the clinical indication. (Fig. 3-43)

14. The abdominal aorta divides into the right and left common iliac arteries at approximately the level of L4.

15. Additional technical considerations for CTA of the aorta may be found earlier, in the section on chest CTA.

16. The primary indications for CTA of the renal arteries are stenosis, aneurysm, and renal transplant evaluation.

17. The renal arteries, which are small structures, are optimally visualized with MDCT section widths of 1.25 mm or less.

18. The general rule for CTA in all body areas is that the section width should be no wider than the diameter of the smallest vessel to be evaluated.

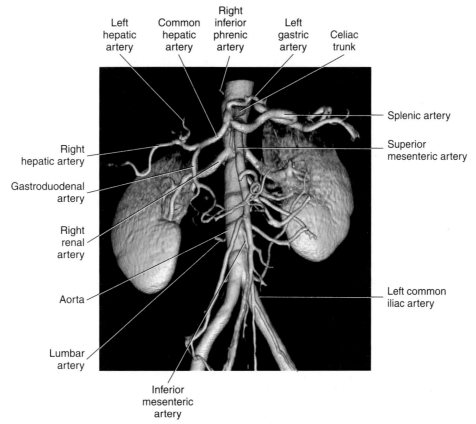

Left hepatic artery

Common hepatic artery

Right inferior phrenic artery

Left gastric artery

Celiac trunk

Right hepatic artery

Gastroduodenal artery

Right renal artery

Aorta

Lumbar artery

Inferior mesenteric artery

Splenic artery

Superior mesenteric artery

Left common iliac artery

FIGURE 3-43 CT angiogram of the abdominal aorta. *(From Kelley L, Peterson C: Sectional Anatomy for Image Professionals, 2nd ed. St Louis, Mosby, 2007.)*

19. CTA evaluation of the mesenteric vasculature includes the superior mesenteric artery (SMA), inferior mesenteric artery (IMA), superior mesenteric vein (SMV), and inferior mesenteric vein (IMV).
20. Also evaluated are the branches of the celiac axis:
    a. Left gastric artery.
    b. Common hepatic artery.
    c. Splenic artery.
21. Dual-phase imaging, which consists of the arterial (20-30 seconds) and portal venous (60-70 seconds) phases, is typically performed for complete evaluation of the mesenteric vasculature.
22. Indications for CTA evaluation of the mesenteric vasculature include:
    a. Assessment of neoplastic invasion (primarily from pancreatic cancer).
    b. Bowel ischemia; occlusion or thrombosis of the mesenteric vessels can result in decreased blood supply to bowel.
    c. Unexplained gastrointestinal bleed.
23. CTA of the hepatic arteries is performed primarily for assessment of the hepatic transplant patient. Additional indications are aneurysm and pretherapy planning for hepatic carcinoma.

24. Protocols for body CTA depend strictly on the area(s) of clinical concern and the technical capabilities of the CT system employed. Example technical parameters using a 64-slice system are:
    a. Water as an oral contrast agent to distend the proximal GI tract.
    b. Initial non-contrast, low-dose acquisition through the area(s) of interest to localize vasculature, evaluate for calcium, intramural hematoma (IMH), or other pathology.
    c. Injection of 75 to 125 mL of a non-ionic contrast agent at 4 mL/sec.
    d. Administration of a saline flush to improve contrast agent dose efficiency.
    e. Test bolus or automated bolus tracking measured at the celiac artery.
    f. Helical CTA acquisition with 0.625-mm detector width.
    g. Scan extent is determined by the area(s) of clinical concern.
    h. 120 kVp, auto mA modulation.
    i. 0.5- to 0.8-second gantry rotation time.
    j. Reconstructed slice thickness of 0.6 to 0.75 mm with 50% overlap.
    k. Use of MPR, MIP, and VR imaging techniques.

B. CT Enteroclysis

1. *CT enteroclysis* is a specialized evaluation of the small bowel whereby a nasogastric catheter is placed into the duodenum under fluoroscopic guidance. 1.5 to 2.0 L of enteral contrast agent is administered directly into the small intestine for maximal opacification.
2. Non-IV contrast, thin-section (0.6-1.25 mm) CT images are acquired through the abdomen and pelvis.
3. Coronal and sagittal MPR images are used to visualize the small intestine in its entirety.
4. Alternatively, CT enteroclysis can be performed with a neutral enteral contrast agent such as water or 0.1% barium sulfate (VoLumen) infused through a nasogastric tube. 125 to 150 mL of an iodinated IV contrast agent is administered at a rate of 3 to 5 mL/sec. CT acquisition occurs at a delay of 45 to 50 seconds, corresponding to the early portal venous phase of optimal intestinal wall enhancement.
5. Clinical indications for CT enteroclysis include Crohn's disease, obstruction, and neoplasms of the small intestine.

C. CT Enterography

1. *CT enterography* is an MDCT scan specifically of the small intestine that is less invasive than CT enteroclysis.
2. Opacification of the small intestine is achieved by the oral administration of a large volume (1.5 to 2.0 L) of low-density (0.1%) barium sulfate solution (VoLumen).
3. Example protocol for oral contrast agent administration is:
   a. 500 mL 60 minutes before scan.
   b. 500 mL 40 minutes before scan.
   c. 250 mL 20 minutes before scan.
   d. 250 mL 10 minutes before scan.
4. An iodinated IV contrast agent is administered at a rate of 3 to 5 mL/sec to a total volume of 125 to 150 mL. CT acquisition occurs at a delay of 45 to 50 seconds, corresponding to the early portal venous phase of optimal intestinal wall enhancement.
5. Thin-section (0.6-1.25 mm) acquisition is made through the abdomen and pelvis.
6. Coronal and sagittal MPR images are used to visualize the small intestine in its entirety.
7. CT enterography avoids the necessity of a nasogastric catheter. However, it may not consistently achieve the level of small bowel distention and opacification possible with CT enteroclysis.

D. CT Colonography

1. *CT colonography* is a primarily screening MDCT examination of the large intestine with the primary goal to identify adenomatous polyps.
2. Beyond routine screening for polyps or malignancy, additional indications for CT colonography (CTC) include:

a. Failed conventional colonoscopy.
b. Patient contraindication to conventional colonoscopy.

3. The properly prepared bowel is distended and scanned utilizing MDCT technology. Dedicated CTC software displays the acquired slice data as a 2D or 3D model with an endoscopic perspective. The viewer has the ability to "fly through" the colon to identify polyps.
4. Proper bowel preparation is crucial to the success of a CTC exam. The components of bowel preparation may be itemized as:
   a. Diet: The patient is restricted to low-residue diet for 2 to 3 days before the exam. On the day before the exam, only clear liquids may be ingested.
   b. Catharsis: Bowel cleansing agents include the standard colonoscopy preparations of polyethylene glycol (PEG) and magnesium citrate. Please consult your department protocol for details regarding bowel cleansing agents and procedures.
   c. Tagging: A dual-agent method consisting of the oral administration of both barium and a water-soluble iodine contrast agent. The barium tags residual stool and coats the surface of polyps. The iodine contrast agent tags residual fluid. Tagged fluid and fecal matter exhibit high CT density and appear "white" on the CTC image. Tagging allows for differentiation of polyp from fecal matter and improves the visualization of polyps that may be surrounded by residual fluid.
5. Adequate distention of the colon is the second important component of a successful CTC examination.
6. Colon insufflation involves the introduction of room air or carbon dioxide (CO_2) into the colon for the purpose of bowel wall distention.
7. Insufflation occurs after a small catheter has been inserted into the rectum with the patient in the left lateral decubitus position.
8. In the manual technique of colon insufflation, room air is manually introduced into the large intestine via rectal catheter.
9. Automated CO_2 delivery also accomplishes insufflation with the use of a mechanical pump that dispenses CO_2 into the colon.
10. The advantages of automatic CO_2 insufflation include better overall distention and lower risk of perforation. Also, owing to the faster absorption rate of CO_2, there is less postprocedural discomfort for the patient.
11. Once insufflation is complete, the patient is placed in the supine position, and a scout (topogram) image is obtained. Additional air or CO_2 is administered until the desired level of distention is reached.
12. Thin-section (1.0-1.25 mm) acquisition of the colon is obtained with the patient supine. Detector collimation ranges between 0.6 mm and 2.5 mm, depending on the capabilities of each particular MDCT system.

13. The patient is then turned prone, and the scan is repeated.
14. If the patient is unable to tolerate the prone position, a decubitus or oblique position may be substituted.
15. Two positions are a necessity to ensure maximal distention of the various segments of the colon and to differentiate between fixed polyps and mobile feces and fluid.
16. Dedicated CT colonography software reformats the acquired data into 2D and 3D endoluminal displays of the interior walls of the colon.
17. Electronic stool extraction software may be employed to remove retained fecal matter from the display and reduce false-positive interpretations.
18. Images are best displayed in a "lung-type" window setting, for example, WL −400, WW 1600.
19. Screening CTC is typically performed without the use of an iodinated IV contrast agent.
20. Dose reduction is vital for the screening CT-colonographic exam. Owing to the high-contrast nature of soft tissue polyps surrounded by air, very low mA settings are possible with minimal image quality loss due to noise. Effective mAs can be manually set at 50 or lower. Automated tube current modulation techniques may also be used to limit patient radiation dose during CT colonography.

E. CT Cystography

1. *CT cystography* is a specialized CT examination of the bladder in which an iodinated contrast agent is directly administered under gravity into the bladder via Foley catheter.
2. Indications include:
   a. Trauma.
   b. Fistula formation between the bladder and adjacent organs.
   c. Postoperative leakage.
   d. Neoplasms.
3. Technical considerations for CT cystography include:
   a. An iodinated contrast agent, mixed with normal saline, is introduced to fully distend the bladder. Total volume of fluid ranges between 250 and 300 mL.
   b. Thin-section (<1 mm) acquisition is performed through the bladder.
   c. Multiple acquisitions—contrast administration, post–contrast administration, and post–drainage—may be obtained.
   d. Sagittal or coronal MPR and 3D volume-rendered reconstructions are performed.

MUSCULOSKELETAL SYSTEM

1. Despite the superiority of MRI in most clinical applications, CT of the musculoskeletal system remains a valuable modality option.
2. Mainly because of its superior speed, CT remains the primary imaging choice for evaluation of the patient with trauma. CT has become the first choice for assessment of spinal injury in the emergency setting. Fractures and dislocations of the complex components of the spine, joints, and so on, are imaged superbly with MDCT. The cortex of bony structures is particularly well demonstrated on CT.
3. Also, patients with orthopedic hardware, incompatible implanted devices, or other contraindications to magnetic resonance imaging may benefit from CT evaluation of the musculoskeletal system.
4. Each CT examination of the musculoskeletal system must be individualized to meet the clinical needs of the patient. There are many vital considerations that need to be tailored to any given examination, including:
   a. Optimal patient position.
   b. Extent of the area to be scanned.
   c. Necessity of IV contrast agent and the administration details.
   d. Technical parameters such as slice thickness, imaging planes, and 3D applications.

Technical Considerations

A. Spine

1. The articulation between successive vertebrae consists of the intervertebral disc and two posterior facet (zygapophyseal) joints.
2. An intervertebral disc separates each two vertebrae, beginning at the C2-C3 space. There is no disc space between C1 and C2.
3. Each disc consists of a soft center called the *nucleus pulposus*, which is surrounded by the firmer, outer *anulus fibrosus*. The disc is connected to the superior and inferior surfaces of the respective vertebral bodies at the end plate.
4. The *spinal cord* extends inferiorly from the brain's medulla and terminates at approximately the level of T12-L1. At its distal end, the spinal cord tapers into the *conus medullaris*. The *cauda equina* is the nerve bundle extending inferiorly from the spinal cord.
5. The intervertebral discs are homogeneous in appearance with attenuation values ranging between 50 and 100 HU.
6. Clinical indications for CT evaluation of the spine include:
   a. Trauma: CT of the spine has become routine and has replaced radiographic evaluation in many trauma centers. The lower cervical spine (C6-C7) and the thoracolumbar junction (T12-L2) are the most common sites of spine fracture.
   b. Degenerative disease, including the evaluation of neck or back pain and the associated neurologic symptoms of degenerative disc disease. Degenerative processes include:
      • *Herniated disc*: Disc herniation may appear as a slight bulge, a moderate protrusion, or a more severe disc extrusion, whereby the

nucleus pulposus tears through the anulus fibrosus. A *sequestered disc* or *free fragment* occurs when a portion of the disc's nucleus completely breaks free and migrates from its normal position.

- *Facet joint disease:* The *facet joints* are formed by the articulation between the inferior articular processes of one vertebra and the superior articular processes of the next. Degenerative changes due to arthritis or abnormal facet growth (hypertrophy) are common.
- *Spondylosis:* A condition of hypertrophy (overgrowth) of the facets that can lead to spinal stenosis.
- *Spinal stenosis:* Consists of narrowing of the bony canals that contain the spinal cord, nerve roots, or both. Compression of the spinal cord or nerve roots may result in the referred limb pain commonly referred to as *sciatica.* Additional causes are disc herniation, tumor, and the formation of osteophytes (abnormal bone growths).
- *Spondylolysis:* A defect in the pars interarticularis commonly caused by osteophyte formation. The *pars interarticularis* is the area of a vertebra between in the inferior and superior articular processes (the neck of the "scotty dog").
- *Spondylolisthesis:* Forward "slipping" of an upper vertebral body over the lower due to degenerative changes of the facet joints. This disorder is best demonstrated on sagittal MPR images of the spine.

c. Neoplasm: Although primary tumors readily occur, the majority of neoplasms involving the spine are metastatic in origin. Metastatic spinal lesions from breast, lung, or prostate cancer are the most prevalent.

d. Infectious processes such as osteomyelitis and abscess.

e. Inflammatory disorders, including rheumatoid arthritis and ankylosing spondylitis.

f. Postoperative assessment: in general, CT undergoes less image degradation from metallic hardware compared with magnetic resonance imaging.

7. The patient is positioned supine and head-first for CT examinations of the cervical, thoracic, or complete spine. During CT evaluation of the lumbar spine only, positioning the patient supine and feet-first may improve comfort by limiting how much of the patient's body enters the gantry.

8. For the nontraumatic CT examination of the cervical spine, the patient should be instructed to relax the shoulders downward to reduce streak artifact from the broad upper trunk. The patient's hands may be positioned underneath the body or

stabilized with appropriate, comfortable immobilization straps.

9. For nontraumatic examinations of the thoracolumbar spine, the legs should be slightly elevated and flexed at the knees, and supported on pillows or an appropriate positioning cushion to alleviate pressure on the lower back.

10. The trauma patient undergoing CT evaluation of the musculoskeletal system must be positioned with minimal manipulation.

11. Acquisition with 16–detector row (or higher) MDCT systems typically utilize detector collimation within the range of 0.625 to 1.25 mm, with images reconstructed at widths based on the anatomy or pathology in question.

12. For general studies of the thoracic and lumbar spines, slice reconstruction at widths of 3 to 5 mm are sufficient. Section widths of 1 to 2 mm or less are preferable for imaging the cervical spine. For trauma situations and in anticipation of 3D and multiplanar reconstructions, the thinnest possible detector collimation should be utilized, with overlapping slices at thicknesses ranging from 0.75 to 1.25 mm.

13. Cervical spine acquisition usually includes at least C3 through T1 for general indications; the cervical spine in its entirety (C1-C7) should be included for trauma (Figs. 3-44 and 3-45).

14. For CT evaluation of the thoracic spine, the specific area of clinical concern is acquired, including at least one vertebral level both above and below. The entire thoracic spine may be covered, offering the availability of comprehensive sagittal and coronal reformation for evaluation of vertebral alignment, degenerative disease, and so on.

15. Most degenerative disease processes affect the lumbar spine beginning at the level of L3-L4. Scanning from L2 to S1 is typically sufficient, with expansion of coverage for trauma situations (Figs. 3-46 to 3-48).

16. All CT examinations of the spine should consist of a contiguous, volumetric acquisition. Individually angled scans through each disc space are unnecessary because of the isotropic nature of MDCT.

17. ATCM techniques should be utilized to minimize patient radiation dose.

18. Acquisition is performed with a large SFOV (48-50 cm). Targeted reconstructions are made using a DFOV between 10 and 15 cm. Larger DFOV reconstructions may be used to retrospectively display a greater anatomic area as the clinical indication dictates.

19. Separate data reconstructions using soft tissue and bone algorithms (kernels) may be required to display pathology optimally.

20. Dual window settings are used for bone and soft tissue evaluation. Sample WL and WW settings for optimal image display are:

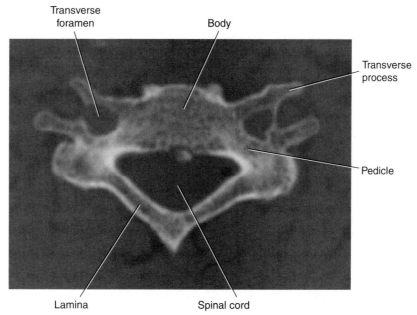

FIGURE 3-44 Cervical spine—axial image.

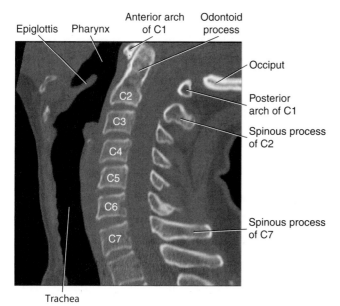

FIGURE 3-45 Cervical spine—sagittal multiplanar reformation (MPR) image.

    a. Soft tissue: WL 50, WW 400.
    b. Bone: WL 300, WW 2000.
21. IV administration of a contrast agent is typically not indicated for CT examination of the spine. Exceptions include assessment for metastatic disease, soft tissue mass, infection, or abscess. An IV contrast agent may also be indicated in the patient with a history of prior spine surgery, in an effort to differentiate scar tissue from recurrent disc disease.
22. When indicated, 100 to 125 mL of a non-ionic contrast agent may be administered at a rate of 2 to 3 mL/sec with scanning during the portal venous phase.

23. For trauma settings, injury to the vertebral arteries may be evaluated with administration of an IV contrast agent and the inclusion of a CT angiographic study of the affected spinal area. Higher injection rates (4-5 mL/sec) are used and arterial phase or dual-phase imaging is performed.
24. MPR, MIP, and 3D volume-rendered techniques are routinely used for CT spine evaluation.
25. Thin-section MDCT offers less streak artifact from metallic hardware when than conventional single-detector CT (SDCT), leading to better imaging of the postoperative spine.

B. Upper and Lower Extremities
1. Trauma is the primary indication for CT evaluation of the musculoskeletal system. CT provides demonstration of fractures and identification of bony fragments.
2. CT of the musculoskeletal system is used to identify and characterize bony neoplasms such as cysts, benign and malignant tumors, and metastatic deposits.
3. Benign tumors of the skeletal system include enchondroma, chondroblastoma, osteoid osteoma, and osteochondroma.
4. Malignant tumors of the skeletal system include osteosarcoma, chondrosarcoma, and multiple myeloma.
5. Multiple myeloma is the most common malignant primary tumor of the skeletal system. It is a systemic malignancy involving the plasma cells found within bone marrow.
6. The degenerative changes to bone due to arthritis are well demonstrated on CT.
7. Infection of a bone, or *osteomyelitis*, may be assessed with CT imaging.

Inferior vena cava

Aorta

Intervertebral disk

Psoas major muscle

Cauda equina

Inferior articular process

Superior articular process

Zygapophyseal (facet) joint

Spinous process

FIGURE 3-46 Lumbar spine—axial image displayed using a bone window.

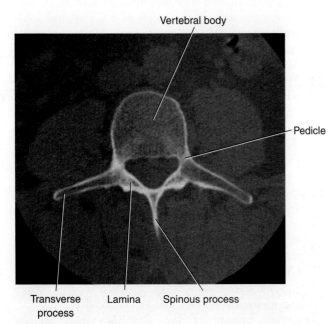

Vertebral body

Pedicle

Transverse process

Lamina

Spinous process

FIGURE 3-47 Lumbar spine—axial image displayed using a bone window.

8. Inflammatory and infectious processes involving the soft tissues of the extremities, such as cellulitis, fascitis, and abscess, may also be amenable to CT assessment.

9. Isotropic data acquisition allows for the production of high-quality multiplanar reformation (MPR) images. Isotropic multiplanar imaging is the hallmark of quality MDCT evaluation of the musculoskeletal system and is accomplished by applying two key concepts:

   a. Choose the thinnest detector collimation available to produce the thinnest slices available.

   b. Reconstruct the acquired data with the smallest DFOV possible for the part of interest.

10. Thin section acquisition and the use of reduced DFOV settings may result in an increase in patient radiation dose. In cooperation with the interpreting physician, the CT technologist must balance the image quality requirements of the study against the responsibility to reduce patient dose to a minimum.

11. Thin-section (<1.25 mm) volumetric acquisition is made in the axial plane. Scan is acquired perpendicular to the long axis of the part to maximize the number of slices obtained. The extent of the scan is determined by the clinical indication.

12. Images are reconstructed using at least a 50% overlap to improve the quality of 3D and MPR images.

13. With isotropic data acquisition, resolution of the MPR images is equal to that of the axial scan. This capability eliminates the need for an additional scan in a second plane for most clinical situations.

14. A high spatial frequency algorithm (kernel) is used for image reconstruction to maximize bony detail. Additional reconstruction with a soft tissue algorithm can be utilized as clinically warranted.

15. Dual window settings are used for bone and soft tissue evaluation. Sample WL and WW settings for optimal image display are:

   a. Soft tissue: WL 50, WW 400.

   b. Bone: WL 300, WW 2000.

Lumbar vertebral
body

Dorsal
root ganglion

Cauda
equina

Spinous
process

Ligamentum   Lamina
flavum

FIGURE 3-48 Lumbar spine—axial image displayed using a soft tissue window.

16. Scout (topogram) images should be acquired in both anteroposterior and lateral projections. Scout images are carefully evaluated to ensure proper patient position and minimize the scanning coverage.

17. Patient positioning during CT studies of the extremities varies with the part to be scanned and the clinical indication. The challenge is to obtain the proper position while maintaining a sufficient level of comfort for the patient throughout the exam.

18. Ensuring patient comfort is vital, because movement severely compromises scan quality.

19. The primary goal of patient positioning during scanning of the upper extremity is to comfortably place the part of interest free of superimposition with the rest of the body.

20. The "superman" position places the patient prone with the affected arm above the head. This position allows the hand, wrist, forearm, and elbow to be scanned without superimposition with the patient's head and trunk.

21. The patient's hand is usually pronated for studies of the hand, wrist, and forearm. When not contraindicated, the patient's hand is supinated for scans of the elbow, a position that places the humeral epicondyles parallel to the CT table.

22. When the "superman" position is unattainable, acquisition may be obtained with the patient supine and the affected arm at the side in a neutral position. This position results in unavoidable streaking artifact from the patient's body.

23. Assessments of fracture and dislocation are the primary indications for CT of the elbow, forearm, wrist, and hand.

24. The wrist's scaphoid bone is a common location for complex fracture. Axial CT imaging with coronal and sagittal MPR images of the scaphoid are extremely valuable in their ability to demonstrate small fractures and non-union, which may not be easily identified on conventional radiographs (Fig. 3-49).

Fourth   Fifth
metacarpophalangeal joint   metacarpal base

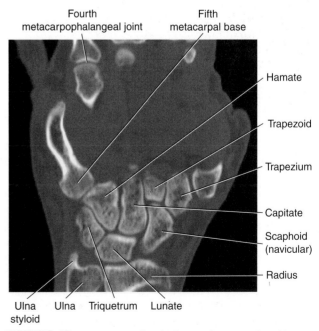

Hamate

Trapezoid

Trapezium

Capitate

Scaphoid
(navicular)

Radius

Ulna   Ulna   Triquetrum   Lunate
styloid

FIGURE 3-49 Wrist—coronal multiplanar reformation (MPR) image.

FIGURE 3-50 Foot—axial image.

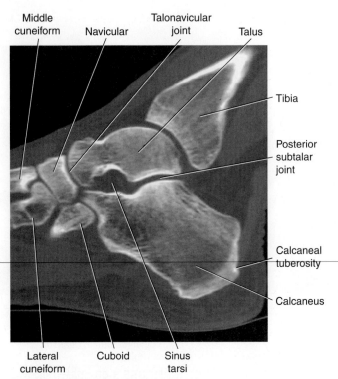

FIGURE 3-51 Ankle—sagittal multiplanar reformation (MPR) image.

25. The foot may be clinically divided as:
    a. *Forefoot:* Metatarsals and phalanges.
    b. *Midfoot:* Navicular, cuboid, cuneiforms.
    c. *Hindfoot:* Talus and calcaneus.
26. Imaging planes for the foot and ankle for both direct acquisition and MPR reconstruction may be described as follows:
    a. Direct axial: The plane parallel to the foot's plantar surface. Scanning in the direct axial plane is performed with the patient's foot flexed and the toes pointing straight up. Gantry angulation may be used to achieve correct scan plane when it is not otherwise possible (Fig. 3-50).
    b. Oblique axial: Parallel to the metatarsals, approximately 20 to 30 degrees caudal from the direct axial plane. MPR images along this plane are used to assess the tarsal-metatarsal joint.
    c. Sagittal: Divides the foot and ankle from medial to lateral. Sagittal MPR images provide detailed visualization of the tarsal and metatarsal bones and joints (Fig. 3-51).
    d. Coronal: Divides the foot and ankle from posterior to anterior. Provides visualization of the ankle joint with an anteroposterior perspective (Fig. 3-52).
27. Examinations of the midfoot and forefoot are usually performed with the patient supine, knee slightly flexed, with the affected foot flat on the scan table. The unaffected foot should be removed from the scan plane through greater flexing of the unaffected leg. Removing the other extremity from the field allows for DFOV optimization and minimizes streak artifact.
28. Thin-section (<1.5 mm) volumetric acquisition is made in the oblique coronal plane. The scan plane

FIGURE 3-52 Ankle—coronal multiplanar reformation (MPR) image.

is perpendicular to the long axis of the metatarsals to maximize the number of slices obtained. The gantry may be angled to achieve the proper scan acquisition plane. The extent of the scan is determined by the clinical indication.

29. The ankle and hindfoot are typically scanned with a thin-section (<1.5 mm) volumetric acquisition in the direct axial plane, perpendicular to the tibia. The patient's feet are flexed 90 degrees (toes up) and supported on a box or cushion. The scan

should begin above the syndesmosis—the articulation between the distal tibia and fibula—and should extend through the entire calcaneus.

30. *Tarsal coalition* refers to the abnormal union of adjacent bones of the ankle. It is most common at the talocalcaneal and calcaneonavicular joints.

31. The *Lisfranc joint* is the articulation between the tarsals and metatarsals. CT is used to evaluate fractures, subluxations, and dislocations of the Lisfranc joint.

32. Examinations of the distal femur, knee, and proximal tibia are performed with the patient in a relaxed, supine position. When possible, the other leg may be flexed at the knee and/or raised to bring it out from direct superimposition with the part of interest. (Fig. 3-53)

33. CT examinations of the knee may also be performed at varying degrees of flexion (0, 30, 45, 60, and 90 degrees) to demonstrate patellar tracking abnormalities.

34. Tibial plateau fractures are particularly well suited to evaluation by CT.

35. The *bone length study* involves the use of the CT system to acquire digital scout radiographs of the lower extremities. Both anteroposterior (AP) and lateral scout views are obtained using a low-dose technique. Scout views include from above the hip joint through the ankle joint. Analytical system software is used to measure and compare the length of each extremity for size discrepancy.

36. Most CT studies of the musculoskeletal system do not require IV administration of a contrast agent.

37. The indications for the use of an IV contrast agent are:
    a. Identification of bony or soft tissue infection and abscess.
    b. Inflammatory processes involving muscle, which may be better demonstrated with a contrast agent because of the tendency of infected muscle to enhance to a lesser degree than normal musculature.
    c. Assessing the vascularity of a musculoskeletal neoplasm.
    d. CTA evaluation in trauma situations.

C. Shoulder Girdle and Sternum

1. The *shoulder girdle* consists primarily of the glenohumeral, acromioclavicular, and sternoclavicular joints.

2. The clinical indications for and technical aspects of CT studies of the shoulder girdle are similar to those for studies of the distal extremities.

3. The patient is typically positioned supine with the arms down at the side.

4. Studies of patients with wide shoulders may suffer from *out-of-field artifacts*, in which the shoulders extend beyond the limits of the SFOV. This streaking artifact can be avoided by positioning the side of interest more toward the center of the gantry. The out-of-field artifact will still occur but will not appear in the small DFOV chosen to target the shoulder of interest.

5. When not contraindicated, the unaffected arm may be raised above the head to reduce streaking due to the dense shoulder area.

6. The patient should be instructed to suspend respiration during CT acquisition through the sternum, sternoclavicular joints, or clavicle to avoid motion artifact.

7. For the shoulder, thin-section (<1.25 mm) axial scans are volumetrically acquired through the glenohumeral joint, extending from above the humeral head inferiorly through the proximal humerus (Fig. 3-54).

8. The isotropic dataset may then be reformatted into coronal and sagittal images through the glenohumeral joint. Surface- and volume-rendered 3D images may be reconstructed.

9. The scan prescription for studies of the clavicle, acromioclavicular joints, sternoclavicular joints, clavicle, sternum, scapula, and humerus is adjusted accordingly.

D. Pelvic Girdle

1. Bony structures of the *pelvic girdle* include the sacrum, coccyx, sacroiliac joints, and hips.

2. The clinical indications for and technical aspects of CT studies of the sacrum and coccyx are similar to those in the remainder of the spine.

3. Trauma is the chief clinical indication for CT evaluation of the articulation between the femoral head and acetabulum (hip joint). Dislocations and fractures of the hip joint are well-demonstrated on CT.

4. The *acetabulum* comprises the ischium, the ilium, and the pubis.

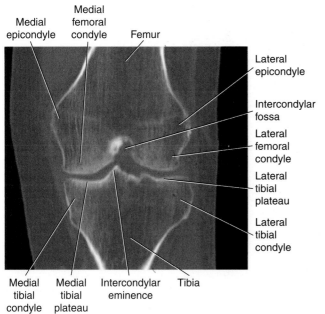

FIGURE 3-53 Knee—coronal multiplanar reformation (MPR) image.

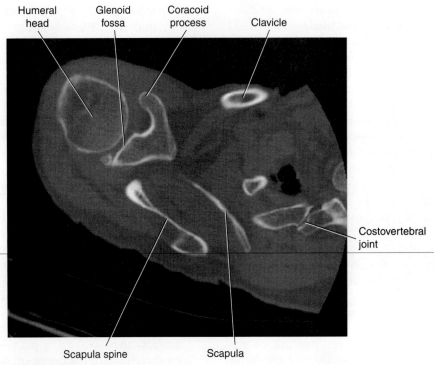

FIGURE 3-54 Shoulder—axial image.

5. MPR and 3D reconstructions provide excellent views of the acetabulum and femoral head. CT is an important imaging tool for the diagnosis of fracture in these areas (Figs. 3-55 and 3-56).

6. Additional clinical indications for CT of the hips include:

   a. Postoperative evaluation of prosthesis for hip fracture.

   b. Developmental dysplasia of the hip.

7. The technical considerations for CT studies of the pelvic girdle are similar to those for studies of the distal extremities.

FIGURE 3-55 Hips—axial image.

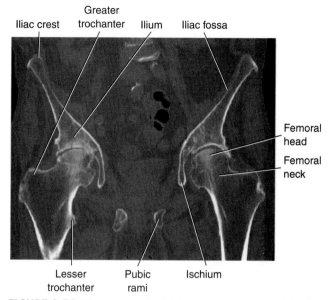

FIGURE 3-56 Hips—coronal multiplanar reformation (MPR) image.

8. The patient is scanned in the supine position, feet-first in the gantry. The hands and arms are raised above the acquired field.
9. Contrast-enhanced MDCT acquisitions of the post-traumatic pelvis may include CTA evaluation for vascular injury as well as assessment of the bladder via CT cystography.

Special Procedures

A. CT Arthrography

1. *CT arthrography* is CT evaluation of a joint after the intra-articular injection of an iodinated contrast agent.
2. This evaluation offers additional detail of the soft tissue structures of the joints, including ligaments, tendons, cartilage, and menisci.
3. The single-contrast technique involves the direct administration into the joint space of a small amount (approximately 0.5-10.0 mL, depending on the joint) of a contrast agent diluted with saline before thin-section CT acquisition.
4. In the double-contrast technique, a small amount of room air is also introduced into the joint along with the contrast medium.

B. CT Myelography

1. The intrathecal administration of a contrast during a myelogram improves visualization of the spinal cord, nerve roots, and surrounding soft tissue structures. An iodinated contrast agent is administered directly into the subarachnoid space surrounding the spinal cord.
2. Post-myelography CT examinations of the spine are commonly performed to take advantage of the intrathecal contrast agent administration.

C. Peripheral CT Angiography

1. Peripheral CT angiography, the angiographic assessment of the peripheral arterial tree from the renal arteries through the feet, is commonly referred to as a "CT runoff."
2. The speed, greater volume coverage, and isotropic spatial resolution of MDCT make the acquisition of the entire peripheral arterial system of the lower extremities possible.
3. The abdominal aorta bifurcates into the left and right common iliac arteries at about the level of L4.
4. Each iliac artery further bifurcates at about the level of L5-S1 into internal and external iliac arteries.
5. The internal iliac arteries are the major blood suppliers to the pelvis. The external iliac arteries supply blood to the lower limb as the femoral arteries (Fig. 3-57).
6. Appropriate IV contrast agent administration is the key to performing high-quality peripheral CTA examinations. Acquisition must occur during the period of peak opacification of the arterial tree:
   a. The time it takes for contrast agent to reach the peripheral arteries from the injection site varies widely among patients. The contrast media transit time—the time needed for an IV contrast agent to reach the aorta—in patients with vascular disease ranges from 12 to 40 seconds. Accurate scan delay should be obtained by either a test bolus or automated bolus-tracking techniques.
   b. Acquisition speeds range from 35 mm/sec in 4-slice MDCT systems to upwards of 92 mm/sec or greater with 64-slice systems and beyond. The scan delay chosen must coincide with the acquisition time to ensure that scanning occurs during the period of peak arterial opacification. Faster scanners run the risk of "outrunning" the bolus by completing the acquisition before the entire contrast agent volume has been administered. Faster scanners, therefore, require longer preparation delays.
   c. The duration of scan acquisition is based on the anatomic length of the study and the capabilities of the particular CT system in use. The following formula may be used as a guide to determine injection rate and contrast agent volume specific to the required scan time:

   Bolus duration = Scan time − 5 seconds

   d. The subtraction of 5 seconds allows the scanner to keep pace with the contrast agent as the latter moves down the aorta and results in the cessation of contrast agent administration just (5 seconds) before the end of data acquisition.
   e. The calculated bolus duration is attained with injection rates between 3 and 5 mL/sec for total contrast agent volumes between 125 and 175 mL (2 mL/kg maximum).

Ascending branch
Left profundus femoris artery
Left lateral circumflex artery
Right lateral circumflex femoral artery
Left medial circumflex artery
Descending branch
Perforating branches of profundus femoris
Left femoral artery

FIGURE 3-57 Three-dimensional CT angiography of the femoral arteries. *(From Kelley L, Peterson C: Sectional Anatomy for Image Professionals, 2e, St Louis, Mosby, 2007.)*

f. A biphasic injection technique, in which a higher rate is followed by a lower rate, may be used to widen the period of optimum peripheral arterial enhancement.

g. The use of a saline flush may also assist in broadening the peak enhancement window and improving the efficiency of contrast agent utilization.

7. The technical parameters of peripheral CTA vary according to departmental protocol. A few generalizations can be outlined as follows:

a. The patient is positioned supine and feet-first into the gantry. The feet are immobilized with the legs carefully aligned in a neutral, comfortable position to limit motion.

b. The detector collimation and subsequent slice thickness values depend on scanner capability. For systems at 16 slices and above, 0.6 to 0.75 mm detector collimation with 0.75 to 1.0 mm reconstructions is used.

c. Overlapping reconstructions are used for high-quality volume-rendered 3D and MIP images.

d. Acquisition is made from just below the diaphragm to below the ankles (approximately 1200 to 1400 mm of coverage) in a single scan.

e. Reduction of kVp to 100 and the utilization of the ATCM technique effectively manage patient radiation dose levels. Lowering the kVp setting from the standard 120 down to 100 also has the added benefit of increasing the image contrast provided by the iodine administration.

f. DFOV is kept as small as possible to improve resolution of the peripheral vasculature while including the wider-appearing abdominal vessels in the display.

g. Evaluation of peripheral artery disease (PAD) is the primary indication for peripheral CTA.

h. *Claudication* refers to the condition of intermittent cramping pain in the legs due to poor circulation. Arterial stenosis and occlusion are typically the causes of the vascular insufficiency.

i. Additional indications for peripheral CTA include:
   - Acute ischemia from thrombosis.
   - Vascular trauma.

- Lower extremity aneurysm.
- Postoperative evaluation of endovascular repair.

D. Interventional CT

1. CT provides precise localization for interventional procedures, such as percutaneous biopsy, abscess drainage, and radiofrequency ablation.
2. CT interventional guidance is used during procedures involving the lungs, mediastinum, adrenals, liver, pancreas, kidneys, retroperitoneum, and pelvis.
3. The most common indication for CT-guided percutaneous biopsy is to confirm the malignancy of a mass.
4. Protocol and procedures for CT-guided biopsy are department-specific. Details regarding the technical aspects of any given CT-guided biopsy vary greatly, depending upon the clinical indication, anatomic area of interest, and individual physician preferences.
5. Generalizations regarding the role of CT during percutaneous biopsy procedures are as follows:
   a. Diagnostic CT exam of the area is performed and reviewed to determine the optimal patient position for the biopsy.
   b. The patient is positioned (supine, prone, decubitus) according to plan, and the area of interest is scanned for re-localization of the mass.
   c. The z-axis location for biopsy is determined and marked through use of the laser lighting system of the CT unit.
   d. CT system software is used to measure the distance between the lesion and skin entrance point and determine the optimum angle for needle insertion.
   e. Once the biopsy pass is made, additional scans are obtained to ensure proper location of the needle tip within the lesion. The needle tip is often readily identified as an area of black shadow artifact in the immediately adjacent soft tissue of the lesion.
   f. Upon removal of the biopsy sample, additional CT acquisition is performed through the area to detect postprocedural complications such as pneumothorax and hemorrhage.
   g. CT guidance for fluid aspiration and drainage is similar in concept to that for percutaneous needle biopsy.
   h. Abscess drainage and cyst aspiration are the most common indications for CT imaging guidance.
   i. Percutaneous abscess drainage often involves the placement of a catheter within the fluid collection for drainage.
   j. Before catheter removal, a repeat CT scan is typically performed to confirm resolution of the fluid collection.
   k. CT-guided radiofrequency ablation (RFA) involves the placement of a probe into a tumor under CT imaging guidance.
   l. Once the probe is positioned precisely within a tumor, radiofrequency waves are passed through the probe to heat and destroy malignant tissue.
   m. The most common indication for CT-guided RFA is treatment of a hepatic neoplasm.

E. CT Fluoroscopy

1. *CT fluoroscopy* is the use of real-time CT imaging for CT-guided interventional procedures.
2. It allows for continuous monitoring of needle insertion to ensure proper path, angle, and depth.
3. A disadvantage of CT fluoroscopy is the added radiation dose for both patient and staff.
4. The patient dose can be reduced by employing the lowest possible mA station and minimizing the fluoroscopic time of the procedure.
5. Techniques employed to reduce occupational exposure during CT fluoroscopy–guided interventional procedures include:
   a. Low mA and kVp, limited CT fluoroscopy time, and increased distance from source.
   b. Use of the "last-image hold" feature to reduce the need for continuous CT fluoroscopy.
   c. Use of appropriate lead shielding, including apron, thyroid shield, glove, and glasses.
   d. Draping of a lead shield over the patient area that is not involved in the interventional procedure, to reduce scatter radiation.
   e. Use of a needle holder to keep the operator's hands out of the CT fluoroscopy field.

F. CT and Positron Emission Tomography

1. *Positron emission tomography* (PET) is a functional nuclear medicine study utilizing fludeoxyglucose F 18 (FDG) as a radiopharmaceutical.
2. Malignant cells demonstrate an increase in metabolic activity and glucose utilization. Once administered, FDG mimics glucose and is taken up by normal and abnormal tissues. The amount of FDG uptake is directly proportional to an area's metabolic activity. Malignant cells take up a disproportionate amount of FDG in comparison with metabolically normal tissue.
3. Annihilation photons are emitted from the radionuclide FDG that has been taken up by the tumor cells. PET detectors absorb the emitted photons, measuring the activity of a given area of potential malignancy.
4. The emitted photons are attenuated as they travel along their path toward exit from the patient. Photons that travel longer distances undergo greater attenuation and a reduction in energy. The process of *attenuation correction* utilizes the transmission data acquired in the corresponding CT analysis to account for this change in energy.
5. PET provides a map of normal and abnormal tissue function. It offers excellent sensitivity for malignancy

but suffers from an inability to accurately localize tumor activity. Fusion of PET with CT provides such precise anatomic localization.

6. The combined PET-CT scanner provides a single exam, fusing the individual technologies. PET-CT fusion yields cross-sectional images displaying functional abnormalities and accurately registered to precise anatomic locations.

7. A combined PET-CT system contains separate CT and PET hardware within a single gantry.

8. Patients have usually fasted for 6 to 12 hours before a PET-CT exam to maximize FDG tumor uptake. Fasting is necessary to control the blood glucose level.

9. The patient's blood glucose level may be measured before the injection of FDG. It should be below 150 mg/dL to prevent inhibition of FDG uptake by glucose circulating in the bloodstream.

10. A typical dose is 10 to15 millicuries (mCi) of FDG administered intravenously.

11. Strenuous physical activity can cause abnormal physiologic uptake of the FDG in muscle. Therefore, the patient is instructed to avoid such activity before the injection and during the delay for imaging. In addition, all patient activity and speech are limited for up to 60 minutes following the injection of FDG.

12. After this 1-hour uptake period, the patient is positioned within the scanner.

13. Scout (topogram) images are obtained for the region(s) of clinical interest after the patient is given the appropriate instructions regarding limiting motion, breath-holds, and so on.

14. CT images are first acquired, both for anatomic localization of structures and to provide the attenuation correction information necessary for accurate PET data.

15. PET scan acquisition for the same area along the z-axis is then obtained after automatic translation of the patient table into the PET portion of the gantry apparatus.

16. Once the scans are completed, images are available for review either separately or fused together.

17. The major clinical applications for PET-CT are in oncology and neurology.

18. PET-CT now plays an important role in the diagnosis and management of cancers of the head, neck, lung, breast, and GI system. Patients with lymphoma and melanoma are also monitored with PET-CT.

19. The characterization of solitary pulmonary nodules is an additional important clinical application of PET-CT.

20. Neurologic disorders such as Alzheimer's disease, dementia, and epilepsy may be evaluated by PET-CT.

G. Radiation Therapy Planning

1. Advanced imaging may be used to provide volume and localization information for tumors to improve the accuracy of radiation delivery for therapy purposes.

2. 3D tumor localization aids planning in shaping the dose to maximally irradiate the tumor volume while reducing the radiation dose to the surrounding normal tissue.

3. *CT simulation, or virtual simulation,* describes the process of obtaining anatomic information with CT imaging that is used to calculate the beam arrangement during radiotherapy.

4. The CT simulator consists of a standard CT system with the following additions and modifications:
   a. A flat table-top, similar to that used during radiotherapy.
   b. Immobilization devices to position the patient in a fashion equal to the therapy procedure.
   c. A large bore dimension to accommodate multiple patient positions and to ensure the inclusion of the entire patient anatomy utilizing a large SFOV.
   d. Virtual simulation software for treatment planning.

Review of Physics and Instrumentation in Computed Tomography

COMPUTED TOMOGRAPHY SYSTEM OPERATION

1. The fundamental principle of computed tomography (CT) may be summarized as follows: An image of an object may be reconstructed on the basis of the attenuation that occurs as x-radiation is transmitted through it.
2. The x-ray beam is rotated around the patient, exposing a given volume of tissue from all directions. Detectors measure the radiation that is transmitted through the patient. An image is reconstructed on the basis of the magnitude of x-ray attenuation that occurs at spatially distributed points within the patient.
3. The general process of CT imaging may be divided into several steps:
   a. *Data acquisition*—the measurement of the attenuation that occurs along each path through the patient from x-ray tube to detector.
   b. *Data reconstruction*—the computerized processing of the transmission measurements into the CT image.
   c. *Multidimensional image display*—display of the reconstructed gray-scale image in two-dimensional (2D) and/or three-dimensional (3D) format; a representation of the attenuation that occurred across the scanned volume of tissue.
   d. *Image archival and communication*—display as well as storage, both short-term and long-term (archival), of images on computer workstations (Fig. 4-1).

A. Scan Modes

1. The most basic scan mode utilized by a CT system is scout image acquisition (Fig. 4-2). This survey scan is a digital radiograph obtained by keeping the x-ray tube and detector array in a fixed position while the patient bed is translated through the gantry.

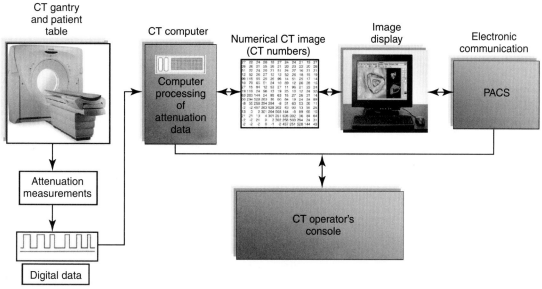

FIGURE 4-1 The main components of CT image production, display, and archival. *(From Seeram E: Computed tomography: physical principles, clinical applications, and quality control, ed 3, St Louis, 2009, Saunders.)*

Lateral scout of the head used for CT examinations of the brain, sinuses, orbits, mastoids, and so on.

Antero posterior (AP) scout of the chest, abdomen, and pelvis used for various CT examinations of the trunk.

FIGURE 4-2 The CT scout image or scanogram is typically the first image acquired during any CT examination.

2. Also referred to as a *scanogram*, a scout image may be produced in the anteroposterior (AP), posteroanterior (PA), lateral, or oblique projection through adjustments in the positions of the x-ray tube and detectors.

3. The angle of the tube and detectors in relationship to the patient position during scout acquisition is referred to as the *azimuth*.

4. The scout image, the initial image acquired during a CT examination, is used as a localizer for the prescription of the subsequent cross-sectional CT acquisition(s).

5. Historically, conventional axial, or step-and-shoot CT scanning consisted of the complete revolution of the x-ray tube around the patient, acquiring a single data set at a precise anatomic location. During the data acquisition process, the patient table would not move. The data would then be mathematically reconstructed into a single image. The thickness of the reconstructed image was controlled by the extent to which the beam was collimated. To acquire the next CT image, the table would translate (index) a predetermined amount to the next anatomic position, and the system would again rotate around the patient. This process would repeat until the area of clinical interest was completely evaluated.

6. The CT system itself is generally composed of a powerful computer and display system, a patient bed, and the gantry components (Fig. 4-3).

7. The CT gantry houses the majority of the mechanical components of CT system operation, including the generator, x-ray tube, assorted collimators, the data acquisition system (DAS), slip-rings, and the detectors.

8. The x-ray and detector components of a CT system were originally limited by hard-wired cables, which prevented continuous rotation within the gantry. At the end of each rotation of the x-ray tube and/or detectors, the system would need to reverse course and travel in the opposite direction because the cables were of finite length.

9. *Slip-ring technology* eliminates the need for cables by utilizing a system of contact brushes that supply electricity to power the system and enable the passage of transmission data to the computer system.

10. The addition of slip-ring technology allows for the continuous helical acquisition that has become the standard in modern CT imaging.

11. The technical elements of helical CT acquisition include:
    a. Continuous rotation of the gantry components (slip-ring technology).

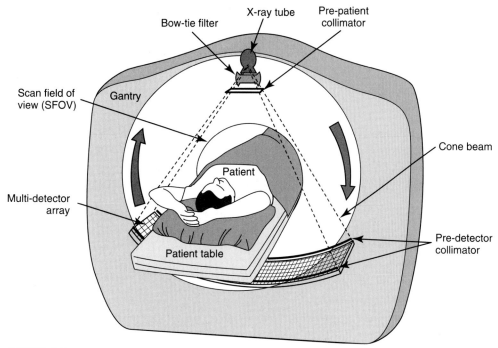

FIGURE 4-3 General schematic diagram of a multislice CT (MSCT) system.

b. A powerful x-ray tube capable of long exposure output.

c. Continuous movement of the patient bed.

d. Specialized mathematical reconstruction techniques.

12. Helical geometry allows for volumetric data acquisition. The reconstruction of CT sections at any point along the scanned volume is possible. The section width must be the same, however, and is controlled by the collimation (slice thickness) chosen prior to data acquisition.

13. The development of multislice CT (MSCT) advances the helical acquisition principle. Multidetector arrays enable CT sections of varying widths to be reconstructed at any point along the acquired volume.

B. X-Ray Tube

1. CT employs a glass- and/or metal-enclosed x-ray tube consisting of a cathode and a rotating anode disc.

2. Dual filaments allow for a choice of two focal spot sizes ranging from 0.5 to 1.2 mm in diameter. Depending on the vendor, the choice of foci may be controlled by the user through the selection of milliamperage (mA) setting, scan field of view (SFOV), and so on.

3. Smaller focal spots improve the geometric efficiency of the x-ray beam, leading to greater spatial resolution.

4. *Flying focal spot technology* involves the electromagnetic steering of the electron beam emitted from the cathode. The beam of electrons is directed toward two separate locations on the rotating anode, resulting in two sources of x-radiation.

5. As the tube rotates around the patient, the number of data samples is essentially doubled owing to the electronic switching between the two focal spots. This oversampling technology can be used to improve the system's temporal and spatial resolution.

6. The long acquisition times and relatively high exposure rates of helical single-slice CT (SSCT) and MSCT require an x-ray tube with very high heat storage capacity.

7. The x-ray tube must be very efficient at dissipating the tremendous heat generated during a CT examination. Several methods, including oil- and air-cooling, increased anode diameter, and conduction by tube rotation, have been utilized to improve heat capacity.

8. The modern CT x-ray tube has specific characteristics that enable it to achieve the performance demanded by state-of-the art MSCT:

a. High heat rating—must have the ability to absorb tremendous heat, while dissipating it quickly.

b. Small size, lightweight—must be capable of rotating within the CT gantry at a high rate of speed.

c. Stable and long-lasting—must be capable of withstanding huge centrifugal forces with an extended useful life.

9. Milliampere (mA) setting can vary widely from 30 mA to upwards of 800 mA. Selection of mA setting depends on a number of factors, including the clinical indication for the CT study, patient size/density,

and required signal-to-noise ratio (SNR) for adequate exam quality.

10. The mA setting for a given study may be manually selected on the basis of the aforementioned criteria. Automatic tube current modulation (ATCM) programs adjust the mA throughout an acquisition to reduce patient radiation dose to a minimum. ATCM automatically alters the applied mA according to a predetermined noise index that is acceptable for appropriate image quality.

11. Exposure time for a given CT acquisition varies and is determined by anatomic extent, detector configuration, table speed, and so on. Each acquisition may reach upwards of 30 to 60 seconds in length, with total scan times equal to the sum of all acquisitions occurring during the study.

12. The mA setting in coordination with the scan time (seconds) gives the constant milliampere-seconds (mAs) value for a CT acquisition. The mAs value directly controls the quantity of x-radiation, or *photon fluence*, directed toward the patient.

13. The rate at which the photon fluence passes through a unit area over unit time is termed the *photon flux*.

14. The mAs value for a given acquisition is directly proportional to patient radiation dose and inversely proportional to image noise.

15. *Effective mAs* describes the calculated mAs value per acquired slice. The main controlling factor of effective mAs is table speed. The pitch selected for a given acquisition determines the speed at which the patient translates through the gantry for each tube revolution, as shown by the following formula:

$$\text{effective mAs} = \frac{\text{mAs}}{\text{pitch}}$$

As illustrated by the formula, as pitch increases, the mAs applied to each acquired slice decreases.

16. *Peak kilovoltage* (kVp) controls the quality of the x-ray beam with regard to its overall penetrating capabilities. Higher kVp settings produce x-ray beams with greater penetrating power.

17. The use of lower kVp decreases the patient radiation dose and may improve contrast, particularly during CT angiography (CTA) procedures.

18. Higher kVp settings are utilized to decrease the streak artifact that may occur as the beam passes through very dense parts, such as those found in the posterior fossa during head imaging.

19. The CT x-ray tube is extremely efficient and capable of generating an x-ray beam using peak voltages typically within the range of 80 to 140 kVp.

20. Dual-energy CT systems are capable of applying multiple x-ray energies during a single CT acquisition. Transmission data are acquired from tissue interaction with both high- and low-kVp radiation.

Differentiation and characterization of tissue composition are made possible by the difference in attenuation between the two x-ray spectra.

21. Complex voltage-switching systems may be employed to achieve *dual-energy CT scanning*. As the single tube rotates around the patient, the applied peak kVp is switched at an extremely high rate for each successive projection.

22. Alternatively, *dual-source CT systems* utilize two completely separate x-ray tubes and detector arrays positioned 90 degrees from each other within the gantry. The two x-ray tubes acquire data simultaneously at different kVp values.

23. Dual-energy CT has expanded clinical opportunities, including:
   a. Improved resolution of soft tissue structures (ligaments, tendons) during musculoskeletal imaging.
   b. The ability to visualize atherosclerotic plaque within contrast-enhanced vasculature during cardiac CT studies.
   c. Contrast medium subtraction techniques for the demonstration of pre-contrast images from a single scan acquired after the IV administration of iodinated contrast media.
   d. Characterization of the biochemical composition of urinary tract calculi.

24. Even with single-slice CT, the beam that emerges from the x-ray tube consists of photons with varying energy.

25. This polyenergetic x-ray beam undergoes filtration in an effort to remove low-energy x-ray photons. These are photons with insufficient energy to complete the path from source to patient to detector and would go unmeasured, adding solely to patient radiation dose.

26. Additionally, a monoenergetic beam is less susceptible to artifacts from a process known as *beam hardening*. As the beam traverses the patient, low-energy photons are absorbed first, increasing the average intensity of the beam as it travels along its path. This change in the beam quality can have an artifactual result on the CT image.

27. The CT x-ray tube contains both inherent and added filtration in an effort to improve the energy quality of the x-ray beam.

28. The tube housing, cooling oil, and so on, constitute the inherent filtration, which amounts to approximately 3.0 mm of aluminum-equivalent filtration.

29. Minimal additional filtration in the form of thin (0.1-0.4 mm) copper sheets and bow-tie filters are also added to improve beam utilization efficiency.

30. *Bow-tie filters*, which are thicker at the ends than in the middle, help shape the beam to reduce patient radiation exposure. Because most body parts are circular or cylindrical, less radiation is necessary at the periphery than in the center. Bow-tie filters

reduce beam intensity toward the outer margins, resulting in a lower patient radiation dose.

31. Each CT unit will have a proprietary standard procedure for proper tube warm-up prior to patient scanning. Tube warm-up prevents damage to the x-ray system and prolongs tube life.

32. This procedure will may also involve a series of calibration scans programmed to include a wide range of the many combinations of kVp, mA, and collimation settings available.

C. Generator and Transformers

1. Current CT scanners utilize high-frequency generators. These modern and efficient units are small enough to be housed within the CT gantry.

2. The CT generator includes a high-voltage transformer necessary to convert the low-frequency/low-voltage alternating current supplied to the unit into the high-frequency/high-voltage current required for efficient x-ray production.

3. Power output is vendor-specific, within a typical range of 60 to 100 kilowatts (kW).

D. Collimation

1. Once straightforward, the concept of collimation has become more complex with the advent of multi-slice CT (MSCT).

2. CT collimation for MSCT can be divided into two distinct components:
   a. Beam collimation.
   b. Detector (section) collimation.

3. A review of detector collimation can be found later, in the section on detector configuration.

4. The general purpose of beam collimation in CT is to restrict the radiation exposure to the area of interest, reducing patient radiation dose and improving image quality.

5. SSCT incorporates a fan-shaped beam with a transverse (x-y) dimension corresponding to the size of the detector array and the maximum scan field of view (SFOV).

6. The length of detector coverage in the transverse dimension is determined by the fan angle of the emitted beam. A wider fan angle extends coverage of the detector array along the x- and y-axes.

7. Along the longitudinal, or z-axis, the beam is collimated to the anticipated slice thickness. Located just outside the tube housing, the mechanical aperture responsible for beam restriction is termed the pre-patient collimator.

8. Pre-patient beam collimation in SSCT directly controls the amount of tissue exposed to x-radiation as the tube rotates about the patient.

9. For example, acquisition of 5-mm slices during a SSCT examination is obtained with a beam collimation of 5 mm: The collimator aperture is mechanically set to an opening 5 mm wide along the z-axis. The width of tissue exposed at the center of beam rotation is 5 mm. Beam collimation of 5 mm results in the reconstruction of 2D images that each represent 5 mm of tissue.

10. No further adjustments to slice thickness are possible after the slice data have been acquired (retrospectively) during SSCT.

11. SSCT beam collimation consists of:
    a. Pre-patient collimation: A mechanical device controls the aperture dimension at the x-ray tube, directly limiting the beam to the desired section width.
    b. Post-patient collimation: The radiation transmitted through the patient is controlled by pre-detector collimators. Post-patient (pre-detector) collimators are used to improve image quality by limiting scatter radiation before it reaches the detectors.

12. There are two components of pre-patient collimation:
    a. The tube housing itself acts as an initial collimator. The tube aperture roughly shapes the primary beam into a fan or cone shape, for SSCT or MSCT, respectively. The beam emerges from the tube housing at a specific fan angle, corresponding to the in-plane length of the detector array.
    b. The primary pre-patient collimator is positioned just beyond the tube housing. It restricts the beam along the z-axis, controlling slice thickness in the SSCT system.

13. Multislice CT (MSCT) systems also utilize pre- and post-patient collimation for reasons similar to those described for SSCT.

14. During MSCT, the beam may be limited, prior to reaching the patient, according to the desired section width and the number of detector rows to be utilized for image formation.

15. Post-patient collimation occurs through a high-resolution comb placed over the detector array. Functioning like a grid, this comb removes unwanted scatter radiation and off-axis photons that result from the more divergent nature of the MSCT beam.

16. MSCT utilizes a cone-shaped beam, which is incident upon an expanded array of detectors. The detector array consists of multiple rows of individual detector elements.

17. As the number of detector rows in an MSCT system increases, the divergence of the cone beam needed for coverage also increases.

18. The MSCT beam is collimated to the total width of the slices acquired with each gantry rotation.

19. At a maximum, the MSCT cone beam may be colli-mated to a dimension equal to the entire multi-row detector array. For example, in a 64-slice system with 0.625-mm detectors, the cone beam is calcu-lated as follows:

$$64 \times 0.625 \text{ mm} = 40 \text{ mm}$$

In this example, the primary beam is limited by pre-patient collimators to a maximum dimension of 40 mm along the z-axis.

20. Beam collimation in the MSCT system may further restrict the field to expose a smaller portion of the detector array. However, this has only an indirect effect on section thickness, which is controlled pri-marily by detector configuration in the MSCT system.

21. The combination of user-defined beam width and detector configuration ultimately controls the num-ber and thickness of the images acquired during an MSCT examination.

22. The relationship among beam collimation (width), detector size (collimation), and the number of detec-tors is described as follows:

$$d \text{ (mm)} = \frac{D \text{ (mm)}}{N}$$

where d is detector collimation, D is beam collima-tion (width), and N is number of detector rows. From the previous example, a 64-slice system with 0.625-mm detectors:

$$0.625 = \frac{40 \text{ mm}}{64}$$

23. Collimation of the beam in MSCT directly affects the volume of tissue measured for each rotation of the tube. Wider collimation results in greater anatomic coverage with each tube rotation. This allows for an increase in the overall acquisition volume over a given scan time.

24. Compared with SSCT, MSCT allows faster and more extensive coverage along the z-axis while also providing thinner section widths for each gantry rotation.

25. The *section width* (slice thickness) describes the amount of tissue in the longitudinal or z-axis that is represented by the 2D CT image.

26. Section width is controlled directly by beam colli-mation during SSCT. During MSCT, section width is determined by a combination of beam collimation and detector collimation settings.

27. *Detector collimation* describes the process of deter-mining section width in the MSCT system; it is covered further later, in the section on detector configuration.

28. *Section interval* describes the spacing between two adjacent CT images. It is measured as the distance between the center of one section and the center of the next adjacent section.

29. *Contiguous images* are those acquired with equal sec-tion thickness and interval. For example, 5-mm sections reconstructed every 5 mm will completely cover a given volume of tissue, with no unmeasured tissue.

30. *Noncontiguous images* are those acquired with an interval greater than the section width. For exam-ple, 1-mm sections reconstructed every 10 mm would not evaluate the intermittent 9 mm of tissue.

31. *Overlapping images* are reconstructed with a sec-tion interval that is less than the section width. A percentage value may be assigned to the extent of overlap. For example, 1.0-mm-thick images recon-structed every 0.5 mm are said to possess a 50% overlap.

32. Overlapping images are used predominantly to improve the quality of multiplanar reformation (MPR) and 3D reconstructions.

33. Pitch is an important factor during helical SSCT and MSCT studies. *Pitch* describes the relationship between collimation and table movement during scanning (Fig 4-4).

34. The pitch of a helically acquired CT study charac-terizes the amount of longitudinal data acquired for every rotation of the gantry apparatus and the overall acquisition speed.

35. The original definition of pitch for single-slice heli-cal CT (SSCT) stated the following:

$$\text{pitch} = \frac{\text{table feed per rotation}}{\text{section width}}$$

For example, with a section width of 5 mm and a user-defined pitch of 1.5, the table would move 7.5 mm for each gantry rotation.

$$1.5 = \frac{7.5 \text{ mm}}{5.0 \text{ mm}}$$

36. This original definition of pitch may now be referred to as *detector pitch*.

37. Increasing the detector pitch would result in greater table translation with each gantry revolution.

38. Higher detector pitch settings resulted in greater coverage along the z-axis with each revolution of the gantry, at the cost of reduced image quality.

39. In the helical multislice CT (MSCT) system, section width is no longer primarily controlled by beam colli-mation at the x-ray tube. Detector configuration plays a major role in the determination of reconstructed section width.

40. A new adaptation of the pitch principle termed *beam pitch* is required:

$$\text{beam pitch} = \frac{\text{table feed per rotation}}{\text{total collimation}}$$

41. Specific to MSCT, total collimation equals the com-bined thickness of all of the sections that are simul-taneously acquired with each gantry rotation:

$$\text{total collimation} = \text{No. of sections} \times \text{section width}$$

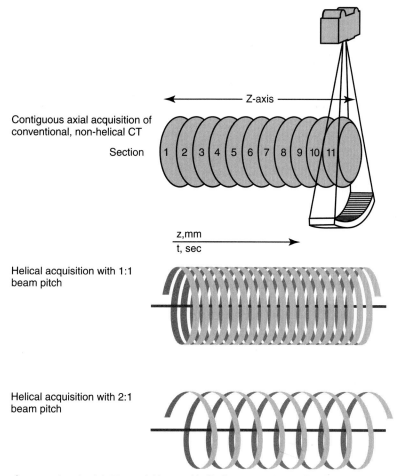

Z-axis

Contiguous axial acquisition of
conventional, non-helical CT

Section 1 2 3 4 5 6 7 8 9 10 11

z, mm
t, sec

Helical acquisition with 1:1
beam pitch

Helical acquisition with 2:1
beam pitch

FIGURE 4-4 A comparison of conventional axial CT acquisition and helical CT acquisition. The diagram also illustrates the geometric change in data acquisition as pitch increases during helical CT scanning.

42. For example, a given MSCT system has an array of 16 detectors, each 1.25 mm wide. The total length of the detector array (along the z-axis) equals 20 mm (16 × 1.25 = 20). A beam pitch set at 1.75 will have the table move 35.00 mm for every gantry rotation:

$$\text{beam pitch} = \frac{\text{table feed per rotation}}{\text{total collimation}}$$
$$= \frac{35.00 \text{ mm}}{(16 \times 1.25)}$$
$$= \frac{35.00}{20}$$
$$= 1.75$$

43. A pitch setting less than one (1) reduces the table speed for each gantry revolution. This increases the acquired data and subsequently improves image quality.

44. However, lower pitch settings also result in higher patient radiation dose. Increasing pitch moves the patient through the gantry faster, exposing tissue to the beam for shorter periods, and reducing dose.

E. Detectors: Design and Scan Geometry

1. The primary physical issue of CT imaging is the measurement of the attenuation exhibited by a volume of tissue. In its most basic form, the reconstructed CT image is a 2-dimensional map of the measured attenuation values.
2. Attenuation itself is defined as the reduction of intensity of a radiation beam as it passes through a substance.
3. During transmission through an object, radiation quanta may be absorbed due to the photoelectric effect. X-ray photons may also suffer a loss of energy and the subsequent change of direction known as Compton scattering.
4. The overall attenuation depends on the beam quality (photon energy) and the atomic density of the imaged tissue. After passing through the patient, the transmitted radiation is incident upon an array of CT detectors.
5. The CT detector is responsible for measuring this transmitted radiation and converting it into a

proportionate electronic signal to be used for image reconstruction.

6. The signal emitted by a detector is proportionate to the intensity of the transmitted radiation incident upon and measured by the detector.

7. The desired qualities of a CT detector include:

   a. High efficiency: The CT detector material must be efficient at absorbing the transmitted x-ray photons and converting them into a proportionate signal. The detectors' absorption efficiency is controlled by factors such as the overall size of the detector and the density and atomic number of the material used. The geometric efficiency of a CT detector is primarily influenced by the amount of interspace material necessary between adjacent detectors. Although valuable in limiting interference (crosstalk) between adjacent detectors, the interspace material reduces geometric efficiency by absorbing transmitted x-ray energy. X-ray photons absorbed by interspace material do not add to the generated signal.

   b. Rapid signal decay: The detector must be capable of measuring transmitted x-ray photons with an excellent response time and limited afterglow. The *response time* of a detector is its ability to quickly measure x-rays and then recover before the next measurement. *Afterglow* refers primarily to the tendency of scintillation crystal detectors to continue to glow in response to x-rays once the exposure source has been terminated.

   c. High dynamic range: The CT detector must be sensitive enough to measure a broad range of x-ray transmission data and accurate enough to modulate signal in response to small changes in radiation transmission.

8. Historically, CT detectors were composed of either gas ionization chambers or scintillation crystals. Gas ionization detectors convert x-ray energy directly into an electrical signal. Solid-state scintillation crystal detectors convert x-ray energy first into light energy, which must then be converted into electrical signal.

9. Gas ionization detectors consist of small high-pressure chambers of xenon gas. Interaction with x-rays causes a proportional amount of ionization of the xenon gas, resulting in the discharge of a small electrical signal. An increase in absorbed x-ray energy would result in an increase in emitted signal.

10. Gas ionization detectors were used primarily for conventional third-generation CT systems, prior to the advent of helical technology.

11. All modern MSCT systems utilize solid state detectors, consisting primarily of a scintillating crystal material.

12. The detector crystal emits a quantity of light energy proportional to the x-ray incident upon an individual detector. The light is measured by a photodiode device and is converted to an electronic signal to be sent for processing by the CT computer system.

13. Crystal materials employed as CT detectors include cesium iodide, cadmium tungstate, bismuth germanate, rare earths such as gadolinium oxysulfide, and scintillating gemstone minerals.

14. Solid state detectors are preferred for MSCT because of their ability to accurately record incident x-ray energy from any angle. This flexibility is important owing to the widened cone beam geometry inherent to MSCT systems.

15. The detector configuration or detector geometry is often used to delineate the major technologic advances in CT imaging. Each generation of CT system is identifiable by its detector geometry, as follows (Fig. 4-5):

   a. First Generation:
   • The prototypical, head-only CT system developed by Sir Godfrey Hounsfield who first put the technology to clinical use in 1972.
   • Consisted primarily of two detectors (paired adjacently along the z-axis) exposed to a tightly collimated pencil beam of x-rays.

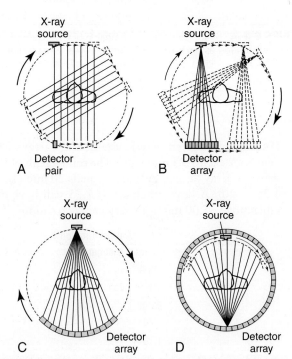

FIGURE 4-5 The geometries of the first four generations of CT scanners. **A,** First-generation scanners: pencil beam, translate and rotate. **B,** Second-generation scanners: fan beam, translate and rotate. **C,** Third-generation scanners: fan beam, rotate only. **D,** Fourth-generation scanners: fan beam, stationary circular detector array. *(Modified from Seeram E: Computed tomography: physical principles, clinical applications, and quality control, ed 3, St Louis, 2009, Saunders.)*

- The tube and detectors would translate across the patient's head, rotate by 1 degree, and then translate back in a method known as rectilinear or translate-rotate scanning.
  b. Second Generation
    - Also utilizes a translate-rotate geometry, but with an increase in the number of detectors, allowing for greater increments of rotation between translations and a reduction in the overall scan time.
    - First use of fan beam to expose a wider detector array.
    - Expanded clinical capabilities beyond head imaging.
  c. Third Generation
    - An expanded curvilinear array of detectors rotates with the x-ray tube around the patient.
    - Rotate-rotate geometry eliminates the need for translation.
    - Larger fan beam is used to expose the expanded detector array.
  d. Fourth Generation
    - Co-evolved with third generation systems and based upon a rotate-stationary geometry.
    - The gantry houses a stationary, circular ring of detectors and the x-ray tube rotates around the patient.
16. Later developments in CT technology have not been consistently labeled as additional "generations." However, there have been substantial advances in detector configuration, which will be outlined below.
17. Electron beam CT (EBCT) utilizes a unique technical configuration devoid of moving parts (Fig. 4-6). As an adaptation of fourth-generation design, EBCT has a stationary-stationary geometry, with both the x-ray source and detectors fixed during scanning.
18. EBCT systems have no x-ray tube. A fan beam of x-radiation is produced by directing a beam of electrons toward stationary target rings of tungsten.
19. Each curved tungsten target emits radiation when bombarded by the electron beam, and x-rays are collimated toward the patient.
20. After passing through, and being attenuated by, the patient, the transmitted radiation is measured by a curvilinear array of stationary detectors, which lie opposite the target portion of each ring.
21. Without moving parts, an EBCT system is capable of extremely short exposure times, on the order of 50 msec or less.
22. Owing to its high-speed capabilities, the primary application of EBCT is cardiac imaging.
23. As discussed earlier, helical or spiral CT scanners utilize slip-ring technology, which removes the necessity of cables to power the assembly and transmit data. With the resulting continuous rotation of the tube and/or detector array, a helix of data is obtained as the patient is transported through the gantry.
24. Helical SSCT systems may have third- or fourth-generation geometries. The helical acquisition is made possible by the addition of slip-ring technology, not by advancement in detector technology.
25. Most helical CT systems utilize solid state detector arrays because of their improved efficiency and stability.
26. The introduction of MSCT was made possible through a complete redesign of the CT detector array.
27. All MSCT systems utilize third-generation geometry and solid state scintillation detectors.

FIGURE 4-6 The essential components of an electron beam CT (EBCT) system. The data acquisition geometry consists of a fan beam of x-rays produced by an electron beam that strikes a tungsten target ring. *(Modified from Seeram E: Computed tomography: physical principles, clinical applications, and quality control, ed 3, St Louis, 2009, Saunders.)*

28. In contrast to the one-dimensional detector array of SSCT, the MSCT detector is said to be 2D. An MSCT system utilizes a curvilinear detector array with multiple rows of individual detector elements segmented along the longitudinal axis, or z-axis.

29. Parallel rows of individual detectors allow for acquisition of multiple sections of scan data with each rotation of the x-ray tube around the patient. This results in a markedly larger coverage area over a given scan time.

30. Of equal importance is the ability of MSCT scanners to reconstruct images of varying thicknesses at any z-axis position within the volume of data acquisition.

31. From the same data set, both thin-section images for maximum resolution and thicker images for ease of display may be reconstructed without additional scanning.

32. In traditional SSCT, the section width was controlled by beam collimation. Pre-patient collimators restricted the primary beam at the center of rotation equal to the desired section width.

33. With MSCT, detector collimation determines the width of the reconstructed section. By electronically adjusting the detector dimension, the operator can control the width of the x-ray beam contributing to a reconstructed section. Beam collimation no longer directly controls section width.

34. Beam collimation still has an important indirect effect on section width. The beam width must be wide enough to encompass the total thickness of the simultaneous sections to be acquired with each gantry revolution.

35. For example, as previously described in the section on collimation, a 64-channel MSCT system acquires 64 slices simultaneously, each 0.625 mm wide along the z-axis. The maximum coverage for each gantry revolution is 40 mm ($64 \times 0.625 = 40$). The beam width must therefore be collimated to 40 mm.

36. In summary, MSCT technology dictates that the width of a CT slice is no longer primarily controlled by pre-patient collimation, but instead is controlled by electronic separation or combination of signals from the individual detector rows.

37. *Detector configuration* refers to the number, length, and organization of the individual detector elements in an MSCT system.

38. The three general formats of MSCT detector configuration are as follows (Fig. 4-7):
    a. Uniform matrix-array: Utilizes multiple detectors in the longitudinal direction, each the same length. For example, a 4-slice MSCT system employs 16 detector elements, each 1.25 mm in length.
    b. Adaptive-array: Detectors are configured with the thinnest widths at the center, surrounded by detectors of incrementally increasing widths along the z-axis. For example, an MSCT with

an adaptive array of 16 rows may be composed of 2 middle detectors of 1.0 mm each (2 mm total), followed by pairs of 1.5 mm (3 mm total), 2.5 mm (5 mm total), and 5.0 mm (10 mm total), moving outward from the center of the array. Added together, the detectors total 20 mm along the z-axis.
    c. Hybrid-array: Consists of two detector sizes. The narrower detectors are positioned midline, flanked by the wider detectors. For example, the central rows of a 16-channel MSCT system are 0.625 mm, with the remaining peripheral rows at 1.25 mm.

39. It is important to keep in mind the distinction between the number of data channels an MSCT system possesses and the quantity/size of its detectors:
    a. The quantity of data channels controls the number of sections the scanner can simultaneously acquire with each gantry rotation. For example, what is commonly referred to as a 16-slice MSCT system has in fact 16 data channels at its disposal. The maximum number of sections that may be reconstructed from each gantry rotation is 16.
    b. The number of detectors in the array is equal to, or greater than, the number of data channels. The 16-slice MSCT system may utilize an adaptive array of 24 detectors (Fig. 4-8, A).
    c. With 16 possible data channels, the maximum number of sections this system can simultaneously acquire is 16. Therefore, when the beam collimation is set to a width of 20 mm, data from the middle 16 detectors (0.625 mm) are combined, or binned, to form 8 sections, each 1.25 mm wide.
    d. Data from the four 1.25-mm detectors from each side of the array contribute an additional 8 sections per gantry rotation, each 1.25 mm thick.
    e. The result is a total of 16 1.25-mm sections acquired for each rotation of the gantry (Fig. 4-8, B).
    f. *Binning* refers to the electronic combination of signal from adjacent detectors to form a reconstructed slice that is thicker than the individual detector width.
    g. The effective section width for the preceding example is 1.25 mm. The minimum section width possible is 1.25 mm. However, it is possible to further apply the concept of binning to reconstruct thicker sections for the same data set.
    h. The preceding examples illustrate the process of detector collimation. The width of the x-ray beam remains the same, but the signal emitted from each detector is manipulated to control section width.
    i. In the example shown in Fig. 4-8, C, signal from pairs of 1.25-mm detectors and quads of 0.625-mm detectors are electronically combined to form 8 2.5-mm-thick sections from data collected during each gantry rotation.

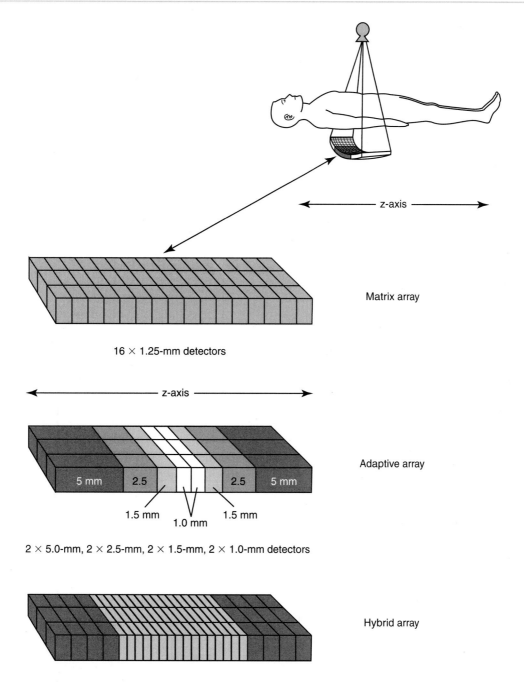

FIGURE 4-7   The predominant types of MSCT detector configurations: matrix, adaptive, and hybrid arrays.

40. The relationship between beam collimation and section width in MSCT can be explored by modifying Fig. 4-8, C as follows:
    a. While utilizing the previously described 16-channel adaptive array MSCT system, the operator can choose to further collimate the primary beam to a width of 10 mm. After transmission through the patient, radiation is now incident upon only the central 16 detectors (0.625 mm × 16 = 10 mm).
    b. In the example shown in Fig. 4-8, D, the minimum effective section width is 0.625 mm. When clinically appropriate, the signal from each detector can be used to reconstruct images that represent 0.625 mm of tissue.
    c. The user may also decide that the large quantity of 0.625-mm images required to cover a given volume of anatomy is not clinically indicated. In this case, signal from adjacent detectors can be electronically combined (binned) to form thicker (1.25-mm) images.

41. It is the combination of beam collimation and detector collimation that controls:

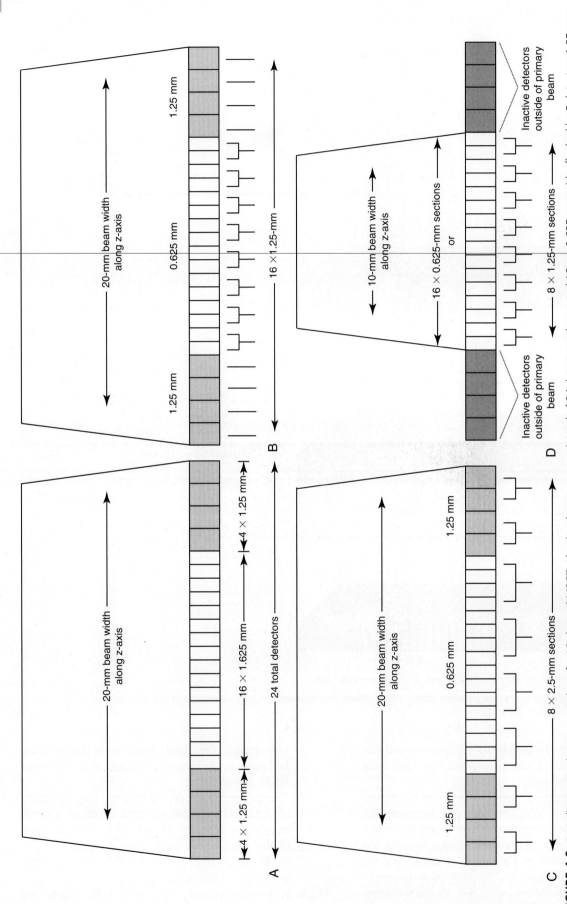

FIGURE 4-8 **A,** A diagrammatic representation of a 16-channel MSCT adaptive detector array. A total of 24 detectors. The central 16 are 0.625 mm wide, flanked by 8 detectors 1.25 mm wide. **B,** With 16 available data channels, data from the 0.625-mm detectors are binned to form 8 1.25-mm sections. The maximum number of sections simultaneously acquired per gantry revolution is 16, each 1.25 mm in width. **C,** In this example, the signal measured by 2 adjacent 1.25-mm detectors is binned, and the signal measured from 4 adjacent 0.625-mm detectors is also electronically combined. The result is the reconstruction of 8 2.5-mm-thick sections from each gantry rotation. **D,** In this example, the beam has been collimated to a width of 10 mm along the z-axis, each 0.625 mm thick; alternatively, binning can result in 8 1.25-mm-thick sections per gantry rotation.

a. The number of sections that can be simultaneously acquired with each gantry rotation.

b. The minimum section width that can be reconstructed from the acquired volumetric data set.

42. The volumetric nature of MSCT data acquisition ensures that regardless of the section width chosen, images may be reconstructed at any point (increment) along the scanned volume.

43. Nonhelical, or axial, data acquisition is also possible with an MSCT system. Axial acquisition offers excellent image resolution and is often used during applications for which the accurate display of small anatomic details is vital.

44. During axial acquisition, the beam is collimated to the maximum desired section width and is incident upon a predetermined number of detectors.

45. For example, a 4-channel MSCT system has an array of 16 detectors, each 1.25 mm wide. During axial acquisition mode, the user selects a beam collimation of 10 mm, exposing the middle 8 detectors to transmitted radiation. For each complete rotation of the gantry around a fixed table location, a maximum of four images may be reconstructed from signal collected from the available four data channels in two ways:

a. Four 2.5-mm sections, each section combining data from two detectors.

b. Two 5.0-mm sections, each section combining data from four detectors.

46. Axial section width is therefore controlled by beam collimation and the summation of signal from a predetermined number of detector elements (Fig. 4-9).

47. *Cine CT acquisition* involves multiple axial scans obtained at a single anatomic level over a predetermined period. The primary clinical applications of cine CT acquisition involve dynamic imaging of physiologic processes such as respiration, swallowing, and the cardiac cycle as well as for CT perfusion studies.

48. Cine CT is also utilized during automated bolus tracking for optimal contrast enhancement. Multiple axial scans are acquired at a selected level—usually the vessel or organ of interest—and the helical acquisition is triggered once a predetermined level of contrast enhancement is reached.

49. At the time of publication of this book, the most widely accepted, studied, and published standard for detector configuration is the 64-slice MSCT system.

50. The latest developments include 256-slice and 320-slice volumetric acquisition MSCT systems.

51. Further advancement of multidetector technology continues in an effort to improve spatial and temporal resolution and to reduce patient radiation dose. Future directions for technologic improvements include smaller detectors, more detector rows, and better detector efficiency.

52. Flat-panel detector technology and its application for expansive volumetric data acquisition is another potential direction for CT.

53. Flat-panel detectors are essentially larger area detectors used in place of the segmented detector rows found in MSCT systems. The system uses a widely divergent cone beam of radiation to cover the expanded detector.

54. The detector itself consists of a film of scintillating crystals bonded to a matrix of silicon photosensors, similar to a digital radiography image receptor. The matrix array of photodiodes and transistors

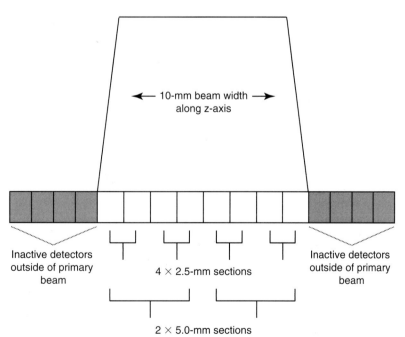

FIGURE 4-9 In this example, axial acquisition may result in the reconstruction of four 2.5-mm sections or two 5.0-mm sections. The maximum number of sections acquired per gantry rotation is governed by the number of available data channels. The detectors that lie outside the collimated beam do not measure transmitted radiation or contribute signal to the reconstruction process.

generates an electronic signal proportionate to the light emitted from the scintillating sheet.

55. A prototypical flat-panel detector has a dimension of 40 × 30 cm. For each gantry revolution, z-axis coverage up to 18 cm is possible.

56. The extensive volumetric scan coverage with each gantry rotation makes possible the acquisition of entire organs in a single axial scan.

57. Flat-panel detector systems also provide improved resolution through extremely thin reconstructed sections. Initial flat-panel CT detectors have achieved sections with sensitivity profiles as thin as 150 μm (0.15 mm).

58. The wide 2D field of view made possible by a single, large area detector also allows such a system to operate as a conventional fluoroscopic device. This type of real-time CT fluoroscopy may have substantial applications for interventional CT and may offer a true dual-purpose radiographic imaging system.

59. C-arm systems with flat-panel CT capabilities have numerous applications during surgical procedures. A further application, termed an O-arm, incorporates a telescoping gantry that enables the acquisition of 3D CT images in addition to standard fluoroscopy.

60. Additional clinical applications of flat-panel detector CT systems include:
    a. Ultra-high resolution of bony structures.
    b. Dynamic cardiac imaging.
    c. Whole-organ perfusion studies.

F. Data Acquisition System

1. The DAS consists of electronic components responsible for measuring the transmitted x-radiation absorbed by the detectors.

2. Electronic amplifiers condition and boost the electronic signal that the detectors transmit in response to radiation absorption.

3. The analog-to-digital converter (ADC) is the component of the DAS responsible for converting the electronic signal into digital form. This digital data are then transmitted to the system computer for image reconstruction.

4. The vast range of tissue densities inherent in CT imaging results in extremely small fluctuations in attenuation. The ADC must be enormously sensitive to a vast range of signal intensities.

5. During MSCT, the DAS is responsible for controlling the signal emitted from the activated detectors exposed to the collimated x-ray beam.

6. The DAS of a multislice CT system has a maximum number of data channels used to transmit data from the detectors to the computer system for image reconstruction.

7. The number of data channels controls the number of slices the system can acquire with each gantry rotation.

8. The following example may be used to illustrate the relationship between beam collimation, data channels, quantity of detectors, and the number of sections an MSCT system can acquire per gantry rotation:
   a. The DAS of a four-channel MSCT system has four z-axis data channels.
   b. The system's detector array contains 16 detectors, each measuring 1.25 mm along the z-axis (20 mm total).
   c. When the beam collimation is set to 20 mm, all detectors measure transmitted radiation and produce proportional signal to be collected by the DAS.
   d. Because only four z-axis data channels are available, the signal from four detectors may be combined, or binned, to form images that are 5 mm thick (4 × 1.25 mm = 5.0 mm).
   e. Therefore, with a beam collimation of 20 mm, this system is capable of producing four CT images per gantry rotation with a minimum thickness of 5.0 mm each (Fig. 4-10, A).
   f. If the beam is further collimated to 10 mm, the transmitted radiation exposes only the center 10 mm of the detector array, corresponding to the middle 8 detectors out of the total of 16 (8 × 1.25 mm = 10 mm).
   g. The four channels are now capable of producing 4 CT sections per gantry rotation, each 2.5 mm in thickness and representing the combined data from two detectors (2 × 1.25 mm = 2.5 mm) (Fig. 4-10, B).
   h. Beam collimation to 5 mm on this system would result in the possible reconstruction of four 1.25-mm-thick images for every gantry rotation (Fig. 4-10, C).

G. Computer System

1. An in-depth analysis of the function of the CT computer system is beyond the scope of clinical practice and this review book.

2. However, the CT technologist should have a basic understanding of the fundamental operation of the CT computer system and should be able to identify the major technical components.

3. Fast and efficient data processing and extremely large data storage capacity are the most important characteristics of CT computer systems.

4. The central processing unit (CPU) is capable of performing multiple tasks simultaneously, a function called *parallel processing*.

5. *Pipelining* is an additional feature of CT computers systems that further improves the speed and efficiency with which it can perform multiple simultaneous functions, including detector signal pre-processing, convolution, post-processing, and image manipulation.

6. The primary data processing component of the CT system is the array processor. A separate computer with its own CPU, the array processor is connected to the main host computer of the CT system.

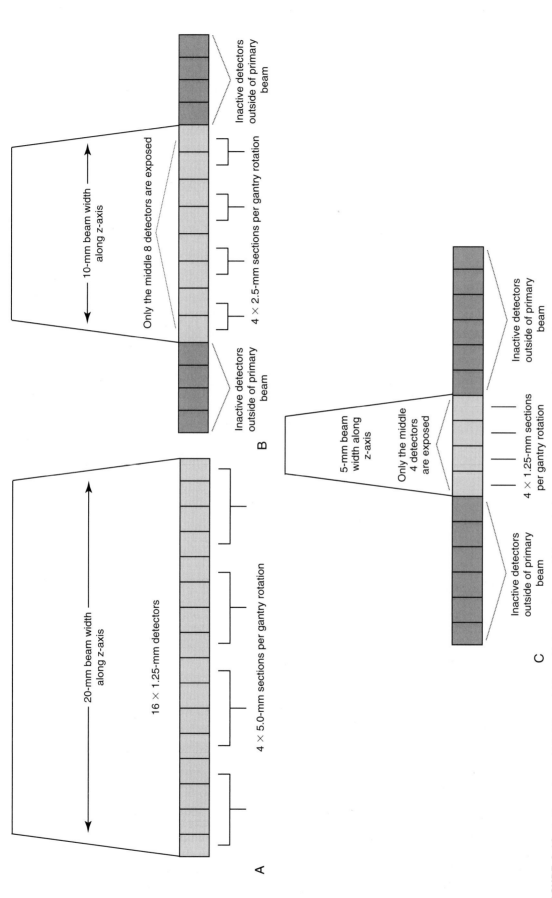

FIGURE 4-10 A, Four-channel MSCT acquisition with 20-mm beam width. For each gantry rotation at this selected beam width, the system is capable of reconstructing a maximum of four 5.0-mm CT sections. The data from four adjacent detector elements (1.25 mm each) are binned, or electronically combined. **B,** Four-channel MSCT acquisition with 10-mm beam width. With only the central eight detectors exposed to transmitted radiation, a maximum of four 2.5-mm CT images may be reconstructed for each gantry rotation. The detectors that lie outside the collimated beam do not measure transmitted radiation and do not contribute signal to the reconstruction process. **C,** Four-channel MSCT acquisition with 5.0-mm beam width. With only the central four detectors exposed to transmitted radiation, a maximum of four 1.25-mm CT images may be reconstructed for each gantry rotation. The detectors that lie outside the collimated beam do not measure transmitted radiation or contribute signal to the reconstruction process.

7. The array processor is responsible for receiving scan data from the host computer, performing all of the major processing of the CT image, and returning the reconstructed image to the storage memory of the host computer.
8. The hard disk drive is the common choice for mass storage of CT computer system data.
9. The hard disk drive is a rewritable, nonremovable storage system that must be capable of storing a tremendous amount of data. It also must be able to transfer data quickly, in a manner quantified by the data transfer rate.
10. The operating system (OS) is the main software of the CT computer. It controls the utilization of the hardware resources, such as the available memory, CPU time, and disk space.
11. Common types of operating system software include Windows, MS-DOS, OS/2, and UNIX.
12. The remaining software of the CT computer system may be organized as follows:
    a. Pre-processing software, processes the signal data collected from the detectors and conditions it by applying appropriate correction factors for beam hardening, detector malfunction, and so on.
    b. Reconstruction software is responsible for mathematically constructing the raw data into image data using algorithms for the processes of convolution, back projection, data frequency filtering, and so on.
    c. Post-processing software manipulates the image data for review and interpretation. This software controls the image visualization and analysis tools of the CT system, including applications such as windowing, image display filters, 3D/MPR reformation, and analytic functions (region of interest, distance).

IMAGE PROCESSING AND DISPLAY

A. Image Reconstruction

1. The data acquisition process can be outlined as follows:
    a. The x-ray tube rotates around the patient while emitting a constant beam of x-radiation. The quantity of radiation is controlled primarily by the mA setting, and the beam quality (penetrability) is controlled primarily by the kVp.
    b. As the x-ray photons pass through the patient, some are absorbed completely and others lose a portion of their energy and change direction as scatter radiation. This process, termed *attenuation,* can be described as the reduction in intensity of the x-ray quantum as it travels along from tube to detector.
    c. The extent of attenuation depends on multiple factors, including the x-ray energy and the atomic structure and density of the exposed tissue.

d. Attenuation values are calculated by mathematically comparing the radiation incident upon the patient (I_0) to the radiation transmitted through and measured by the detector (I).
e. The logarithmic relationship is mathematically described by the formula:

$$\text{Relative transmission} = \log \frac{\text{Intensity of x-ray at the source}(I_0)}{\text{Intensity of x-ray at the detector}(I)}$$

f. The portion of the x-ray beam transmitted through the patient and incident upon a single detector is termed a *ray.* Each ray undergoes a specific quantity of attenuation based on its particular path through the patient.
g. The measurement of transmitted radiation made by an individual detector is called a *ray sum.* It equals the total attenuation occurring along a straight-line path from tube to detector.
h. The ray sum, or transmission measurement, equals the total attenuation of all materials along the ray.
i. The detector emits an electronic analog signal in proportionate response to the transmitted radiation it absorbs. As the detector array rotates about the patient, the signal varies according to the measured x-ray energy flux.
j. During the process of data acquisition, ray sum measurements are made by the DAS hundreds of times per second. The term *view* is used to describe each data sample made by the DAS. A view contains transmission measurements made along multiple rays, each corresponding to a particular detector (ray sums).
k. The sampling rate may be quantified as *views per rotation* (VPR). The VPR determines the quantity of samples, and therefore transmission data, acquired during each gantry rotation.
2. The analog transmission values (signal) acquired by the DAS are digitized by the ADC and sent to the computer for processing as raw data.
3. From the thousands of ray sum measurements acquired, the computer system generates an attenuation map, spatially localizing the degree of attenuation that occurs across a given section of anatomy.
4. The large magnitude of data samples acquired during scanning allows for precise localization of attenuation values for each pinpoint area of tissue within a given section.
5. The ability of an object to attenuate the x-ray beam is assigned a value termed the *linear attenuation coefficient* (μ).
6. If the intensity of radiation incident upon an object is known, the magnitude of attenuation occurring as the x-ray beam passes through an object can be calculated by measuring the intensity of radiation transmitted.
7. The Lambert-Beer equation illustrates the relationship between radiation intensity and object density,

and allows for the calculation of an object's linear attenuation coefficient (μ):

$$I = I_0 e^{-\mu x}$$

where e is Euler's constant (2.718) and x is object thickness.

8. The Lambert-Beer equation is valid only for homogeneous pencil-beam radiation sources, such as the first-generation CT system developed by Hounsfield.

9. The situation becomes much more complicated by the heterogeneous nature of the x-ray beam and the additional difficulties inherent in the cone beam geometry of modern MSCT systems. Nevertheless, the Lambert-Beer equation neatly demonstrates how the attenuation coefficients contained within a sample (section) of patient anatomy can be calculated.

10. The reconstructed CT image displays a 2D map localizing the attenuation that occurs throughout each section of tissue.

11. The primary goal of CT image reconstruction is to spatially distribute the attenuation data recorded by the detector array.

12. The mathematical process primarily responsible for CT image reconstruction is called *back-projection*. During this reconstruction method, the ray sum data acquired from each projection (data sample) is projected back onto a matrix.

13. A *matrix* is a 2D grid of numbers arranged in rows and columns.

14. The acquisition of an extremely large number of projections for each gantry rotation results in a detailed but relatively blurry digital representation of the object(s) in study.

15. An additional process called *convolution* is applied to reduce image unsharpness. An algorithm or convolution kernel acts as a mathematical filter, modifying the ray sum data and removing the unwanted burring effect of the back-projection.

16. The appearance of the CT image may be altered by the application of different algorithms to manipulate the signal during image reconstruction. For example, a soft tissue algorithm yields a smooth image, which is preferable for the evaluation of soft tissue structures. A bone algorithm sharpens edges and improves the demonstration of bony detail with high-resolution CT images.

17. This back-projection of ray sum data onto a matrix combined with mathematical filtration constitutes the current method for image reconstruction in the modern MSCT system—*the filtered back projection*.

18. However, additional techniques are necessary to eliminate unwanted image degradation due to patient movement during helical data acquisition.

19. Conventional CT data acquisition consists of incremental, slice-by-slice scanning. For each 360-degree rotation of the gantry components, the patient/table remains stable and transmission data are recorded. The bed then moves to the next location, determined

by the chosen section interval, and the process is repeated until the desired anatomic coverage is achieved.

20. Helical, or spiral scanning refers to the volumetric data acquisition process whereby the gantry and bed undergo continuous motion. The acquired data are described as having a helical, or spiral geometry.

21. During helical data acquisition, the patient bed is continuously feeding through the gantry as the tube and detector array rotate. Therefore, no single slice of patient anatomy is ever exposed to a full 360 degrees of evaluation.

22. *Interpolation* is the mathematical process whereby data from tube rotations just above and just below a given slice position are used for image reconstruction.

23. Interpolation allows for the reconstruction of a thin, motion-free image from a volumetric data set acquired from a moving patient.

24. The technique known as 360-degree linear interpolation (*360LI*) uses two sets of projection data acquired 360 degrees apart to form an image at a precise z-axis location.

25. More commonly used for current MSCT image reconstruction is the 180-degree linear interpolation technique (*180LI*).

26. The 180LI technique interpolates data acquired at a distance only 180 degrees away from the reconstructed slice location. For every one-half rotation of the gantry during scanning, a complimentary ray is acquired, at the point where the x-ray tube and detectors are in exact opposite positions from those in the previous, complimentary view.

27. Data acquired from the complimentary ray are used to form an image at a precise z-axis location.

28. Interpolation of data from a shorter distance away along the z-axis reduces blurring and improves image quality.

29. Multidetector row CT systems utilize an additional process called *z-filtering* during image reconstruction. Z-filtering allows for thin sections to be reconstructed at any point along the acquired z-axis volume. This reconstruction method utilizes multiple complimentary rays beyond those immediately above and below the particular slice plane.

30. Image reconstruction for MSCT helical acquisition is complicated further by the addition of cone beam geometry.

31. The widened 2D detector array of MSCT systems requires a more divergent x-ray beam. The rays measured from a more divergent beam arrive at the detector at an oblique angle, which must be compensated for during the reconstruction process.

32. As the number of detector rows and subsequent beam divergence increase, the situation may arise in which not all of the rays measured by the detectors have passed through a given section plane. Rays that are positioned at the periphery of the

cone beam may never pass through a midline section as it relates to the total data acquired from a single gantry rotation.

33. Special cone beam reconstruction algorithms are used to overcome this issue. Examples are the Feldkamp-Davis-Kress (FDK) and advanced single-slice rebinning (ASSR) algorithms. The mathematical theory and function of these specialized algorithms are beyond the scope of both the clinical practice of CT and this review book.

34. Once the reconstruction process is completed, the raw data (ray sum or transmission measurements) is displayed as image data. The resultant images of this initial, or prospective, reconstruction are evaluated by a radiologist, further manipulated in 3D or MPR, archived to long-term storage, and so on.

35. Multiple data reconstructions can be performed retrospectively, with adjustments to the section interval, display field of view, image centering, or algorithm (kernel). MSCT systems also allow changes in section width through adjustment of the detector collimation.

36. The projection (raw) data must be available within the system to perform such retrospective reconstructions. Each CT system is capable of storing a finite amount of raw data for retrospective reconstruction.

B. Image Display

1. *Digital image* is used to describe an image of an object that is numerically based. To review:
   a. The CT image is a digital image made up of numerical values acquired from a conversion of analog signal.
   b. The signal is generated by detectors that measure the attenuation of radiation by an object (patient).
   c. A numerical value called the linear attenuation coefficient (μ) is assigned to a sample of tissue quantifying its degree of attenuation.
   d. The digital CT image is therefore based on numerical values that quantify x-ray attenuation.

2. The digital CT image is displayed on an arrangement of numerical values called a matrix. The matrix is made up of a series of *picture elements*, arranged in rows and columns, called pixels (*pi-x-els*).

3. The number of pixels contained in a matrix varies throughout digital imaging but is 512 across and 512 down (512 × 512) in most CT systems.

4. As presented on a display screen or a sheet of film, the CT image is two-dimensional. However, each pixel actually represents a volume of tissue. The volume data are referred to as a voxel, for *volume element* (*vo-x-el*) (Fig. 4-11).

5. The longitudinal dimension of the voxel corresponds to the z-axis of scanning, with a voxel depth equal to the reconstructed section width. For example, sections reconstructed at a 1.25-mm width have voxel lengths (z) of 1.25 mm.

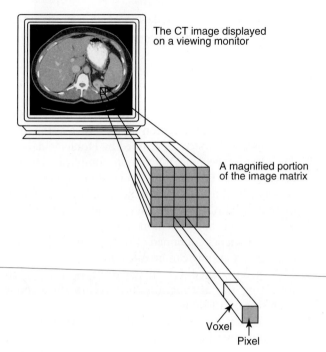

The CT image displayed on a viewing monitor

A magnified portion of the image matrix

Voxel

Pixel

FIGURE 4-11 The digital CT image is displayed upon a matrix, which is composed of rows and columns of pixels. Each pixel represents a three-dimensional volume element called a *voxel*.

6. Each voxel digitally represents a quantity of scanned patient tissue. The tissue within the voxel has exhibited some measure of attenuation, and a corresponding linear attenuation coefficient (μ) is assigned to the pixel. The μ of each pixel represents the average attenuation exhibited by the tissue spatially localized within the voxel.

7. The calculated μ for each pixel is not an absolute value and can vary for an identical voxel scanned on a different CT system or at a different moment in time. This variation is due to naturally occurring fluctuations in the photon energy produced by the x-ray system.

8. The conversion of the linear attenuation value (μ) into a CT number normalizes the voxel attenuation and corrects for this potential variation in pixel number. The *CT number* is a relative value that standardizes the attenuation value (μ) of a tissue by comparing it with the attenuation of water for a particular CT system.

9. The mathematical relationship between linear attenuation coefficient (μ) and CT number is given as follows:

$$\text{CT number} = \frac{\mu_t - \mu_w}{\mu_w} \bullet K$$

where μ_t is the linear attenuation coefficient of the pixel/voxel in question, μ_w is the linear attenuation of water for a given CT system, and K is a constant value of 1000 termed the *contrast factor*.

10. The calculated CT number is given in Hounsfield units (HU), named for the inventor of CT technology, Sir Godfrey Hounsfield.

11. For example, during a body CT scan, a particular voxel of tissue has a total linear attenuation coefficient (μ) of 0.189. The μ of water for this scanner is known to be 0.181. The CT number for this pixel can be calculated as follows:

$$\text{CT number} = \frac{\mu_t - \mu_w}{\mu_w} \bullet K$$
$$= \frac{0.189 - 0.181}{0.181} \bullet 1000$$
$$= 0.044 \bullet 1000 = 44 \text{ HU}$$

12. This pixel value corresponds to a typical HU for soft tissue structures such as musculature and abdominal organ parenchyma.

13. Another voxel from the same section location has a total linear attenuation coefficient (μ) of 0.008. The CT number for this pixel can be calculated as follows:

$$\text{CT number} = \frac{\mu_t - \mu_w}{\mu_w} \bullet K$$
$$\text{CT number} = \frac{0.008 - 0.181}{0.181} \bullet 1000$$
$$\text{CT number} = -0.956 \bullet 1000 = -956 \text{ HU}$$

14. The HU for this pixel is a negative number because the tissue it represents has an attenuation value less than that of water. This pixel value corresponds to a typical HU for an air-filled structure such as the lungs or GI tract.

15. This relationship also clearly illustrates why the CT number for a voxel containing water is at or around 0 HU:

$$\text{CT number} = \frac{\mu_t - \mu_w}{\mu_w} \bullet K$$
$$\text{CT number} = \frac{0.181 - 0.181}{0.181} \bullet 1000$$
$$\text{CT number} = 0 \bullet 1000 = 0 \text{ HU}$$

16. Table 4-1 lists approximate linear attenuation coefficients (μ) and relative Hounsfield values for assorted body tissues.

17. To review, the pixel value, given in Hounsfield units, is a numerical representation of the attenuation of a voxel of tissue as compared with that of water for an individual CT system.

18. The CT image is most accurate when a voxel represents only one tissue type. *Partial volume averaging* occurs when multiple types of tissue are represented by a single voxel. The attenuation coefficients for each tissue type are averaged, yielding a single pixel value whose HU attempts to represent the entire contents of the voxel.

19. Partial volume averaging can be reduced by minimizing the voxel dimension. Small voxels have a greater propensity to contain only one tissue type, thereby improving accuracy.

20. The simplest method of reducing voxel dimension is to reduce reconstructed section width. A thinner

TABLE 4-1	Approximate Lin... Coefficients (μ) a... Hounsfield Value... Tissue Types	
Tissue	**Linear Attenuation Coefficient (μ)***	
Dense bone	0.528	+1500 to +2000
Muscle	0.237	+50 to +65
White matter	0.213	+40 to +46
Gray matter	0.212	+35 to +40
Blood	0.208	+30 to +35
Cerebrospinal fluid	0.207	+15
Water	0.206	0
Fat	0.185	−50 to −100
Lungs	0.093	−550 to −950
Air	0.0004	−1000

*The listed values for μ are at 100 kVp or approximately 60 keV mean x-ray energy. Modified from Bushong Sc: Radiologic science for technologists, ed 9, St Louis, 2008, Mosby.

slice (section) is produced from voxels with shorter lengths along the z-axis. Thinner section widths reduce the partial volume effect.

21. The volume of a voxel may also be reduced by decreasing the pixel dimension. The pixel dimension, d, is given by the following formula, in relation to the display field of view (DFOV):

$$d = \frac{\text{DFOV (mm)}}{\text{matrix size}}$$

22. The matrix size is relatively standard in CT imaging at 512^2, or 512 pixels across by 512 pixels down.

23. The scan field of view (SFOV) is one of two fields of view described in CT imaging. SFOV is determined by the size (x- and y-axes) of the detector array. SFOV controls the diameter of the circular data acquisition field within the CT gantry:

   a. Most modern MSCT systems have an SFOV within the approximate range of 48 to 52 cm. Therefore, the maximum circular field of data acquired is between 48 and 52 cm.

   b. A CT system allows for a reduction in SFOV for certain clinical applications by reducing the number of activated detectors during data acquisition.

   c. Most CT systems have multiple SFOV choices. Common examples are large SFOV (50 cm) and small SFOV (25 cm).

   d. The selection of SFOV may also involve additional filtration and corrective algorithms for certain clinical applications. For example, CT systems typically offer some version of a specific SFOV for the head. It utilizes an acquisition diameter of 25 cm but also includes specific adaptations within the reconstruction process to improve the quality of CT images of the head.

display field of view (DFOV) is chosen by the CT operator on the basis of the part size in question. The selected DFOV determines what portion of the acquired data will be displayed across the matrix:

a. For example, during a CT examination of the abdomen, the operator chooses a large SFOV (50 cm) to ensure that the entire patient circumference is included within the data acquisition field.

b. The DFOV for image reconstruction is selected on the basis of the dimension of the anatomic area the operator selects to display across the image matrix. The size of the DFOV equals the size of the part of interest.

c. Continuing with the example, a DFOV of 38 cm displays a reconstructed circle whose diameter equals 38 cm. A DFOV of 12 cm would display only 12 cm of the acquired 50 cm of scan data across the image matrix.

d. Choosing a smaller DFOV, or targeting:
   - Limits the anatomic area displayed.
   - Increases the size of the displayed anatomy and, most importantly, reduces the pixel dimension and the volume of each voxel (Fig. 4-12).

e. As a geometric cuboid, the volume of a voxel may be calculated as follows:

voxel volume $(mm^3) = d^2 (mm^2) \bullet$ section width (z, mm)

25. To review, the pixel dimension and voxel volume are controlled by three technical parameters:
    a. Matrix size
    b. Display field of view (DFOV)
    c. Section width (z)

26. An important concept to keep in mind is that the actual size of the pixel does not change. A 512 × 512 matrix always has pixels of a consistent dimension. What changes is the amount of tissue spatially localized into each voxel and subsequently represented by each pixel's CT number.

27. Less tissue in each voxel reduces the partial volume effect and improves image quality (Fig. 4-13).

28. In addition to the size of a reconstructed image, the image centering may also be altered with use of an application of the Cartesian coordinate system:

a. The x-y axis is located within the rotational plane of the CT gantry.

b. The x-axis runs from right to left (or vice versa) when one is viewing an axial image.

c. The y-axis runs from anterior to posterior (or vice versa) when one is viewing an axial image.

d. The z-axis runs parallel to the movement of the CT table, in and out of the gantry. The z-axis corresponds to the plane running superior to inferior (or vice versa) when one is viewing sequential axial CT images of the head, neck, and trunk.

e. When one is imaging the upper or lower extremities, the z-axis runs parallel to the long axis of the part, from proximal to distal (or vice versa).

f. This coordinate system is sometimes referred to as RAS (for *right*, *anterior*, and *superior*) coordinates.

g. The clinical images in Fig. 4-14 illustrate the display effects of DFOV reduction and targeting.

29. In contrast to targeting, the displayed CT image may also be electronically magnified.

30. Magnification is an electronic feature of the system software and display monitor. The process of image magnification results in a larger displayed image but has no effect on pixel/voxel dimension (Fig. 4-15).

31. Once image reconstruction is complete, the CT image exists as a digital matrix. Each pixel is assigned a Hounsfield value on the basis of the attenuation of the tissue localized in its corresponding voxel.

32. For visual display, the numerical data are converted into an image based on a gray scale. Each pixel is assigned a shade of gray according to its CT number.

33. *Windowing* is used to describe the process of gray-scale mapping of the CT image. A basic understanding of computer language is helpful in comprehending how gray-scale mapping of the CT image is accomplished.

34. Like any other computer system, the CT computer utilizes a binary system (0, 1) based on discrete units termed *bits*.

35. The bit depth of a digital imaging system defines the number of information bits contained within each pixel. The bit depth controls the maximum number of CT Hounsfield values that may be assigned to any one pixel, as illustrated by the following relationship:

Pixel CT # $= 2^k$

where k is the bit number.

36. The CT computer system is typically capable of displaying 12 bits of data per pixel and is therefore able to display any of up to 4096 (or 2^{12}) Hounsfield values for each pixel.

37. The typical range of Hounsfield scale CT numbers is −1024 HU to +3071 HU. This range equals the 4096 different values possible with a 12-bit system ($2^{12} = 4096$).

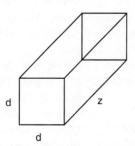

FIGURE 4-12 Dimensions of a voxel. Pixel dimension (*d*) is controlled by the image matrix and the selected display field of view (DFOV). The voxel depth (*z*) is controlled by the section width.

$$d = \frac{DFOV(mm)}{matrix} = \frac{380}{512} = .74 \text{ mm}$$

.74 mm · .74 mm · 3 mm

Section width = 3 mm
Voxel volume = $.74^2 \cdot 3.0 = 1.64 \text{ mm}^3$

38 cm DFOV

SFOV = 50 cm

12 cm DFOV

$$d = \frac{DFOV(mm)}{matrix} = \frac{120}{512} = .23 \text{ mm}$$

.23 mm · .23 mm · 3 mm

Section width = 3 mm
Voxel volume = $.23^2 \cdot 3.0 = 0.16 \text{ mm}^3$

FIGURE 4-13 The combination of matrix, DFOV, and section width determines the amount of tissue that is spatially localized into each voxel. The pixel value (CT number) represents all of the tissue localized within a single pixel.

38. During display of the CT image, each pixel is assigned a shade of gray on the basis of its CT number (HU). In theory, up to 4096 different shades of gray could be assigned to a given pixel.

39. Display monitors used for CT image evaluation possess a dynamic range of about 8 bits and can display 256 individual shades of gray.

40. Because the human eye is capable of differentiating only about 60 to 80 individual shades of gray, the 256 levels possible with an 8-bit system are more than sufficient.

41. Gray-scale mapping, or windowing, occurs when the display system assigns a shade of gray to an individual pixel on the basis of its CT number (HU).

42. The image window determines the range of pixel values that will be assigned a particular shade of gray. Any pixel with a value outside the image window will not be assigned a shade of gray, but will appear either white or black.

43. The specifics of the displayed pixel range are determined by a user-selected *window level* (WL) and *window width* (WW).

44. The range of displayed pixels is controlled by the image window width. For example, for a WW of 150, a range of 150 pixel values are assigned individual shades of gray. Only pixels with Hounsfield values that fall within the set range are assigned one of the available 256 shades of gray.

45. Any pixel with a CT number lower than the set range appears black. Any pixel with a CT number higher than the set range appears white.

46. There are 256 shades of gray available to display 4096 possible pixel numbers. The selected window width determines how many consecutive CT Hounsfield values will be displayed by a single shade of gray.

47. Narrow WW values assign fewer pixel values to each step along the gray scale. Wide WW values assign more pixel values to each shade of gray.

48. In the most basic example, a WW of 256 (WW/256) will display a single pixel value for each shade of gray. A WW of 2560 (WW/2560) assigns 10 consecutive pixel values for each step along the gray scale.

DFOV = 48 cm

DFOV = 24 cm

Targeted DFOV = 24 cm

FIGURE 4-14A-C A, A 5.0-mm axial CT section of the abdomen acquired with a large scan field of view (SFOV) of 50 cm. The display field of view (DFOV) is set at 48 cm, so almost all of the acquired data are displayed on the image matrix. The volume of each voxel equals $(480/512)^2 \bullet 5 = 4.39^3$ mm. **B,** The same 50 cm of raw data retrospectively reconstructed with a DFOV of 24 cm. The volume of each voxel now equals $(240/512)^2 \bullet 5 = 1.10^3$ mm. Each voxel represents significantly less tissue in this targeted reconstruction. **C,** An additional retrospective reconstruction with new RAS coordinates centering the targeted 24 cm DVOV over the spine.

Image magnified by a factor of 2.

FIGURE 4-15 The image from Fig. 4-14,A is shown here magnified by a factor of 2. The DFOV remains at 50 cm, and the voxel volume is still 4.39 mm. The image has been electronically magnified on the display monitor and demonstrates a loss of sharpness in comparison with the targeted image in Fig. 4-14, C.

49. The window width is centered on a middle pixel value termed the *window level*.

50. The window level is the pixel value, given in Hounsfield units (HU), at the center of the window width. The window level is generally set at or near the Hounsfield value of the primary tissue of interest.

51. For example, if the previously cited window width of 150 (−25 to +125 HU) is centered at a CT number of +50 HU, the window may be graphically illustrated as shown in Fig. 4-16.

52. In this example, only pixels with values between −25 HU and +125 HU will appear as some shade of gray. Any pixel with a Hounsfield value less than −25 HU will appear black. Any pixel with a Hounsfield value greater than +125 HU will appear white.

53. Fig. 4-17 provides an example of an axial CT image of the abdomen displayed with this window.

54. A window with a WL of −500 HU and a WW of 1000 may be graphically illustrated as shown in Fig. 4-18.

FIGURE 4-16 Pixels with values between −25 HU and +125 HU are each assigned a shade of gray. Pixels with values less than −25 HU are black, and those with values greater than +125 HU are white.

55. In this example, only pixels with values between −1000 HU and 0 HU will appear as some shade of gray. Any pixel with a Hounsfield value less than −1000 HU will appear black. Any pixel with a Hounsfield value greater than 0 HU will appear white.
56. Fig. 4-19 is an example of an axial CT image of the abdomen displayed with this window.
57. A window with a WL of +500 HU and a WW of 2000 may be graphically illustrated as shown in Fig. 4-20.
58. In this example, only pixels with values between −500 HU and +1500 HU will appear as some shade of gray. Any pixel with a Hounsfield value less than −500 HU will appear black. Any pixel with a Hounsfield value greater than +1500 HU will appear white.
59. Fig. 4-21 provides an example of an axial CT image of the abdomen displayed with this window.
60. Keep in mind that most CT imaging systems routinely have the ability to assign up to 4096 (2^{12}) Hounsfield values to any one pixel. With only 256 shades of gray

FIGURE 4-17 An axial CT image of the abdomen displayed with a window level (WL) of +50 HU and a window width (WW) of 150. This narrow window setting results in a high-contrast image. There are many "black" and "white" pixels, with fewer pixels assigned shades of gray because of the narrow window setting.

FIGURE 4-18 Pixels with values between −1000 HU and 0 HU are each assigned a shade of gray. Pixels with values less than −1000 HU are black, and those with values greater than 0 HU are white.

available for display, pixels with similar Hounsfield values may be group-assigned a single shade of gray. The extent to which this grouping of pixel shade occurs depends on the window width.

61. For example, with a wider window setting, such as 4000, very few pixels if any will fall outside the display range and appear white or black. Groups of pixels whose CT numbers are similar will be assigned the same shade of gray (Fig. 4-22).

62. In general terms, the window width controls the contrast of a CT image, and the window level controls its brightness.

63. Specific window width and level settings depend primarily on the visual preferences of the user.

Some general guidelines to CT window settings can be found in Table 4-2.

64. The mathematical basis and digital display of the CT image may be summarized as follows:
   a. During data acquisition, a numerical value called the linear attenuation coefficient (μ) is assigned to a sample of tissue, quantifying its degree of attenuation.
   b. The pixel value, given in Hounsfield units, is a numerical representation of the attenuation of a voxel of tissue relative to that of water.
   c. During image display, each pixel is assigned a shade of gray on the basis of its CT number (Fig. 4-23).

65. Once the image is displayed on a computer monitor, CT software systems are capable of various analysis features including:
   a. *Image display filters*: Different from the algorithms utilized during image reconstruction, these display filters are used to visually enhance the CT image during certain clinical applications. Some are used to smooth the CT image for improved low-contrast resolution. Edge-enhancing filters sharpen the CT image during high-resolution imaging applications of the lungs and dense bones. Image filters do not affect the process of raw data reconstruction; rather, they alter the display characteristics of an image after the reconstruction process.
   b. Analytic functions: Quantitative software applications for evaluation of disease processes or other anatomic abnormalities:
   • *Region of interest* (ROI) provides a quantitative analysis of the Hounsfield values of a specific anatomic area. A graphic outline in the shape of a circle, square, freeform design, and so on is placed over an area of the image. System software calculates the average CT number in HU within the defined ROI. The average ROI measurement provides

FIGURE 4-19 The image from Fig. 4-14 is displayed here with a window level (WL) of −500 HU and a window width (WW) of 1000. This combination of settings would typically be referred to as a "lung window," because it offers good detail of the visualized lung parenchyma. Denser structures such as bone and soft tissue appear white because their pixel values are greater than 0 HU.

Window level (WL) = +500 HU
Window width (WW) = 2000

FIGURE 4-20 Pixels with values between −500 HU and +1500 HU are each assigned a shade of gray. Pixels with values less than −500 HU are black, and those with values greater than +1500 HU are white.

information about tissue characteristics that may be helpful for clinical diagnosis.

- *Linear distance measurement* is a graphic used for precise size determination, distance for interventional procedures, and so on (Fig. 4-24).

c. *Cine viewing mode* allows the user to review large quantities of CT images at a high rate. The images are viewed in a motion loop, the speed of which can be controlled by the user. Cine viewing is particularly beneficial when one is reviewing the enormous image sets generated during MSCT studies.

FIGURE 4-21 The image in Fig. 4-14 is displayed here with a window level (WL) of +500 HU and a window width (WW) of 2000. This combination of settings would typically be referred to as a "bone window," because it offers good detail of the dense bony structures. The window is centered on a higher window level, resulting in pixels with greater Hounsfield values assigned shades of gray.

TABLE 4-2	Sample Window Settings for Common Clinical Applications	
Window Name	Window Level (WL)	Window Width (WW)
Abdomen	+40 HU	350
Brain	+40 HU	100
Subdural	+50 HU	150
Stroke	+35 HU	35
Lung	−600 HU	1300
Vocal cords	−300 HU	1000
Liver	+50 HU	150
Trabecular bone	+250 HU	2000
Cortical bone	+350 HU	3000

C. Post-Processing

1. One of the major benefits of ... produce superior MPR and 3D ... ment is made possible by the ... data sets.
2. *Isotropic* describes voxels ... along the x-, y-, and z-axes. ... approached by applying two ...
   a. Choosing the thinnest detector collimation available to produce the thinnest slices available reduces voxel dimension in the z-axis.
   b. Reconstructing the acquired data with the smallest DFOV allowed on the basis of the part of interest reduces pixel dimension along the x- and y-axes.
3. For example, an abdominal CTA acquisition with a 64-slice MSCT system is made with a detector collimation of 0.6 mm. If images are reconstructed on a 512 matrix with a DFOV of 32 cm, the pixel dimension may be calculated as follows:

$$d = \frac{DFOV}{matrix}$$

$$= \frac{320}{512}$$

$$= 0.625 \text{ mm}$$

4. In the example, the pixel dimension along the x- and y-axes is roughly equal to the z-axis dimension

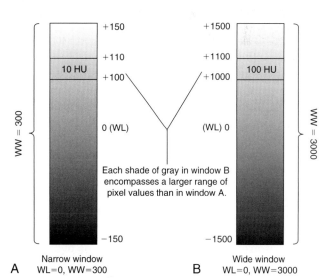

FIGURE 4-22 The effects of window width settings on image contrast. Window *A* results in a narrow range of pixel values displayed as shades of gray. Small steps in pixel number are represented by large steps in gray shade. The image appears higher in contrast because of the predominance of white and black pixels with values that fall outside the window width. Window *B* offers a more gradual change in gray shade as pixel number changes. Larger steps in pixel number are required to elicit large steps in gray shade. The image appears lower in contrast owing to the predominance of gray pixels with values that lie within the "wide" window.

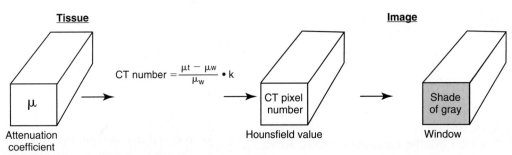

FIGURE 4-23 The numerical basis of the CT image. Linear attenuation coefficient (μ) is converted to CT pixel number (HU), which is then assigned a shade of gray for image display.

FIGURE 4-24 CT software systems are capable of various analysis features. ROI #1 calculates an average pixel value of 14.35 HU. ROI #2 calculates an average pixel value of 16.34 HU. Because of their relatively low (<20 HU) attenuation values, both renal masses most likely represent benign cystic masses. Each measurement also includes the statistical standard deviation (SD) of the pixel numbers within the ROI and the geometric area of the ROI. The linear distance indicated by graphic #3 can be utilized to measure size and/or angle.

of the reconstructed section width (0.6 mm). This isotropic data set would result in high-quality MPR and 3D images.

5. Reconstruction of such isotropic, overlapping, thin-section CT images greatly reduces the step artifact that can negatively affect the quality of MPR and 3D CT images.

6. An isotropic volumetric data set yields high-quality images with equal resolution in any reconstructed plane. It eliminates the need for data acquisition in two planes, as had been the norm for many applications, such as CT of the sinuses and small parts such as the wrist and ankle (Fig. 4-25).

7. *Multiplanar reformation* (MPR) describes the process of displaying CT images in a different orientation from the one used in the original reconstruction process.

8. Unlike retrospective reconstruction, reformation does not change the makeup of the image voxels.

Reformation merely alters the viewing perspective of the images into a different anatomic plane.

9. The reformatted image is 1 voxel thick, with the pixels facing the viewer each representing the average attenuation occurring within the represented voxels.

10. MPR images are typically formed from a vertical stack of contiguous, helically acquired axial CT images. They are usually displayed in planes that are perpendicular, or orthogonal, to the original plane of data acquisition.

11. *Orthogonal planes* are at right angles to each other.

12. Because most CT examinations acquire data in the transverse, or axial plane, the most common orthogonal MPR planes are (Fig. 4-26):

   a. Coronal, the vertical plane that divides the part into anterior and posterior portions.

   b. Sagittal, the vertical plane that divides the part into right and left portions.

FIGURE 4-25 Isotropic voxels. The x- and y-axis dimensions of the CT image pixel are determined by the selected display field of view (DFOV) value and reconstruction matrix. The width of the reconstructed section determines the voxel length along the z-axis. Isotropic resolution is achieved when the selected factors result in equal dimensions for the x-, y-, and z-axes.

13. Reformats may also be constructed in a nonperpendicular or nonorthogonal plane, as follows:
    a. Oblique: any plane that is tilted from the coronal, sagittal or axial plane
    b. Curved: graphically designed reformation that samples an anatomic structure along points placed by the user. Curved reformations are common through areas such as blood vessels, pancreas, mandible, and spinal cord.
14. MPR images were historically displayed with a thickness equal to the acquired section width, i.e., one voxel thick. The truly volumetric acquisition made possible with MSCT allows for the display of MPR slabs of variable thickness, which average the attenuation values of multiple voxels.
15. Multiplanar reformations may also be thickened to represent slabs of tissue with alternative techniques such as maximum intensity projection (MIP) and minimum intensity projection (min-IP).
16. MIP images display only the maximum pixel value along a ray traced through the object to the viewer's

assumed perspective in front of the viewing monitor. Tissues with lower attenuation values are not displayed, leaving high-attenuation structures such as bone and contrast-enhanced soft tissue structures free of superimposition.
17. As the viewer faces a MIP image, each pixel represents the maximum attenuation that occurs in the associated voxel. The voxel length is determined by the user as the slab thickness.
18. For example, MIP images are valuable in demonstrating contrast-enhanced blood vessels during CT angiography and for the opacified urinary tract during CT urography.
19. Similar in principle, min-IP images display the minimum pixel value along each ray to the viewer. Min-IP reformations are used primarily during the evaluation of the biliary tree, colon, lungs, and trachea.
20. *Three-dimensional* (3D) *CT* describes the process of displaying volumetrically acquired CT data with a perception of 3D depth on a computer monitor or recording film.

FIGURE 4-26 Multiplanar reformation (MPR) and anatomic planes. A, anterior; R, right; S, superior; P, posterior; L, left; and I, inferior.

21. The CT system composes a 3D model using the stack of acquired CT images displayed with definable shading, lighting, and rendering.

22. *Rendering* uses 3D algorithms to provide a specific perspective to the construction of the 3D model:

    a. *Surface render*ing, also termed shaded-surface display (SSD): A technique that uses the concept of *thresholding* to limit the displayed volumetric data. The threshold allows the user to select the range of pixel values rendered in the 3D model. For example a higher, bone threshold (>300 HU) can be chosen to build a skeletal model of the patient's skull. Decreasing the threshold to include voxels with soft tissue attenuation values results in a 3D model with the patient's skin intact.

    b. *Volume rendering* (VR) adjusts the opacity of voxels included in the 3D model according to their tissue characteristics. Unlike the thresholding

concept used for SSD rendering, volume rendering does not exclude voxels, but instead alters their appearance so that the 3D model contains the entire volume dataset.

23. Rendering applications are also used to control the perspective of the viewer evaluating the 3D model, as follows:

    a. *Orthographic volume rendering* is the method of externally viewing a 3D reconstructed object. The viewer's perspective is one of being outside the object and looking at its surface.

    b. *Perspective volume rendering* provides a viewpoint of being within the lumen of the object, similar to an endoscopic view. Also referred to as *immersive rendering*, this type of 3D reconstruction is commonly utilized during CT colonography and CT bronchography.

24. The quality of MPR and 3D images can be improved by adhering to several basic principles:

a. Utilize the thinnest section width possible for the anatomical area, the clinical indication, and the need to keep patient radiation dose to a minimum. Thicker, anisotropic sections result in MPR images in which the separation of each axial section is apparent on the reformation. Commonly referred to as *step artifact*, this unwanted result can be avoided with an isotropic acquisition.

b. The section interval should be less than the reconstructed section width. Overlapping the reconstruction reduces the appearance of separate individual axial sections on the reformatted image. A 50% level of overlap is suggested for optimal reformatted image quality, for example, 1.0-mm sections reconstructed every 0.5 mm.

c. Optimize patient comfort to minimize motion. Movement during data acquisition severely degrades the quality of reformatted images. Patient motion can cause blurriness in the reformation and/or severe step artifact at the point of motion.

IMAGE ARCHIVAL AND COMMUNICATION

1. Once reconstructed, the CT image is displayed on a computer display for further manipulation, review, and evaluation. The images are stored locally on the hard drive of the CT system.

2. The CT system has limited short-term storage capabilities, and the images must then be transferred for long-term safekeeping as part of the patient's medical record.

3. Each CT image reconstructed on a 512^2 matrix is approximately 0.5 megabytes (MB) in digital size. Each CT examination can contain thousands of individual CT images. The long-term archival of CT data requires substantial physical and financial resources.

4. *Image compression* is a complex computer technique that reduces the size of digital CT image data. Compression of CT images reduces the storage requirements and increases the speed at which CT images may be transmitted among computer systems.

5. The technical details of digital image compression are well beyond the scope of clinical CT practice and of this review book. However, the CT technologist should at least be familiar with the two main types of digital image compression:

    a. Lossless (reversible) compression, in which the image is digitally compressed without loss of data and is identical to the original.

    b. Lossy (irreversible) compression, in which data are lost during the compression process and the image does not exactly match the original. Lossy compression results in the loss of data but is capable of much higher compression rates than lossless compression.

6. All CT images are networked and stored in accordance with a standard protocol known as the Digital Imaging and Communications in Medicine (DICOM) standard. The DICOM standard confirms the process of recording, storing, printing, and transmitting medical image data.

7. The DICOM standard was cooperatively developed in 1985 by the American College of Radiology (ACR) and the National Electrical Manufacturers Association (NEMA). The DICOM standard is continuously updated and augmented to meet the changing needs of medical imaging and CT.

8. The purpose of DICOM conformance is to ensure that all medical image files can be conveniently archived and transmitted along various systems and networks, regardless of the manufacturing vendor.

9. Medical images must exist in DICOM file format and must be transferred along networks conforming to a DICOM communications protocol.

10. Archival or storage of the CT image data can be divided into two main options:

    a. *Hard copy*, which is storage of CT image data on digital image film. Laser imager systems record CT images on light-sensitive film in multiple formats (12:1, 6:1, and so on). Hard copy films allow for convenient viewing on view boxes but are limited by physical space-occupying demands for long-term storage.

    b. *Soft copy*, by which CT image data are stored in digital file format. Mass storage devices, such as hard drives, magnetic tape drives, and magnetic optical disks (MODs), can be used to archive the CT image data for long-term storage.

11. Common digital media such as CD-ROM and DVD are actually optical disks and may also be utilized for CT image storage and transfer. These storage devices have become particularly important because of the dramatic increase in volume of image data with the advent of MSCT and advanced CT procedures. As an alternative to laser film, entire CT examinations can be stored on such media for long-term storage and for communication to patients, referring physicians, surgeons, and so on.

12. Optical discs can be characterized according to their storage capabilities:

    a. *Read-only* discs contain image data for review only; the data cannot be modified or added to.

    b. *Write-once, read-many times* (WORM) discs, which allow the initial storage of large quantities of digital image data and subsequent unlimited viewing, without the ability to reuse the discs. Writable CDs (CD-R) and DVDs (DVD-R) are common examples of WORM media.

    c. *Rewritable discs* allow data to be recorded multiple times. Magnetic optical disks (MODs) and rewritable CDs (CD-RW) and DVDs (DVD-RW) are examples of rewritable media.

13. *Picture archival and communications system* (PACS) are computerized networks charged with the responsibility of storing, retrieving, distributing, and displaying CT and other digital medical images.
14. A PACS consists of several key components:
    a. An interface to the CT system and other imaging modalities for transfer of image data from the scanner(s) to the PACS.
    b. Large, expandable digital archive for long-term image storage.
    c. Display workstations for image review and manipulation.
    d. Digital links to the facilities radiology information system (RIS) and/or hospital information system (HIS) for retrieval and archival of demographic information and other pertinent aspects of the patient's electronic medical record.
    e. Additional elements of a PACS may include film digitizers for the archival of hard copy images, dictation/transcription components, CD/DVD burners, printers, and so on.
15. A PACS communicates with the CT system(s) and other modalities and peripherals via a computerized communication system, or *network*.
16. When the network is of sufficient size to support the PACS over limited geographical distance, such as within a radiology department, it is termed a *local area network* (LAN).
17. A wired version of a LAN, commonly known by the proprietary name Ethernet, is routinely used for PACS. Wireless LANs are also available; they are commonly known by the name Wi-Fi (a trademark of the Wi-Fi Alliance that can be used for certified products).
18. *Wide area networks* (WANs) are used to connect multiple LANs over a larger distances, such as

entire medical centers. The Internet or World Wide Web is the largest WAN.
19. *Teleradiology* refers to the ability of a PACS to transmit image data across a LAN or WAN from the imaging facility to an off-site location.
20. Web-based teleradiology systems use the geographically unlimited WAN of the World Wide Web to transmit images for physician review.
21. In accordance with federal requirements regarding the confidentiality of patient information, networks transferring medical record and image data are subject to strict security measures.
22. Safeguards used to secure networked medical image data include:
    a. The use of security software programs and hardware devices such as secure network routers and firewalls.
    b. Digital encryption designed to code the transmitted data in a form decipherable only by software at the destination location.
    c. Privacy and authentication procedures that require the use of log-in and password combinations to access patient information.
23. Fig. 4-27 outlines the processes of image display, data acquisition, data processing, image manipulation and image archival.

IMAGE QUALITY

1. The capacity to define, measure, and assess image quality is a primary responsibility of the CT technologist.
2. This responsibility includes, but is not limited to:
    a. A thorough understanding of the parameters of CT image quality.
    b. Prompt identification of the causes of CT image and study degradation.

FIGURE 4-27 A CT process flow chart illustrating the imaging chain through data acquisition, data processing, image display, image manipulation, and image archival.

e. *Sampling frequency*: The number of views obtained by the CT system during the data acquisition of an image. This sampling rate may also be referred to as *views per rotation* (VPR). The VPR determines the quantity of samples, and therefore transmission data, acquired during each gantry rotation. Inherent to the system design and not adjustable by the user, a higher sampling frequency is obtained by increasing the temporal data sampling rate or by the number of detectors. For example, a very small object (detail) exhibits a very high spatial frequency. The *Nyquist theorem* dictates that the data sampling frequency must be at least twice the object's spatial frequency in order for the object to be resolved by the CT system.

24. *Longitudinal spatial resolution* is a relatively new term in CT image quality. It is introduced as way of describing how patient movement during volumetric acquisition can affect image detail.
25. The longitudinal spatial resolution is usually qualified by the degree of broadening that occurs to the *slice sensitivity profile* (SSP) during volumetric acquisition.
26. The SSP represents the amount of broadening that occurs along the z-axis during volumetric data acquisition.
27. The section width (slice) for a volumetric acquisition may be graphically displayed as an SSP (Fig. 4-30).

28. The SSP of a conventional nonhelical CT image is rectangular. The section represents a known thickness of tissue centered at a specific location along the patient's longitudinal (z-) axis.
29. As a result of the patient/bed translation during scanning, the SSP of a volumetrically acquired image is curved. The increase in partial volume averaging that occurs during helical acquisition slightly widens the slice profile for each image.
30. Effective section width corresponds to the SSP of the reconstructed section in consideration of the widening that occurs during helical data acquisition.
31. The effective section width is defined as the *full width at half maximum* (FWHM) of the SSP. It is measured by examining the SSP at half of its maximum height.
32. SSP broadening may also be evaluated by measuring the illustrated slice profile at a value termed full width at tenth maximum (FWTM).
33. Some CT systems display the effective section width for an acquisition as a function of other selected scan parameters.
34. The factors that affect longitudinal spatial resolution and the SSP are as follows:
    a. *Spiral interpolation algorithm*, an inherent component of the reconstruction process that is not influenced by the operator. This additional algorithm is applied to the image reconstruction of helically acquired images to reduce SSP-broadening effects.

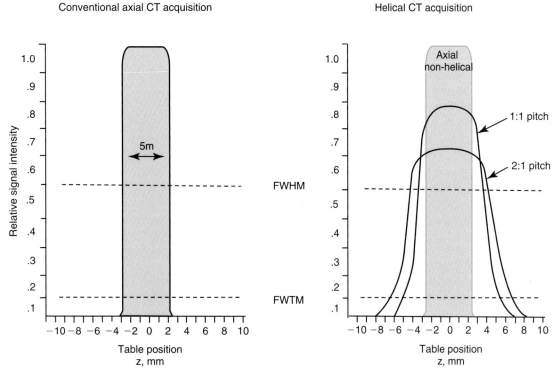

FIGURE 4-30 Slice sensitivity profiles (SSPs) with measurement of section thickness at full width at half maximum (*FWHM*) and full width at tenth maximum (*FWTM*). The SSP of a conventional nonhelical CT acquisition is rectangular. SSP broadening effects are inherent in helical acquisition and worsen with increasing beam pitch.

The 180LI interpolation algorithm is most commonly used. It provides thinner SSP than the 360LI algorithm at the cost of increased image noise.

   b. *Pitch*: For SSCT scanners, increases in detector pitch cause a substantial widening of the SSP and subsequent loss of longitudinal spatial resolution. For MSCT systems, the greater spatial resolution made possible by detector collimation along the z-axis compensates for the negative effects of pitch.

35. Excessive widening of the SSP and a loss of spatial resolution along the z-axis during MSCT examinations may be avoided by using the following general guidelines:

   a. Choose the thinnest beam collimation possible in consideration of patient radiation dose ramifications and the clinical needs of the study, i.e., breath-holds, contrast enhancement patterns, and so on.

   b. Limit pitch by selecting the slowest table translation speed possible. Again, this step must be taken in consideration of patient radiation dose ramifications and the clinical requirements of the study.

   c. Reconstruct images using the thinnest detector collimation possible. Thin-section reconstruction reduces the partial volume effect, reduces or completely eliminates broadening of the SSP, and improves longitudinal spatial resolution.

B. Contrast Resolution

1. The ability of the CT system to detect an object with a small difference in linear attenuation coefficient as compared to the surrounding tissue is called *contrast resolution*.
2. It describes the CT system's ability to differentiate between two adjacent tissues of similar attenuation values and may also be referred to as *low-contrast detectability* or the *sensitivity* of the CT system.
3. Excellent low-contrast resolution remains one of the most important advantages of computed tomography (CT) over other radiographic imaging modalities.
4. MSCT systems are typically capable of differentiating adjacent objects with attenuation differences as small as 3 HU.
5. Contrast resolution is measured by scanning the low-contrast detectability portion of a CT phantom (Fig. 4-31). This insert typically consists of several series of discs or spheres arranged in size order. The discs or spheres exhibit varying contrast from the surrounding material, ranging between 0.3 and 1.0%.
6. Each 1.0% in contrast between adjacent objects amounts to a difference in pixel value of approximately 10 HU.
7. Scans through the insert are performed with various technical factors. Assessment of low-contrast resolution

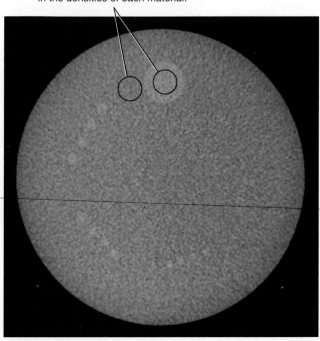

The average pixel values (HU) should demonstrate a difference comparable to the known difference in the densities of each material.

FIGURE 4-31 Low-contrast resolution insert of the American College of Radiology (ACR) phantom, consisting of a series of cylinders of gradually decreasing diameter. Each cylinder is slightly different in density from the background material. The image is visually evaluated to assess the low-contrast sensitivity of the CT system utilizing a range of technical parameters (section width, mA, and so on). ROI measurements can be made to quantify the contrast exhibited between the two slightly different substances.

is made by determining the smallest, lowest contrast circles demonstrated in the image.

8. The technical factors affecting contrast resolution include:

   a. *Inherent subject contrast*: The thickness and atomic density of an object largely determine its image contrast as compared with surrounding tissue. The inherent contrast of an anatomic area can be augmented with the administration of oral and/or IV contrast media. Both negative and positive contrast agents work to alter the inherent contrast of certain tissues.

   b. *Beam collimation*: Scatter radiation reduces contrast resolution. Increasing beam collimation reduces scatter radiation and improves contrast resolution.

   c. *Algorithm selection*: Low spatial frequency algorithms (kernels), such as those used to display soft tissue structures, offer improved contrast resolution.

   d. *Window setting*: A narrow window width can improve contrast resolution by exaggerating the difference in gray shade assignment to pixels with only small differences in attenuation value.

   e. *Detector collimation*: Increased detector collimation results in the reconstruction of thinner sections. As section width decreases, the photon flux for each pixel also decreases. Unless the mA setting is raised to compensate, an increase in noise occurs. Any increase in noise results in a decrease in contrast resolution. In fact, the major limiting factor for contrast resolution is noise.

f. *Noise:* Any change in technical factor resulting in a decrease in noise also results in an improvement to contrast resolution. The factors affecting noise, and therefore contrast resolution, are further discussed later.

C. Temporal Resolution

1. The stop-motion capability of a CT system is referred to as *temporal resolution*. Temporal resolution quantifies the CT system's ability to freeze motion and provide an image free of blurring.
2. The advent of cardiac MSCT has greatly increased the importance of temporal resolution as a CT image quality factor.
3. Historically, the temporal resolution of a CT scanner could be simply equated to the time needed for a complete 360-degree rotation of the gantry. For example, a 1-second scan consisted of a complete gantry revolution in 1 second, yielding a temporal resolution of 1 second.
4. The controlling factors of the temporal resolution of a CT system are the gantry rotation speed and reconstruction method.
5. Current MDCT systems allow complete 360-degree gantry rotations in less than a third of a second (<330 msec).
6. Temporal resolution can be improved by segmenting the data acquisition process into separate components of smaller rotation angles. For example, as described in Chapter 3 in the section on cardiac CT, single-segment or half-scan acquisitions reconstruct data obtained from half of the rotation time. This segmentation results in a 250-msec temporal resolution from a 0.5-sec gantry rotation time.
7. Further improvements in temporal resolution are possible with multisegment reconstructions. At time of publication, state-of-the art temporal resolution has been reduced to well under 200 msec, with dual-slice CT systems reaching as low as 75 msec.

D. Noise

1. In general terms, *noise* in a digital imaging system is any portion of the signal that contains no useful information.
2. Noise can also be described as random (*stochastic*) statistical variations in the signal. Occurring during the computations for each pixel value, these variations interfere with the imaging system's ability to display an accurate image.
3. Noise in the CT image, similar in appearance to the quantum mottle of radiography, manifests as an overall graininess on the reconstructed image.

4. There are three general types of noise in the CT image:
   a. *Quantum* noise, the result of an insufficient x-ray photon flux per voxel. When the CT system attempts to calculate the Hounsfield value for a pixel, but has failed to expose the coinciding voxel to a sufficient amount of x-ray interaction, noise appears on the reconstructed image. The amount of quantum noise is inversely related to the amount of radiation exposed to each voxel. Altering either the voxel dimension or the x-ray flux affects the noise level.
   b. *Electronic system* noise: Signal may be lost and noise introduced to the reconstruction process by the various electronic components of the CT system.
   c. *Artifactual* nose: Artifacts may be viewed as a type of noise. Artifacts can represent a portion of the signal that contains no useful information and may obscure the information present in the image. Please refer to the next section for a detailed review of artifacts.
5. *Signal-to-noise ratio* (SNR) is a descriptive term used to quantify the amount of noise in a displayed CT image. The goal is to produce images with an acceptable noise level—one in which the SNR is high—while maintaining dose and spatial resolution at appropriate levels.
6. As previously mentioned, image noise is the major quality factor affecting low-contrast resolution in the CT image.
7. There are many adjustments to technical factors that improve SNR and contrast resolution while simultaneously decreasing spatial resolution. The inverse of this relationship is also true: Technical factor adjustments that positively affect spatial resolution may negatively affect SNR and contrast resolution.
8. When one is choosing technical parameters for CT protocol design, a compromise must be established between the two. This relationship may be further illustrated by the following formula:

$$D = \frac{SNR^2}{\Delta^3 T}$$

where *D* is radiation dose, Δ is pixel dimension, and *T* is section width

9. This formula mathematically illustrates the following principle: Adjustments made to voxel dimension in an effort to improve spatial resolution must be compensated for with an appropriate increase in dose to maintain SNR and contrast resolution (Fig. 4-32).
10. Noise is most commonly measured by scanning a water-filled phantom with a standardized set of technical factors. The image noise is equal to the standard deviation of pixel values within an ROI measurement of the image (Fig. 4-33).
11. According to relative scale of pixel values, an ROI of a water-filled phantom should measure near 0 HU. However, within the measured ROI, pixel

FIGURE 4-32 The effects of noise on the CT image. Note the "grainy" or "mottled" appearance of **B** as compared to **A**. **A** was reconstructed with a low-spatial frequency algorithm, while **B** is the product of a high-spatial frequency algorithm.

FIGURE 4-33 Water-filled phantom used to measure the noise and uniformity of a CT system. The average CT value of ROI #1 accurately demonstrates a water density of 0.09 HU with an acceptable standard deviation (noise) of 2.87. As a measure of the uniformity of the CT system, the values for ROI #2 and ROI #3 are within acceptable range in comparison with ROI #1.

values range above and below 0 HU. The degree to which this variation occurs is dictated by noise.

12. Noise as standard deviation (σ) can be defined by the following equation:

$$\text{Noise } (\sigma) = \frac{\sqrt{\Sigma(x_i - x)^2}}{n - 1}$$

where x_i is each CT value, x is the average of at least 100 values, n is the total number of CT values in the ROI.

13. This formula is used solely as a guide for understanding the principle of standard deviation as it relates to image noise. The CT system software automatically calculates the standard deviation within a given ROI to be used as a measure of noise for a given set of technical factors.

14. The technical parameters that most directly affect noise include:

a. *X-ray photon flux,* which equals the rate at which x-ray photons pass through a given unit of tissue over a given unit of time. Any decrease in photon flux causes an increase in image noise. Photon flux is largely determined by the operator-controlled settings of mA and time. Voxel dimension, which also directly affects photon flux, is covered separately later. An increase in either mA setting or scan time increases photon flux, SNR, and patient radiation dose. Raising the kVp value can also increase photon flux, but at an overall cost to contrast resolution due to changes in beam quality.

b. *Voxel dimension:* Noise can be decreased by increasing the dimensions of the voxel. A larger voxel has a greater photon flux and is subject to less noise. Voxel dimension may be increased by increasing the DFOV (decreasing zoom factor), decreasing the matrix size, or increasing the section width. Remember that DFOV and matrix size determine the amount of tissue represented by each pixel. As the pixel dimension increases, it is representative of a greater quantity of photon flux and exhibits less noise. Increases in section width also increase pixel/voxel dimension, with one additional drawback: Any improvement in noise is overshadowed by an overall loss of detail due to the partial volume effect.

c. *Pitch/table speed:* As pitch increases, the speed at which the patient travels through the gantry also increases. For each gantry rotation, scans acquired at a higher pitch expose each voxel to less photon flux. Unless dose is increased, a higher pitch results in greater image noise.

   d. *Detector sensitivity and efficiency:* Improvements in these factors decrease noise and allow for an overall reduction in patient exposure. Beyond the control of the operator, CT detector array sensitivity and efficiency are areas of continuing technical advancement for manufacturers.

   e. *Patient factors:* With patient radiation dose constant, acquisitions of larger patients and of denser parts result in noisier CT images. As a method of balancing SNR and patient radiation dose, ATCM systems adjusts dose according to a predetermined SNR. The acceptable image noise level is predetermined by the user. The CT system automatically adjusts dose to a minimum, while not exceeding the set noise level.

   f. *Algorithm/kernel:* The use of low spatial frequency algorithms (kernels), such as smooth or soft-tissue algorithms, reduce noise. High spatial frequency algorithms increase noise on the reconstructed CT image.

E. Uniformity

1. When imaged, a phantom of uniform material such as water should demonstrate consistent CT values regardless of a pixel's position on the image matrix. Pixels at the center of the image should measure as water density ($\sim$ 0 HU), as should pixels at various other points in the image.
2. Beam hardening occurs as the x-ray beam passes through the object (phantom, patient). The beam exposing the center of the object has a higher average photon energy than the beam exposing the periphery of the object. This beam-hardening effect may slightly alter the pixel values at different points across an image of an object of uniform inherent density.
3. The *spatial uniformity* of a CT system describes its ability to maintain relatively consistent CT values across the entire image of an object of equal density.
4. Uniformity may be evaluated by positioning several ROI measurements at different locations along the center and periphery of an image. The CT values should not differ by more than 2 HU from one location to another (Fig. 4-33).

F. Linearity

1. The relative accuracy between calculated CT numbers and their respective linear attenuation coefficients is termed *linearity*.
2. The CT number for water is 0 HU. According to the formula for the calculation of CT number relative to water discussed previously (see "Image Display"), the CT number for air is −1000 HU, and the CT number for water is 0 HU.

3. The CT system is calibrated according to these two known values. Daily calibration procedures should be performed using a water-filled phantom or a gantry cleared of all objects and exposing only room air.
4. Calibration and routine vendor maintenance procedures work to establish and maintain CT system linearity.
5. Linearity may be periodically evaluated by scanning of a specialized phantom insert containing an assortment of materials—acrylic, polyethylene, water, air, artificial bone, and so on (Fig. 4-34). Known ranges of CT values are compared with those obtained by CT acquisition to ensure system accuracy and linearity.

G. Quality Control Procedures

1. A quality control (QC) program monitors the overall technical performance of the CT system by measuring specific aspects of its function and comparing the measurements with a set standard.
2. Any quality control program consists of two main parts:
   a. *Quality assurance*, the measurement of the scanner's performance through quality testing procedures and evaluation of the test results.
   b. *Quality control*, the implementation of corrective actions to improve any identified performance inadequacies of the CT system.
3. Each facility maintains a CT quality control program that involves daily, weekly, monthly, and annual tests to ensure optimal performance in the following areas:
   a. Accuracy and linearity of CT numbers
   b. Spatial resolution
   c. Contrast resolution/low-contrast detectability
   d. Noise
   e. Uniformity
   f. Section width/SSP
   g. Accuracy of laser light alignment
   h. Table indexing and section localization
   i. Patient radiation dose
   j. Scatter radiation
4. The frequency of the tests is determined by the radiology department's overall QC program and by the requirements of specified accrediting agencies.
5. Consistency in the technical factors utilized for QC testing is imperative. Tests should be performed with the same settings for mA, kVp, section width, DFOV, and so on, to ensure accuracy of results.
6. The hallmarks of a superior QC program are routine frequency of testing, prompt taking of corrective actions as needed, and accurate record-keeping.
7. The QC program in CT is usually a component of a larger, department-wide program in total quality improvement (TQI).
8. The responsibilities for implementing the facility-specific quality control tests and procedures vary

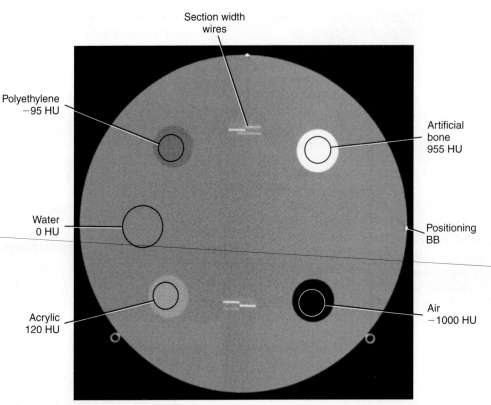

FIGURE 4-34 A linearity phantom containing four inserts of various materials surrounded by water. This American College of Radiology (ACR) phantom also contains two ramps consisting of a series of wires spaced 0.5 mm apart along the phantom's z-axis. The accuracy of the selected section width is evaluated by counting the number of wires visible in cross section. The phantom image in this figure was acquired at a section width of 1.25 mm. The BBs are used to ensure that the phantom is positioned correctly for true axial sections.

among technologists, physicists, and quality control officers.

9. In 2002, the American College of Radiology implemented an accreditation process for CT departments to become ACR-accredited.

10. ACR accreditation in CT involves the submission of acquired clinical and phantom images, dose measurements, and scanning protocols.

11. Details regarding the process for ACR accreditation in CT are beyond the scope of this review book; they are available on the ACR's website (www.acr.org).

ARTIFACT RECOGNITION AND REDUCTION

1. Errors during the measurement of transmitted radiation by the detectors can result in a form of noise on the image termed an *artifact*.

2. An artifact contains no useful information and can severely disrupt the quality of an image by interfering with anatomic detail contained on the CT image.

3. CT image artifacts can take many forms and shapes, including streaks, bands, rings, and shading errors.

4. It is a primary responsibility of the CT technologist to identify artifacts, diagnose their origins, and implement appropriate corrective actions when possible.

A. Beam Hardening

1. As previously described, the average photon energy of the beam increases as it traverses an object (patient). Lower-energy photons are absorbed along the path of each measured ray.

2. The beam that interacts with the center of an object (patient) has a higher average photon energy than the beam that exposed the periphery of the object (patient).

3. An artifact appears when the degree of beam hardening exceeds the CT system's ability to correct during the reconstruction process.

4. Beam-hardening artifacts typically manifest as areas of light and dark streaking bands across portions of the image.

5. The dense bony areas of the posterior fossa of the skull are especially prone to beam-hardening artifacts. The term *Hounsfield bar* is commonly used to describe this particular artifact (Fig. 4-35).

6. Unfortunately, beyond the mathematical corrections included in the image reconstruction process, there is little that can be done technically to resolve beam-hardening artifacts.

7. The use of higher kVp techniques (120-140 kVp) may help to slightly reduce this phenomenon, particularly in the area of the brain's posterior fossa.

—Hounsfield bar

—Streak artifact

FIGURE 4-35 Beam-hardening artifact in the posterior fossa of the skull. Extremely dense regions at the temporal bone and the internal occipital protuberance cause beam-hardening artifact in the form of "streaking" and the Hounsfield bar.

B. Partial Volume Averaging

1. The *partial volume effect* is an unavoidable phenomenon in CT imaging. The complex anatomic structures under examination do not easily lend themselves to representation by series of cubes arranged in matrix form.
2. The attenuation values for an object are often spread over large numbers of voxels. Each voxel also contains values for multiple tissue types. The values are averaged together to yield a single pixel value attempting to represent an assortment of different materials.
3. *Partial volume artifact* occurs when a structure is only partly positioned within a voxel and the attenuation for the object is not accurately represented by a pixel value (Fig. 4-36).
4. Partial volume artifact typically appears as a generalized unsharpness or haziness of the borders of objects. Contrast of the object from its surroundings is compromised.
5. The posterior fossa and the interface between the diaphragm and the abdominal contents are common locations for the appearance of partial volume artifact.
6. The cupping artifact that occurs at the superior portion of the skull is another form of partial volume artifact, which is also heavily influenced by the phenomenon of beam hardening. Here the dense skull table averages with the low-attenuating brain tissue, causing an artifact in which the brain parenchyma may appear abnormally dense.
7. Also, areas of potential pathology, such as small masses, nodules, and fractures, may not be sharply demonstrated owing to the partial volume effect.

8. The use of thin sections is the main method of reducing or eliminating partial volume artifact. Thin sections improve accuracy in the calculation of the pixel's CT number by reducing the voxel volume and limiting the contents of the voxel to fewer varying tissue types.
9. Use of overlapping sections may also improve the reconstructed voxel's position with respect to an object of interest. If the object is well-centered within a single voxel, its attenuation is better represented in the calculation of the pixel's Hounsfield value.

C. Motion

1. Any significant motion on the part of the patient during data acquisition causes noticeable image degradation in the form of a motion artifact.
2. Blurring and streaking are common manifestations of motion artifact on the CT image. Patient motion during volumetric data acquisition may also appear as a step artifact on 3D and MPR images.
3. Patient motion may be involuntary, as with peristalsis, cardiac contraction, and tremors.
4. Technical adjustments to improve the temporal resolution of the CT system may help reduce involuntary motion artifacts. Reductions in scan time (gantry rotation), image segmentation, and physiologic gating can be used to diminish the effects of involuntary motion.
5. Voluntary patient motion, including breathing and swallowing, cause substantial motion artifact on the CT image (Fig. 4-37).
6. There are two basic methods of reducing CT image artifact from voluntary motion:
   a. Communication: Clear and thorough explanation of the patient's responsibilities with regard to suspension or respiration, swallowing, and remaining still.
   b. Immobilization: Appropriate use of positioning and immobilization straps, cushions, holders, and so on.

D. Metallic Artifacts

1. Highly dense metallic objects in and around the patient cause significant image streaking (Fig. 4-38).
2. Objects such as surgical clips, prosthetic devices, guidewires, electrodes, dental fillings, jewelry, zippers, foreign bodies, and dense barium may cause streaking artifacts on the image.
3. Metallic artifacts occur as a result of a combination of errors involving the beam hardening from the metal and the partial volume averaging of the extremely dense object with the less dense surrounding material.
4. In addition, the metallic object may cause severe discrepancies in the obtained projection profiles owing to its abnormally high attenuation.
5. Methods of reducing metallic artifact from CT images include:

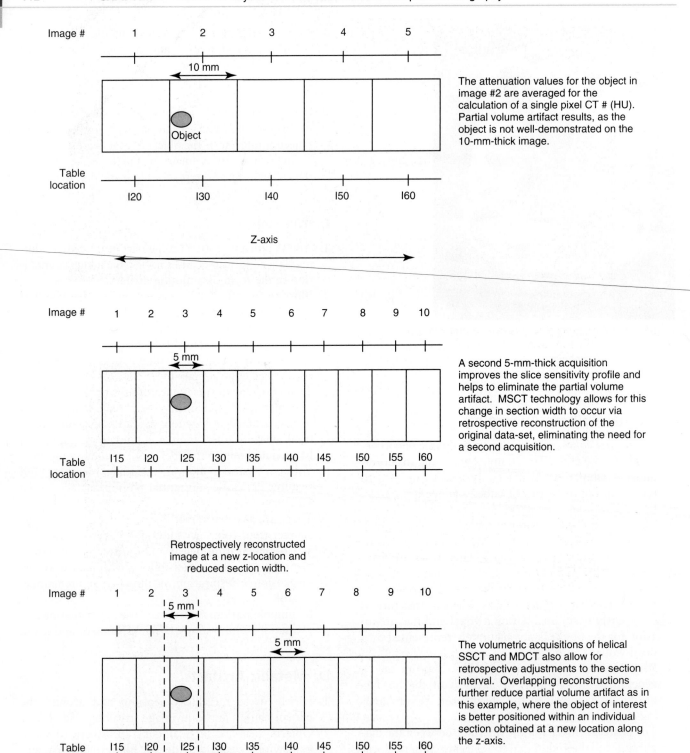

FIGURE 4-36 The partial volume effect that occurs when an object is only partly positioned within a voxel or is much smaller than the overall voxel volume. The object's attenuation is not accurately represented by the pixel value.

a. Removing the metal object from the acquisition whenever possible.
b. Decreasing the section width to reduce partial volume averaging.
c. Increasing the kVp value to improve the beam's penetrability through the object.

d. Adjusting the window width and window level settings, which may slightly reduce the degrading effect of the streak artifact.
e. Reorienting data acquisition to avoid having the metal object in the scanned field. For example, axially acquired sections through the sinuses avoid

FIGURE 4-37 Patient motion during data acquisition, resulting in noticeable image degradation referred to as *motion artifact*. The images shown are examples of image degradation due to voluntary patient movement.

Dental fillings

Portacath device

Intracranial aneurysm clip
displayed in a soft tissue window.

Identical axial brain image
displaying an intracranial aneurysm
displayed in a bone window.

FIGURE 4-38 Examples of metallic streaking artifacts.

the streak artifact caused by dental fillings. Volumetric MSCT axial acquisition through the sinuses allows for high-quality coronal MPR images through the sinuses without metal artifact.

f. CT manufactures may offer metallic artifact reduction (MAR) software in an effort to reduce streaking artifact from metal substances. This continues to be an area of further development in CT image quality.

E. Edge Gradient

1. Streak artifact occurs at the interface between a high-density object surrounded by lower-attenuation material.
2. Edge gradient artifacts are caused by the system's inability to process the high spatial frequency signal that represents the interface between two substances with widely different attenuation values (Fig. 4-39).
3. Common sites for edge gradient artifacts to occur include:
   a. The interface between dense bone and surrounding tissue.
   b. Bowel loops that are densely opacified with oral or rectal contrast media.
   c. Bowel loops distended with air.
   d. Blood vessels that are densely opacified with IV iodinated contrast media.
   e. Areas surrounding biopsy needles during invasive CT procedures.

F. Patient Positioning

1. An *out-of-field artifact* occurs when a portion of the patient has been positioned outside of the scan field of view.

Streaking artifact caused by severe edge gradients between air-filled bowel, with walls coated by dense barium, surrounded by low-density fat in the abdominal cavity.

FIGURE 4-39 Edge gradient artifact occurs at the interface between two objects with a great difference in density.

Patient anatomy lies outside of the scan field of view (SFOV), causing a hyperdense streaking artifact.

Patient anatomy lies outside of the display field of view (DFOV) but within the scan field of view (SFOV). Anatomy is cut off, but no artifact occurs.

FIGURE 4-40 When a portion of the patient is positioned outside the scan field of view, the *out-of-field artifact* occurs. This dense streaking may occur because of improper positioning or when the patient's body extends beyond the limits of the scan field.

2. Hyperdense streaking occurs in the anatomic region that lies outside the scan field (Fig. 4-40).
3. Adjusting patient position from right to left or adjusting the table height relative to the center of the gantry may eliminate the artifact by moving the entire anatomic area into the SFOV.
4. Out-of-field artifacts may be unavoidable when the patient's dimension exceeds the maximum SFOV.
5. The shoulders, abdomen, and lower pelvis are the most common regions where out-of-field artifacts occur.

G. Step Artifact

1. A primary advantage of the volumetric acquisitions of helical SSCT and MSCT is the ability to produce high-quality 3D and MPR images.
2. The step artifact was especially common to older, nonhelically acquired reformations. With step artifact, the image demonstrates the individual sections used to build the reformatted model, and the MPR or 3D image suffers from a lack of overall sharpness and detail (Fig. 4-41).
3. In modern MSCT systems, the highest quality 3D and MPR images are obtained with the acquisition of an isotropic or near-isotropic data set.
4. Near-isotropic acquisitions are attained when the section width (z-axis) is minimized as much as

Stair-step artifact

Coronal reformation of 5-mm-thick axial sections at an interval of 5 mm. Notice the overall lack of sharpness and the obvious stair-step artifact along many of the smooth margins of structures.

Coronal reformation of 2.5-mm-thick axial sections at an interval of 1.25 mm. The stair-step artifact is effectively eliminated, and the reformat exhibits improved anatomic detail and sharpness.

FIGURE 4-41 Step artifact present on a coronal multiplanar reformation (MPR) image of the left kidney.

clinically and technically possible to approach a dimension equal to that of the pixel in the x- and y-axes.

5. True *isotropic acquisitions* occur when the section width equals the pixel dimension and the voxel is cube-shaped. Isotropic data sets have become more commonplace with the greater availability of 64-slice technology.

6. Isotropic data are only one component of high-quality 3D and MPR images. The other equally important piece is an overlapping data set.

7. As previously discussed, overlapping images are those in which the reconstruction interval is less than the section width.

8. Step artifact may still occur in an MSCT system unless thin, overlapping sections are used to build the 3D and MPR images.

H. Equipment-Induced Artifacts

1. Numerous artifacts result from the improper performance of the CT system.

2. Equipment-induced artifacts may be unavoidable and seldom depend on technical selections made by the system operator.

3. The CT technologist must readily identify these types of artifacts and implement appropriate corrective actions to assure their resolution.

4. These types of artifacts include:
   a. *Rings,* which are usually caused by faulty detectors. An error in a detector results in the back-projection of an incorrect ring of density on the reconstructed CT image.
   b. *Streaks:* Detector malfunction and/or misalignment of the tube and detectors may cause the appearance of streak artifact on the CT image.
   c. *Aliasing,* another form of streak artifact caused by an insufficient number of views (data samples) obtained during data acquisition.
   d. *Tube arcing,* which is short-circuiting within the x-ray tube during data acquisition that results in severe streak artifacts in the CT image.
   e. *Cone beam* artifacts are unique to the cone beam geometry of MSCT systems. Cone beam artifacts typically appear similar to partial volume artifacts. In theory, cone beam artifacts worsen as the number of detector rows increases. However, manufacturers address the issue by employing specialized cone beam reconstruction algorithms to compensate for potential errors.
   f. *Windmill,* also referred to as z-spacing or interpolation artifact. This artifact may occur from the use of increased pitch during a volumetric acquisition. The term windmill artifacts comes from the spiraling appearance of shading artifact that appears as a large number of volumetrically acquired images are paged through for review.

PATIENT CARE

1. An average range for activated PTT is:
   a. 10-12 seconds
   b. 17-21 seconds
   c. 25-35 seconds
   d. 43-55 seconds
2. Which of the following is the correct angle of insertion for placing a butterfly needle into a vein for intravenous administration of a contrast agent?
   a. 5 degrees
   b. 15 degrees
   c. 45 degrees
   d. 60 degrees
3. A total volume of 125 mL of an iodinated contrast agent is administered intravenously via automatic injector in 50 seconds. The flow rate for this injection is:
   a. 0.75 mL/sec
   b. 1.25 mL/sec
   c. 1.75 mL/sec
   d. 2.5 mL/sec
4. The acronym CTDI is used to describe which of the following?
   a. a specialized CT imaging technique used to measure bone mineral density
   b. a quality control test that measures the accuracy of the laser lighting system
   c. the radiation dose to the patient during a CT scan
   d. a high-speed CT scanner used for cardiac imaging
5. While one is obtaining a thorough history from a patient prior to the intravenous injection of an iodinated contrast material, which of the following topics should be included?
   1. any prior allergic reactions to contrast media
   2. presence of HIV or hepatitis infection
   3. history of asthma
   a. 1 only
   b. 1 and 2 only
   c. 1 and 3 only
   d. 1, 2, and 3

6. Which of the following factors may affect a patient's calculated glomerular filtration rate (GFR)?
   1. age
   2. sex
   3. race
   a. 1 and 2 only
   b. 2 and 3 only
   c. 1 and 3 only
   d. 1, 2, and 3
7. Which of the following intravenous contrast agent administration methods provides the greatest overall plasma iodine concentration?
   a. drip infusion
   b. bolus technique
   c. biphasic technique
   d. CT portography
8. A patient in shock may exhibit which of the following symptoms?
   1. tachycardia
   2. rapid, shallow breathing
   3. cyanosis
   a. 1 only
   b. 1 and 2 only
   c. 1 and 3 only
   d. 1, 2, and 3
9. The drug SOLU-CORTEF may be classified as which of the following?
   a. anticholinergic
   b. bronchodilator
   c. antihistamine
   d. corticosteroid
10. Which of the following technical factors has a direct effect on patient dose?
    a. matrix size
    b. algorithm
    c. mAs
    d. window level
11. Which of the following is a non-ionic contrast material?
    a. iodamide
    b. iothalamate
    c. iohexol
    d. diatrizoate

12. Which of the following terms is used to describe a patient who is having difficulty breathing?
    a. dyslexia
    b. dyspnea
    c. dysphagia
    d. dysphasia
13. Which of the following devices is used to measure the patient dose from a CT examination?
    a. Geiger counter
    b. proportional counter
    c. ionization chamber
    d. film badge
14. Which of the following describes the situation in which an assumption is made that an unconscious or otherwise physically unable patient consents to medical treatment?
    a. informed consent
    b. witnessed consent
    c. patient proxy
    d. implied consent
15. Complete cardiac diastole corresponds to which portion of the cardiac cycle on an electrocardiogram (ECG)?
    a. P wave
    b. QRS complex
    c. Alpha wave
    d. T wave
16. During CT arthrography, iodinated contrast media is injected directly into the:
    a. joint space
    b. intrathecal space
    c. subarachnoid space
    d. venous bloodstream
17. Which of the following is considered one of the iso-osmolar contrast media (IOCM)?
    a. iodixanol
    b. iopamidol
    c. iohexol
    d. ioversol
18. A common site for the IV administration of iodinated contrast media is the anterior recess of the elbow, otherwise known as the:
    a. brachial fossa
    b. olecranon fossa
    c. retro-ulnar space
    d. antecubital space
19. The potentially serious decline in renal function following the IV administration of contrast material is called:
    a. anaphylaxis
    b. bronchospasm
    c. contrast-induced nephrotoxicity (CIN)
    d. urticaria

20. The quantity of absorbed radiation dose based on the radiosensitivity of a particular tissue type is called:
    a. stochastic dose
    b. kerma
    c. effective dose
    d. CTDI
21. Advantages of a saline flush immediately following the IV administration of iodinated contrast material include:
    1. reduction in required contrast agent dose
    2. reduction in the incidence of contrast-induced nephrotoxicity (CIN)
    3. reduction of streaking artifact from dense contrast agent in the vasculature
    a. 1 only
    b. 3 only
    c. 2 and 3 only
    d. 1, 2, and 3
22. Which of the following medications may be administered to dilate the coronary vasculature prior to a cardiac CT examination?
    a. sublingual nitroglycerine
    b. a β-adrenergic receptor blocking agent (β-blocker)
    c. atropine
    d. albuterol .
23. A normal range for diastolic blood pressure in an adult is:
    a. 40-60 mm Hg
    b. 60-90 mm Hg
    c. 80-120 mm Hg
    d. 95-140 mm Hg
24. Which of the following is a parenteral route of medication administration?
    a. sublingual
    b. intramuscular
    c. transdermal
    d. oral
25. Which of the following methods may be employed to reduce the radiation dose to the pediatric patient undergoing CT?
    1. reduce mA
    2. limit phases of acquisition
    3. increase pitch
    a. 1 only
    b. 1 and 2 only
    c. 1 and 3 only
    d. 1, 2, and 3
26. Radiation exposure and its potentially harmful effects have a relationship that is termed _____ in nature.
    a. stochastic
    b. nonstochastic
    c. negligible
    d. somatic

27. Which of the following types of isolation techniques protects against infection transmitted through fecal material?
    a. acid-fast bacillus isolation
    b. contact isolation
    c. enteric precautions
    d. drainage-secretion precautions
28. Which of the following is considered one of the *ionic* radiopaque contrast media (RCM)?
    a. iohexol
    b. iothalamate meglumine
    c. iopamidol
    d. ioversol
29. The radiation dose index calculation that takes into account the variations in absorption across the field of view due to beam hardening is termed:
    a. $CTDI_w$
    b. $CTDI_{100}$
    c. $CTDI_{vol}$
    d. MSAD
30. Direct contraindications to the administration of iodinated contrast material include:
    1. prior life-threatening reaction to iodinated contrast material
    2. multiple myeloma
    3. diabetes
    a. 1 only
    b. 1 and 2 only
    c. 1 and 3 only
    d. 1, 2, and 3
31. Which of the following units is used to express the total patient dose from a helically acquired CT examination?
    a. roentgens (R)
    b. curies (Ci)
    c. R-cm (roentgens per centimeter)
    d. mGy-cm (milligrays per centimeter)

IMAGING PROCEDURES

32. Components of a comprehensive CT stroke management protocol typically include:
    1. pre-contrast sequence of the brain
    2. CTA of the brain and carotids
    3. CT perfusion (CTP) of the brain
    a. 2 only
    b. 1 and 2 only
    c. 2 and 3 only
    d. 1, 2, and 3

Use Fig. 5-1 to answer questions 33-35.

33. Number 1 on the figure corresponds to which of the following?
    a. left pulmonary artery
    b. ascending aorta
    c. inferior vena cava
    d. descending aorta
34. Which number on the figure corresponds to the superior vena cava?
    a. 2
    b. 3
    c. 4
    d. 5
35. The abnormal density located in the posterior portion of the left lung field on the figure has an average attenuation value of +5.0 Hounsfield units. This density most likely represents:
    a. pneumothorax
    b. hemothorax
    c. atelectasis
    d. pleural effusion

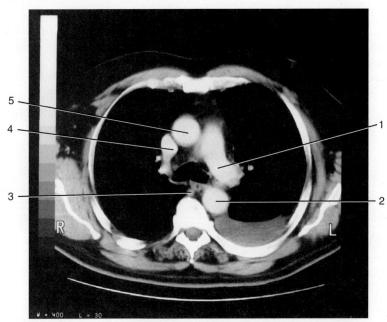

FIGURE 5-1

36. Simple cysts of the kidney have average attenuation values in the range of:
    a. −40 to 0 Hounsfield units
    b. 0 to +20 Hounsfield units
    c. +30 to +50 Hounsfield units
    d. above +60 Hounsfield units
37. After initiation of rapid bolus administration of an iodinated contrast agent, the arterial phase of hepatic contrast enhancement occurs at approximately:
    a. 15-20 seconds
    b. 25-35 seconds
    c. 60-70 seconds
    d. 120-180 seconds

Use Fig. 5-2 to answer questions 38-40.

38. Number 2 on the figure corresponds to which of the following?
    a. left internal jugular vein
    b. left external carotid artery
    c. left internal carotid artery
    d. left external jugular vein
39. Number 5 on the figure corresponds to which of the following?
    a. right internal jugular vein
    b. right external carotid artery
    c. right internal carotid artery
    d. right external jugular vein
40. Number 1 on the figure corresponds to which of the following?
    a. vocal cords
    b. uvula
    c. aryepiglottic fold
    d. epiglottis

41. The abdominal aorta bifurcates at the level of:
    a. T10
    b. T12
    c. L2
    d. L4
42. On an ECG of the complete cardiac cycle, at which portion of the R-R interval is the heart muscle in diastole?
    a. 10%-20%
    b. 35%-50%
    c. 55%-75%
    d. 85%-95%
43. The accumulation of gas within a degenerating intervertebral disc is called the:
    a. aeration effect
    b. vacuum phenomenon
    c. oxygen saturation point
    d. carbonization sign
44. During a spiral or helical CT examination, the scanner acquires data:
    1. continuously as the patient travels through the gantry
    2. one section at a time
    3. in the form of a complete volumetric data set
    a. 1 only
    b. 2 only
    c. 1 and 3 only
    d. 2 and 3 only
45. Which of the following CT studies of the head is typically performed without a contrast agent?
    a. CT angiogram for circle of Willis
    b. coronal scan to rule out (R/O) pituitary tumor
    c. CT of brain to R/O subdural hematoma
    d. CT of brain to R/O metastatic disease
46. Which of the following phases of renal contrast enhancement best demonstrates transitional cell carcinoma (TCC) of the bladder?
    a. early arterial
    b. corticomedullary
    c. nephrographic
    d. excretory

FIGURE 5-2

Use Fig. 5-3 to answer questions 47-50.

47. Number 5 on the figure corresponds to which of the following?
    a. transverse colon
    b. stomach
    c. duodenum
    d. hepatic flexure

48. Which of the following most likely describes the patient position during the formation of the image in the figure?
    a. supine
    b. prone
    c. left lateral decubitus
    d. right lateral decubitus

49. CT examinations of the abdomen are often performed in the position on the figure to demonstrate the relationship between the:
    a. ureters and renal collecting systems
    b. duodenum and pancreatic head
    c. large and small colon
    d. liver and gallbladder

50. Number 3 on the figure corresponds to which of the following?
    a. right ureter
    b. inferior vena cava
    c. renal calculi
    d. right renal artery

51. Which of the following sets of section width and spacing would be most suitable for a general survey CT of the neck?
    a. 0.75 mm thick every 0.75 mm
    b. 3 mm thick every 5 mm
    c. 3 mm thick every 3 mm
    d. 10 mm thick every 10 mm

52. The still viable ischemic cerebral tissue that surrounds the infarct core in a patient with an acute stroke is termed the:
    a. thrombolytic zone
    b. hemorrhage focus
    c. ischemic penumbra
    d. stroke volume

53. Complex fractures of the wrist are most common in which of the following carpal bones?
    a. hamate
    b. scaphoid
    c. capitate
    d. triquetrum

54. A complete CT study of the orbits should include:
    a. 5 mm × 5 mm axial sections only
    b. 10 mm × 10 mm axial and coronal sections
    c. 3 mm × 3 mm coronal sections only
    d. 2.5 mm × 2.5 mm axial and coronal sections

55. High-resolution computed tomography (HRCT) is most commonly used for the evaluation of the:
    a. pancreas
    b. brain
    c. lungs
    d. pelvis

FIGURE 5-3

56. Which of the following technical maneuvers may be used to remove unwanted pulsation artifacts from cardiac motion during a CTA of the chest for pulmonary embolism?
    a. automated bolus tracking
    b. automatic tube current modulation
    c. retrospective ECG gating
    d. saline flush

57. During a general CT examination of the abdomen, an intravenous contrast agent is indicated and is administered with the aid of an automatic injector. Which of the following ranges of flow rate should be used?
    a. 0.2-1.0 mL/sec
    b. 1.0-3.0 mL/sec
    c. 4.0-6.0 mL/sec
    d. 7.0-10.0 mL/sec

58. Diffuse fatty infiltration of the hepatic parenchyma may be referred to as:
    a. chromatosis
    b. steatosis
    c. cirrhosis
    d. lipomatosis

Use Fig. 5-4 to answer questions 59-62.

59. Which of the following corresponds to the low-attenuation area indicated by Number 3 on the figure?
    a. renal cortex
    b. renal pelvis
    c. renal calyx
    d. renal pyramid

60. The data for this reformatted image of the abdomen was most likely acquired in which of the following renal enhancement phases?
    a. pre-contrast
    b. corticomedullary
    c. nephrographic
    d. excretory

61. Number 2 on the figure corresponds to which of the following?
    a. hepatic vein
    b. suprarenal lymph node
    c. adrenal gland
    d. common bile duct

62. Number 6 on the figure corresponds to which of the following?
    a. psoas muscle
    b. omentum
    c. piriformis muscle
    d. erector spinae muscle

63. CT images of the chest should be acquired with the patient:
    a. at full inspiration
    b. breathing quietly
    c. at full expiration
    d. breathing normally

64. During CT scanning of the head, the gantry should be angled:
    a. 15 degrees above the infraorbital-meatal line (IOML)
    b. 10 degrees below the IOML
    c. 0 degrees
    d. 20 degrees above the skull base

65. During CT examination of the larynx, the patient is often instructed to phonate the letter "E" in order to properly evaluate the:
    a. epiglottis
    b. uvula
    c. trachea
    d. vocal cords

FIGURE 5-4

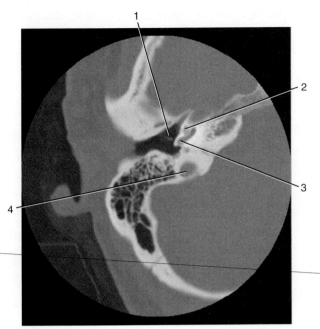

FIGURE 5-5

Use Fig. 5-5 to answer questions 66-69.

66. Number 2 corresponds to which of the following?
    a. carotid canal
    b. incus
    c. cochlea
    d. vestibule
67. Number 4 corresponds to which of the following?
    a. external auditory meatus
    b. internal auditory canal
    c. vestibule
    d. carotid canal
68. Which of the following display field of view (DFOV) values was most likely used to display the image?
    a. 9.6 cm
    b. 18.0 cm
    c. 25.6 cm
    d. 51.2 cm
69. Number 3 on the figure corresponds to which of the following?
    a. vestibule
    b. semicircular canal
    c. cochlea
    d. incus
70. During a CT examination of a female pelvis for a suspected malignancy, ascites may be present in an area posterior to the uterus and ovaries known as:
    a. the cul-de-sac
    b. Morison's pouch
    c. the space of Retzius
    d. the prevesical compartment

71. Which of the following pathologic processes may be considered an interstitial disease of the lungs?
    a. bronchiectasis
    b. mediastinal lymphadenopathy
    c. pulmonary metastasis
    d. bronchogenic carcinoma
72. An enterovesical fistula is an abnormal communication between the bowel and the:
    a. uterus
    b. bladder
    c. vagina
    d. umbilicus
73. Prior to a CT colonography, the patient may undergo a process of bowel cleansing termed:
    a. purgation
    b. hydration
    c. catharsis
    d. fasting
74. Positioning the patient with the knees flexed over a foam cushion during a CT examination of the lumbar spine assists in:
    1. decreasing the kyphotic curvature of the lumbar spine
    2. making the patient more comfortable throughout the exam
    3. decreasing the lordotic curvature of the lumbar spine
    a. 1 only
    b. 2 only
    c. 3 only
    d. 2 and 3 only
75. The imaging plane that is parallel to the foot's plantar surface is called the:
    a. coronal plane
    b. sagittal plane
    c. axial plane
    d. oblique axial plane
76. The condition of intermittent cramping pain in the legs due to poor circulation is called:
    a. varices
    b. claudication
    c. stenosis
    d. thrombosis

FIGURE 5-6

Use Fig. 5-6 to answer questions 77-80.

77. The pathologic process indicated by number 3 on the figure most likely corresponds to:
    a. atelectasis
    b. lymphadenopathy
    c. pleural effusion
    d. ground-glass opacity
78. Number 1 on the figure corresponds to which of the following?
    a. right atrium
    b. pulmonary trunk
    c. ascending aorta
    d. right ventricle
79. This HRCT image of the chest was most likely acquired with a section width of:
    a. 1 mm
    b. 5 mm
    c. 7 mm
    d. 10 mm
80. Number 2 on the figure corresponds to which of the following?
    a. left mainstem bronchus
    b. anterior segment of left upper lobe bronchus
    c. posterior segment of left upper lobe bronchus
    d. anterior segment of left lower lobe bronchus

81. The pituitary gland is best demonstrated during CT in which of the following imaging planes?
    a. axial
    b. coronal
    c. sagittal
    d. transaxial
82. The most common site of organ injury due to blunt abdominal trauma is the:
    a. liver
    b. kidney
    c. spleen
    d. pancreas

Use Fig. 5-7 to answer questions 83-85.

83. Number 7 on the figure corresponds to which of the following?
    a. duodenum
    b. pancreatic head
    c. jejunum
    d. gallbladder
84. Number 2 on the figure corresponds to which of the following?
    a. superior mesenteric vein
    b. superior mesenteric artery
    c. renal artery
    d. portal vein
85. Number 8 on the figure corresponds to which of the following?
    a. duodenum
    b. descending colon
    c. jejunum
    d. ascending colon

FIGURE 5-7

86. The adult spinal cord ends at what vertebral level?
    a. T11-T12
    b. L1-L2
    c. L3-L4
    d. superior portion of the coccyx
87. Which of the following protocols would provide the best image quality for a 3D disarticulation study of the hip?
    a. 10 mm × 15 mm sections, standard algorithm
    b. 10 mm × 10 mm sections, bone algorithm
    c. 1.5 mm × 1.0 mm sections, bone algorithm
    d. 5 mm × 7 mm sections, standard algorithm
88. Which of the following terms is used to describe a fibroid tumor of the uterus?
    a. leiomyoma
    b. cystic teratoma
    c. endometriosis
    d. corpus luteum

Use Fig. 5-8 to answer questions 89-91.

89. Number 1 on the figure corresponds to which of the following?
    a. sphenoid sinus
    b. ethmoid sinus
    c. frontal sinus
    d. maxillary sinus
90. The section thickness that would demonstrate the greatest detail of the paranasal sinuses is:
    a. 3 mm
    b. 5 mm
    c. 7 mm
    d. 10 mm

91. Which number on the figure corresponds to the zygomatic bone?
    a. 3
    b. 1
    c. 2
    d. 6
92. Which of the following anatomic organs is located within the peritoneal cavity?
    a. pancreas
    b. kidneys
    c. uterus
    d. liver
93. Which of the following may be included as part of a routine preparation for a general contrast-enhanced CT examination of the abdomen and pelvis?
    1. instructing the patient to take nothing by mouth (NPO) for 4 hours prior to exam
    2. 1200 mL of oral contrast agent administered 90 minutes prior to exam
    3. having the patient drink 4 liters of polyethylene glycol (PEG) 24 hours prior to exam
    a. 1 only
    b. 2 only
    c. 1 and 2 only
    d. 1 and 3 only
94. During a complete CT scan of the pelvis, sections should be obtained from the:
    a. iliac crests to the pubic symphysis
    b. kidneys through the bladder
    c. bottom of the kidneys to the pubic symphysis
    d. iliac crests to the lesser trochanter

FIGURE 5-8

95. The recommended scan field of view (SFOV) for a CT examination of the cervical spine is:
    a. 9.6 cm
    b. 15.0 cm
    c. 25.0 cm
    d. 50.0 cm

Use Fig. 5-9 to answer questions 96-99.

96. Number 4 on the figure corresponds to which of the following?
    a. navicular
    b. cuboid
    c. calcaneus
    d. talus

97. Which of the following best describes the type of image displayed in the figure?
    a. sagittal maximum intensity projection (MIP)
    b. direct sagittal acquisition
    c. sagittal multiplanar reformation (MPR)
    d. volume-rendered 3D

98. Number 6 on the figure corresponds to which of the following?
    a. navicular
    b. cuboid
    c. calcaneus
    d. talus

99. Number 1 on the figure corresponds to which of the following?
    a. navicular
    b. cuboid
    c. calcaneus
    d. talus

100. Because of its inherent iodine concentration, the thyroid gland appears _____ on CT images.
    a. hypodense
    b. isodense
    c. hyperdense
    d. mottled

101. Air trapping within the trachea and bronchial tree may be optimally demonstrated with multiplanar volume reconstructions (MPVRs) of the thorax known as:
    a. maximum intensity projections (MIPs)
    b. 3D volume renderings
    c. shaded-surface displays (SSDs)
    d. minimum intensity projections (min-IPs)

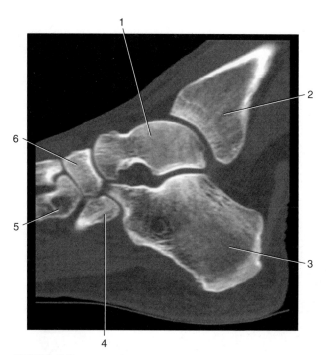

FIGURE 5-9

Use Fig. 5-10 to answer questions 102-104.

102. Which number on the figure corresponds to the anterior horn of the lateral ventricle?
    a. 1
    b. 5
    c. 3
    d. 2

103. Number 3 on the figure corresponds to which of the following?
    a. caudate nucleus
    b. thalamus
    c. third ventricle
    d. pineal gland

104. Which number on the figure corresponds to the septum pellucidum?
    a. 2
    b. 3
    c. 4
    d. 5

105. Which of the following is NOT a portion of the small bowel?
    a. duodenum
    b. jejunum
    c. ileum
    d. cecum

106. Which of the following is used as the IV-administered radiopharmaceutical during a PET-CT fusion examination?
    a. technetium Tc 99m
    b. iodine I 131
    c. fludeoxyglucose F 18 (FDG)
    d. strontium chloride Sr 89

107. The specialized CT examination of the bladder in which an iodinated contrast agent is directly administered under gravity into the bladder via Foley catheter is termed:
    a. CT IVP
    b. CT urogram
    c. CT enteroclysis
    d. CT cystography

PHYSICS AND INSTRUMENTATION

108. Which of the following best describes the shape of the x-ray beam utilized in MDCT?
    a. pencil beam
    b. fan-shaped
    c. electron beam
    d. cone-shaped

109. Collimation of the CT x-ray beam occurs:
    1. at the x-ray tube, regulating slice thickness
    2. just beyond the patient, focusing off-axis transmitted radiation
    3. before the detectors, limiting the amount of scatter radiation absorbed
    a. 1 only
    b. 1 and 2 only
    c. 1 and 3 only
    d. 1, 2, and 3

FIGURE 5-10

110. CT numbers are usually provided in the form of:
    a. Hounsfield units
    b. EMI numbers
    c. Cormacks
    d. μ

111. The mathematical technique allowing the reconstruction of motion-free images from helically acquired CT data is called:
    a. convolution
    b. radon transformation
    c. interpolation
    d. Fourier reconstruction

112. The full width at half maximum (FWHM) of a CT scanner is used to describe:
    a. spatial resolution
    b. contrast resolution
    c. noise
    d. calibration accuracy

113. A first-generation CT scanner consists of an x-ray tube and two detectors that translate across the patient's head while rotating in 1-degree increments for a total of:
    a. 45 degrees
    b. 90 degrees
    c. 180 degrees
    d. 360 degrees

114. Which of the following abbreviations is used to identify a computerized network that stores, retrieves, communicates, and displays digital medical images?
    a. WORM
    b. PACS
    c. DICOM
    d. HIPAA

115. The CT "window" controls the _____ of the CT image as it appears to the viewer.
    a. density and detail
    b. spatial and contrast resolution
    c. contrast and brightness
    d. attenuation coefficient and Hounsfield value

116. Voxels with equal dimensions along the x-, y-, and z-axes are referred to as:
    a. prospective
    b. isotropic
    c. retrospective
    d. anisotropic

117. Which of the following artifacts is not affected by the CT technologist?
    a. motion
    b. partial volume
    c. edge gradient
    d. ring

118. When one is viewing a multiplanar reformation (MPR) image, each pixel represents:
    a. the maximum attentuation occurring within the voxel
    b. the average attenuation occurring within the voxel
    c. the minimum attenuation occurring within the voxel
    d. all attenuation occurring within the voxel above a set threshold value

119. Statistical noise appears as _____ on a CT image.
    a. decreased contrast
    b. increased brightness
    c. concentric circles
    d. graininess

120. An acquisition is made on a 64-slice MSCT system in which each detector element has a z-axis dimension of 0.625 mm. With a selected beam width of 40 mm and the beam pitch set at 1.50, how much will the table move with each rotation of the gantry?
    a. 20 mm
    b. 40 mm
    c. 60 mm
    d. 80 mm

121. The component of the CT computer system responsible for the data processing of image reconstruction is the:
    a. pipeline memory
    b. array processor
    c. hard disk drive
    d. RAM microprocessor

122. For single-slice CT (SSCT) systems, which of the following statements regarding retrospective image reconstruction is FALSE?
    a. The algorithm, matrix size, and DFOV may all be changed.
    b. The slice thickness and SFOV may be changed.
    c. Scan (raw) data must be available.
    d. Retrospective image reconstruction may be used to adjust the center of the image.

123. The loss of anatomic information between contiguous sections due to inconsistent patient breathing is called:
    a. cupping artifact
    b. misregistration
    c. overshoot artifact
    d. out-of-field artifact

124. Before a CT image can be reconstructed by a computer, the transmission signal produced by the detectors must be converted into numerical information by a(n):
    a. kernel
    b. analog-to-digital converter (ADC)
    c. array processor
    d. digital-to-analog converter (DAC)

125. A CT image is formed in part by projecting back all of the attenuation values recorded during data acquisition onto a:
    a. pixel
    b. voxel
    c. matrix
    d. reformat

126. Which of the following archival media is capable of storing the largest number of CT images?
    a. floppy disk
    b. magnetic tape
    c. VHS tape
    d. optical disk

127. Areas of a CT image that contain abrupt changes in tissue density are electronically represented by which of the following?
    a. positive CT numbers
    b. high spatial frequencies
    c. negative CT numbers
    d. low spatial frequencies

Use Fig. 5-11 to answer questions 128-130.

128. Which of the following components of CT image quality are being evaluated in the figure?
    1. low-contrast detectability
    2. noise
    3. uniformity
    a. 2 only
    b. 1 and 2 only
    c. 1 and 3 only
    d. 2 and 3 only

129. The differences in Hounsfield value exhibited in the ROIs measured on this CT image of a water-filled phantom are most likely due to the phenomenon referred to as:
    a. partial volume averaging
    b. noise
    c. beam hardening
    d. detector drift

130. Which region of interest (ROI) on the figure demonstrates the greatest amount of image noise?
    a. 1
    b. 2
    c. 3
    d. impossible to determine from the information provided

131. Which of the following terms is used to describe a set of rules for solving a mathematical problem?
    a. reconstruction
    b. algorithm
    c. function
    d. array

132. Which of the following factors does not affect the dimensions of a voxel?
    a. slice thickness
    b. matrix size
    c. kernel
    d. display field of view

1: ■ 00.09, sd 02.57, a 203.92mm2
2: ■ 00.96, sd 02.63, a 203.92mm2
3: ■ 00.97, sd 02.73, a 203.92mm2

FIGURE 5-11

133. The size of the CT image displayed on a computer monitor can be enlarged by increasing the:
    1. DFOV
    2. SFOV
    3. image magnification
    a. 1 only
    b. 3 only
    c. 1 and 2 only
    d. 1 and 3 only

134. The average photon energy of the primary beam of a CT scanner operating at a tube potential of 120 kVp is approximately:
    a. 50 keV
    b. 70 keV
    c. 100 keV
    d. 120 keV

135. MSCT systems typically employ which of the following detector geometries?
    a. first-generation
    b. second-generation
    c. third-generation
    d. fourth -generation

136. The acquisition of a series of CT images at a single anatomic location over a set period is referred to as:
    a. ultrafast CT
    b. cine CT
    c. conventional CT
    d. temporal CT

137. The rate at which a quantity of x-radiation emitted from a CT tube passes through a unit area over a unit of time is called the:
    a. effective mAs
    b. photon flux
    c. constant mAs
    d. photon fluence

138. An average CT number value for bone is:
    a. +100 HU
    b. +500 HU
    c. +1000 HU
    d. +3000 HU

139. A standard CT image reconstructed on a 512^2 matrix has a digital size of approximately:
    a. 0.5 MB
    b. 3.0 MB
    c. 5.0 MB
    d. 10.0 MB

140. The term used to describe the relationship between the linear attenuation coefficient of an object and the calculated CT numbers is:
    a. linearity
    b. mottle
    c. quantum noise
    d. spatial resolution

141. Quality control measurements to test the accuracy of the CT scanner's calibration should be performed:
    a. daily
    b. weekly
    c. monthly
    d. annually

142. The 3D CT technique that includes all of the acquired voxel information in the reconstructed model with adjustments to its opacity is termed:
    a. surface rendering
    b. maximum intensity projection (MIP)
    c. curved multiplanar reformation
    d. volume rendering

143. Where is the high-frequency generator often located in a modern CT scanner?
    a. inside the gantry
    b. just outside the scan room
    c. beneath the CT table
    d. inside the operator's console

144. The smallest unit of information used in the binary language of computers is the:
    a. bit
    b. chip
    c. base
    d. byte

145. The continuous gantry rotation required by helical CT acquisition is made possible by the application of:
    a. electromagnetic bushings
    b. titanium bearings
    c. slip-rings
    d. oil-cooled couplings

146. The process of applying a mathematical filter to remove blurring from the reconstructed CT image is termed:
    a. convolution
    b. interpolation
    c. iteration
    d. z-filtration

147. Which of the following acquisitions may be characterized as contiguous?
    a. 2.5-mm sections reconstructed every 1.25 mm
    b. 5.0-mm sections reconstructed every 7.5 mm
    c. 3.75-mm sections reconstructed every 3.75 mm
    d. 20-second cine acquisition with 1.25-mm sections

148. Pixels representing tissues with average attenuation coefficients greater than that of water have which of the following types of values?
    a. extremely small
    b. positive
    c. negative
    d. low contrast

149. For a single-slice CT (SSCT) system, which of the following statements regarding pre-patient collimation is true?
    1. An increase in pre-patient collimation increases patient radiation dose.
    2. Pre-patient collimation is used to focus radiation through the section of interest.
    3. Pre-patient collimation directly controls slice thickness.
    a. 2 only
    b. 3 only
    c. 1 and 2 only
    d. 2 and 3 only

150. Digital CT images are networked and archived in accordance with a standardized computer protocol identified by which of the following abbreviations?
    a. HIPAA
    b. HTTP
    c. TCP/IP
    d. DICOM

151. The contrast resolution of a CT scanner is NOT related to which of the following?
    a. focal spot size
    b. section width
    c. reconstruction algorithm
    d. signal-to-noise ratio

Use Fig. 5-12 to answer questions 152-153.

152. The artifact present on the lateral borders of the image in the figure most likely represents which of the following?
    a. edge gradient
    b. out-of-field artifact
    c. tube arcing
    d. beam hardening

153. The image in the figure was produced using the following parameters: large (full) SFOV; maximum DFOV (48 cm); 200 mA, 120 kVp; soft tissue algorithm. Which of the following technical adjustments would serve to reduce the artifact present?
    a. switching to a detail or bone algorithm
    b. using a smaller SFOV
    c. increasing the mA to 240 and the kVp to 140
    d. centering the patient within the SFOV

FIGURE 5-12

154. The average photon energy of the CT x-ray beam can be increased by:
    a. increasing mAs
    b. increasing filtration
    c. increasing collimation
    d. all of the above

155. Which of the following is a solid-state device used to record the light flashes given off by a scintillation crystal?
    a. photomultiplier tube
    b. anode
    c. photodiode
    d. input phosphor

156. Automatic tube current modulation (ATCM) software is used in current MDCT systems to control:
    a. patient radiation dose
    b. cardiac motion
    c. timing of the contrast agent bolus
    d. tissue perfusion assessment

157. The type of MSCT detector array that contains multiple rows of detector elements, each of the same length, is called a(n):
    a. uniform matrix array
    b. adaptive array
    c. hybrid array
    d. stationary array

158. A CT image is displayed in a window with a level of 0 and a width of 500. Which of the following statements is correct?
    a. Pixels with values between 0 HU and 500 HU will appear white.
    b. Pixels with values between −250 HU and +250 HU will be assigned shades of gray.
    c. Pixels with values greater than +500 HU will be black.
    d. Pixels with values less than 0 HU will appear white.

159. Reformatted CT image planes that lie perpendicular to the original plane of acquisition may be described as:
    a. oblique
    b. orthogonal
    c. obtuse
    d. orthographic

160. Segmenting the data acquisition process into separate components of smaller rotation angles may improve which of the following components of CT image quality?
    a. temporal resolution
    b. longitudinal spatial resolution
    c. contrast resolution
    d. in-plane spatial resolution

161. Which of the following image artifacts is unique to multislice CT (MSCT) systems?
    a. step artifact
    b. aliasing artifact
    c. out-of-field artifact
    d. cone beam artifact

162. Which of the following is considered an analytic form of image reconstruction?
    1. iterative technique
    2. Fourier reconstruction
    3. filtered back-projection
    a. 1 only
    b. 1 and 2 only
    c. 2 and 3 only
    d. 1, 2, and 3

163. A 16-slice MSCT system utilizes an adaptive array of 24 detectors, each ranging in size from 0.625 to 1.25 mm. What is the maximum number of sections the system can acquire with each rotation of the gantry?
    a. 8
    b. 16
    c. 32
    d. 64

164. The measurement of transmitted radiation made by an individual detector is called a(n):
    a. attenuation coefficient
    b. Hounsfield value
    c. CT number
    d. ray sum

165. The information included during the 3D reconstruction of a CT scan is controlled by the:
    a. algorithm
    b. window setting
    c. threshold setting
    d. gray-scale map

Simulated Exam Two

PATIENT CARE

1. As related to the cardiac cycle, the term _____ refers to the relaxation of heart muscle.
   - a. diastole
   - b. equilibrium
   - c. systole
   - d. a-fib

2. Which of the following may be considered one of the high-osmolar contrast media (HOCM)?
   1. iothalamate meglumine
   2. diatrizoate sodium
   3. iohexol
   - a. 1 only
   - b. 3 only
   - c. 1 and 2 only
   - d. 1, 2, and 3

3. Which of the following technical changes would serve to decrease patient radiation dose during a CT examination?
   - a. increase in matrix size
   - b. change from soft tissue to bone algorithm
   - c. decrease of tube rotation from 360 to 180 degrees
   - d. decrease in DFOV

4. Which of the following medications may be administered to a patient who is having a severe anaphylactoid reaction to iodinated contrast material?
   1. epinephrine
   2. atropine
   3. diphenhydramine
   - a. 1 only
   - b. 1 and 2 only
   - c. 1 and 3 only
   - d. 1, 2, and 3

5. In an effort to reduce patient radiation dose, the technical factors of the applied CT protocol should be optimized on the basis of:
   - a. age
   - b. sex
   - c. size or weight
   - d. physical condition

6. The escape of contrast material from a needle or blood vessel into the subcutaneous tissues is called:
   - a. infusion
   - b. extraversion
   - c. influxation
   - d. extravasation

7. Thorough explanation of the CT procedure and proper communication with the patient are vital in ensuring that:
   1. breathing instructions are properly followed
   2. motion artifact does not occur
   3. patient anxiety is kept at a minimum
   - a. 1 and 2 only
   - b. 1 and 3 only
   - c. 2 and 3 only
   - d. 1, 2, and 3

8. Which of the following is considered in the calculation of the MSAD for an axial (step-and-shoot) CT examination?
   - a. bed index
   - b. gantry rotation time
   - c. mA setting
   - d. pitch

9. Risk factors for contrast-induced nephrotoxicity (CIN) include:
   1. pheochromocytoma
   2. allergy to shellfish
   3. dehydration
   - a. 2 only
   - b. 3 only
   - c. 1 and 2 only
   - d. 1, 2, and 3

10. During CT examinations, the patient's body should be shielded above and below because of:
    - a. the rotational nature of the x-ray tube
    - b. extremely high kVp techniques
    - c. lack of filtration of the CT beam
    - d. reduced collimation of the CT beam

11. Normal range for oxygen (O_2) saturation is:
    - a. 20%-25%
    - b. 50%-60%
    - c. 80%-85%
    - d. 95%-100%

12. Which of the following laboratory measurements can be used to evaluate the renal function of a patient?
    1. BUN
    2. PTT
    3. creatinine
    a. 1 only
    b. 1 and 2 only
    c. 1 and 3 only
    d. 1, 2, and 3

13. Which of the following would be best suited for intravenous injection of contrast material with a power injector?
    a. butterfly needle
    b. central venous line
    c. 23-gauge spinal needle
    d. angiocatheter

14. Prior to the intravenous injection of iodinated contrast material, patients should be questioned regarding their:
    1. renal function
    2. allergic history
    3. cardiac history
    a. 1 only
    b. 2 only
    c. 3 only
    d. 1, 2, and 3

15. A(n) _____ infection is one that a patient acquires during a stay in a health care institution.
    a. blood-borne
    b. nosocomial
    c. iatrogenic
    d. staphylococcal

16. CTDI$_w$ is a weighted index that approximates radiation dose on the basis of the variations that occur across the field of view because of:
    1. beam hardening
    2. detector configuration
    3. pitch
    a. 1 only
    b. 1 and 2 only
    c. 2 and 3 only
    d. 1, 2, and 3

17. Which of the following sets of values would be considered normal levels for creatinine and BUN, respectively?
    a. 3.1 mg/dL; 1.2 mg/dL
    b. 1.2 mg/dL; 14 mg/dL
    c. 0.7 mg/dL; 39 mg/dL
    d. 5.2 mg/dL; 12 mg/dL

18. Which of the following sizes of butterfly needles allows for the most rapid administration of iodinated intravenous contrast media?
    a. 19 gauge
    b. 21 gauge
    c. 23 gauge
    d. 25 gauge

19. The embryo or fetus is most sensitive to ionizing radiation during which portion of gestation?
    a. first trimester
    b. second trimester
    c. third trimester
    d. the fetus is equally radiosensitive during all trimesters

20. The choice between ionic and non-ionic contrast media should be based on:
    1. the allergic history of the patient
    2. the cost of the contrast material
    3. the age and physical condition of the patient
    a. 1 only
    b. 1 and 2 only
    c. 1 and 3 only
    d. 1, 2, and 3

21. Which of the following is an example of a mild reaction to iodinated intravenous contrast media?
    a. dyspnea
    b. shock
    c. pulmonary edema
    d. vomiting

22. During which of the following CT procedures is the patient required to give informed consent?
    a. non-contrast CT of the chest
    b. renal stone survey
    c. 3D reconstruction of the hip
    d. abdomen scan after IV contrast agent administration

23. The International Normalized Ratio (INR) is calculated to standardize which of the following laboratory values?
    a. prothrombin time (PT)
    b. partial thromboplastin time (PTT)
    c. blood urea nitrogen (BUN)
    d. glomerular filtration rate (GFR)

24. Which of the following infection control techniques is required at the site of an intravenous injection of iodinated contrast media?
    a. contact isolation
    b. surgical asepsis
    c. medical asepsis
    d. enteric precautions

25. In order to uniformly expose the entire detector array in an MDCT system, the primary beam must be expanded beyond the physical extent of the array in a process known as:
    a. interpolation
    b. overbeaming
    c. photon flux
    d. back-projection

26. Which of the following is a common site for the intravenous injection of iodinated contrast media?
    1. cephalic vein
    2. antecubital vein
    3. basilic vein
    a. 1 only
    b. 3 only
    c. 2 and 3 only
    d. 1, 2, and 3
27. An intrathecal injection prior to a CT examination of the lumber spine places iodinated contrast material directly into the:
    a. subarachnoid space
    b. dura mater
    c. vertebral foramen
    d. subdural space
28. Automatic tube current modulation (ATCM) is employed by an MDCT system for the purpose of:
    a. z-axis interpolation
    b. improving 3D and MPR image quality
    c. reducing patient radiation dose
    d. freezing heart motion during cardiac CT
29. The range of serum iodine concentration for adequate tissue opacification during contrast-enhanced CT examinations is:
    a. 2-8 mg/mL
    b. 12-20 mg/mL
    c. 30-42 mg/mL
    d. 75-105 mg/mL
30. Components of the aseptic technique utilized for the IV administration of contrast agents include:
    1. thorough hand washing between patients
    2. wearing of disposable gloves
    3. establishment of a sterile field around the site
    a. 1 and 2 only
    b. 1 and 3 only
    c. 2 and 3 only
    d. 1, 2, and 3
31. The amount of x-ray energy absorbed in a quantity of air is termed:
    a. dose profile
    b. kerma
    c. becquerel
    d. MSAD

IMAGING PROCEDURES

Use Fig. 6-1 to answer questions 32-36.

32. Number 4 in the figure corresponds to which of the following?
    a. spleen
    b. duodenum
    c. left adrenal gland
    d. large colon
33. Number 2 in the figure corresponds to which of the following?
    a. inferior vena cava
    b. common bile duct
    c. portal vein
    d. superior mesenteric vein
34. The abdominal space indicated by number 7 in the figure is commonly referred to as:
    a. Morison's pouch
    b. cul-de-sac
    c. splenorenal recess
    d. subphrenic space
35. Number 6 in the figure corresponds to which of the following?
    a. superior mesenteric vein
    b. superior mesenteric artery
    c. gastric artery
    d. right renal vein
36. Number 3 in the figure corresponds to which of the following?
    a. duodenum
    b. splenic vein
    c. jejunum
    d. pancreas

FIGURE 6-1

37. Abnormalities of the middle and inner ear may be best demonstrated with CT utilizing _____ sections.
    a. 1- to 2-mm
    b. 3- to 4-mm
    c. 5-mm
    d. 10-mm
38. The Lisfranc joint is the articulation between the:
    a. tarsals and metatarsals
    b. tarsals and lower leg
    c. metatarsals and phalanges
    d. metatarsals and tarsals
39. The volume and density of calcium measured in the coronary arteries on MDCT examination are quantified with use of a value called the:
    a. Euler constant
    b. Hounsfield number
    c. Agatston score
    d. Lambert-Beer value
40. Which of the following is/are (a) component(s) of the adnexal area of the uterus?
    1. ovaries
    2. fallopian tubes
    3. vagina
    a. 1 only
    b. 1 and 2 only
    c. 2 and 3 only
    d. 1, 2, and 3
41. A CT angiogram of the neck is performed primarily for the evaluation of the:
    a. carotid veins
    b. jugular veins
    c. carotid arteries
    d. coronary arteries
42. Which of the following contrast media may be utilized during the CT evaluation of the gastrointestinal tract?
    1. diatrizoate meglumine (Gastrografin)
    2. effervescent agents
    3. iopamidol (Isovue)
    a. 1 only
    b. 1 and 3 only
    c. 2 and 3 only
    d. 1, 2, and 3
43. The liver has a dual blood supply and receives 75% of its blood from the:
    a. hepatic artery
    b. superior mesenteric artery
    c. portal vein
    d. superior mesenteric vein

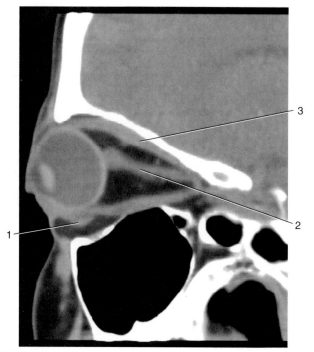

FIGURE 6-2

Use Fig. 6-2 to answer questions 44-47.

44. Number 3 on the figure corresponds to which of the following?
    a. superior rectus muscle
    b. lateral rectus muscle
    c. medial rectus muscle
    d. inferior rectus muscle
45. Number 2 on the figure corresponds to which of the following?
    a. medial rectus muscle
    b. optic nerve
    c. lateral rectus muscle
    d. superior oblique muscle
46. Which of the following best describes the type of image featured in the figure?
    a. direct coronal acquisition
    b. sagittal MIP
    c. coronal MPR
    d. oblique sagittal MPR
47. Number 1 on the figure corresponds to which of the following?
    a. inferior rectus muscle
    b. optic chiasm
    c. inferior oblique muscle
    d. levator palpebrae superioris

FIGURE 6-3

48. Which of the following pelvic bones combine(s) to form the acetabulum?
    1. ilium
    2. ischium
    3. pubis
    a. 2 only
    b. 1 and 2 only
    c. 2 and 3 only
    d. 1, 2, and 3

Use Fig. 6-3 to answer questions 49-52.

49. Number 6 on the figure corresponds to which of the following?
    a. descending aorta
    b. azygos vein
    c. inferior vena cava
    d. brachiocephalic artery
50. Number 4 on the figure corresponds to which of the following muscles?
    a. pectoralis major
    b. pectoralis minor
    c. intercostal
    d. serratus posterior superior
51. Which of the following window settings was used to display the image in the figure?
    a. WL −400, WW 1500
    b. WL 0, WW 150
    c. WL +50, WW 400
    d. WL +275, WW 2500

52. Number 1 on the figure corresponds to which of the following?
    a. superior vena cava
    b. ascending aorta
    c. right brachiocephalic vein
    d. right brachiocephalic artery
53. At what percentage of overlap should CT sections be reconstructed to improve the quality of multiplanar reformation (MPR) images?
    a. 10%
    b. 25%
    c. 50%
    d. 100%
54. A primary responsibility of computed tomography in combined PET-CT is to:
    1. provide precise anatomic location of tumor activity
    2. reduce patient radiation dose
    3. improve radiopharmaceutical uptake
    a. 1 only
    b. 1 and 3 only
    c. 2 and 3 only
    d. 1, 2, and 3
55. The degenerative pathologic process involving the forward slipping of an upper vertebral body over a lower vertebral body is called:
    a. spondylolisthesis
    b. spondylolysis
    c. herniated nucleus pulposus
    d. spinal stenosis

FIGURE 6-4

Use Fig. 6-4 to answer questions 56-59.

56. Number 2 on the figure corresponds to which of the following?
   a. jejunum
   b. sigmoid colon
   c. ileum
   d. cecum

57. Number 3 on the figure corresponds to which of the following?
   a. ureters
   b. cervix
   c. seminal vesicles
   d. vaginal cuff

58. Number 1 on the figure corresponds to which of the following?
   a. rectus abdominis muscle
   b. external oblique muscle
   c. transverse abdominis muscle
   d. internal oblique muscle

59. Number 4 on the figure corresponds to which of the following?
   a. ureteropelvic junction
   b. phlebolith
   c. ureterovesical junction
   d. appendicolith

60. Accurate demonstration of _____ would most likely require the intravenous injection of an iodinated contrast agent during a CT study of the chest.
   a. bronchiectasis
   b. pneumonia
   c. mediastinal lymphadenopathy
   d. pulmonary nodule

61. Which of the following paranasal sinuses is usually the last to fully develop?
   a. frontal
   b. ethmoidal
   c. sphenoidal
   d. maxillary

62. A focused, thin-section axial CT acquisition through just the region of the vocal cords should extend:
   a. from the external auditory meatus inferiorly to the mandible
   b. from the hard palate inferiorly to the hyoid bone
   c. from just above the hyoid bone inferiorly through the cricoid cartilage
   d. from the cricoid cartilage inferiorly through sternoclavicular joint

63. The most common indication for CT-guided percutaneous biopsy is the:
   a. identification of foreign bodies
   b. quantification of bone mineral density
   c. confirmation of a malignancy
   d. measurement of tissue perfusion

64. Axial CT images of the knee may be acquired in four separate series with gantry angulations of 0, 30, 45, and 60 degrees in order to demonstrate the:
   a. tibial plateau
   b. patellofemoral joint
   c. medial and lateral menisci
   d. anterior cruciate ligament

74. The enhancement washout technique for CT characterization of adrenal masses includes:
    1. thin-section pre-contrast acquisition through the adrenals
    2. arterial phase post-contrast acquisition through the adrenals
    3. 10- to 15-minute delayed post-contrast acquisition through the adrenals
    a. 1 and 2 only
    b. 1 and 3 only
    c. 2 and 3 only
    d. 1, 2, and 3

75. Bowel obstruction due to loss of normal contractile motion in an area of intestine is termed:
    a. dyspepsia
    b. intussusception
    c. ileus
    d. adhesion

Use Fig. 6-7 to answer questions 76-79.

76. Number 5 on the figure corresponds to which of the following?
    a. ascending colon
    b. descending colon
    c. sigmoid colon
    d. cecum

77. Number 3 on the figure corresponds to which of the following?
    a. inferior vena cava
    b. common iliac artery
    c. abdominal aorta
    d. superior mesenteric artery

78. Which of the following reformation techniques best describes the image in the figure?
    a. Multiplanar reformation (MPR)
    b. Volume-rendered 3D
    c. Maximum intensity projection (MIP)
    d. Minimum intensity projection (min-IP)

79. Number 6 on the figure corresponds to which of the following?
    a. uterus
    b. rectum
    c. bladder
    d. sigmoid colon

80. CTA of the renal arteries should be performed using a section width of:
    a. 1.25 mm or less
    b. 2-3 mm
    c. 3-5 mm
    d. 5-7 mm

81. The third ventricle of the brain communicates with the fourth ventricle through the:
    a. anterior commissure
    b. septum pellucidum
    c. cerebral aqueduct
    d. fornix

FIGURE 6-7

82. Complete CT examinations of the chest for investigation of bronchogenic carcinoma should include sections from the:
    a. mandible through the liver
    b. apices to the diaphragm
    c. top of the apices through the liver
    d. clavicles through the adrenals

83. The mediastinum includes which of the following anatomic structures?
    1. superior vena cava
    2. stomach
    3. ascending aorta
    a. 1 only
    b. 1 and 2 only
    c. 1 and 3 only
    d. 1, 2, and 3

84. The proper scan field of view (SFOV) for a CT of the abdomen of a patient who measures 42 cm is:
    a. head (25 cm)
    b. small (25 cm)
    c. medium (35 cm)
    d. large (48 cm)

85. The kidneys are located in the retroperitoneum and are bound by a band of fibrous connective tissue called:
    a. Cooper's ligament
    b. Camper's fascia
    c. linea alba
    d. Gerota's fascia

86. After initiation of rapid bolus administration of an iodinated contrast agent, the portal venous phase of hepatic contrast enhancement occurs at approximately:
    a. 15-20 seconds
    b. 25-35 seconds
    c. 60-70 seconds
    d. 120-180 seconds

Use Fig. 6-8 to answer questions 87-90.

87. Number 1 on the figure corresponds to which of the following?
    a. splenium of the corpus callosum
    b. internal capsule
    c. body of the corpus callosum
    d. genu of the corpus callosum

88. Number 6 on the figure corresponds to which of the following?
    a. anterior cerebral artery
    b. falx cerebri
    c. callosal marginal artery
    d. middle cerebral artery

89. Which number on the figure corresponds to the internal capsule?
    a. 1
    b. 2
    c. 4
    d. 5

90. Number 3 on the figure corresponds to which of the following?
    a. pineal gland
    b. middle cerebral artery
    c. fourth ventricle
    d. aqueduct of Sylvius

91. The prone position may be used for a post-myelogram CT examination of the lumbar spine in an effort to:
    a. reduce the lordotic curve
    b. decrease patient gonadal radiation dose
    c. reduce metrizamide pooling
    d. increase the lordotic curve

92. The bolus duration of any IV contrast agent administration can be calculated as the product of injection flow rate and:
    a. scan time
    b. osmolality
    c. cardiac output
    d. contrast agent volume

93. During the use of CT fluoroscopy for guided interventional procedures, which of the following technical considerations may be used to reduce occupational radiation exposure?
    1. increased kVp
    2. lead shielding
    3. use of a needle holder
    a. 2 only
    b. 1 and 2 only
    c. 1 and 3 only
    d. 2 and 3 only

FIGURE 6-8

FIGURE 6-9

Use Fig. 6-9 to answer questions 94-97.

94. Number 4 on the figure corresponds to which of the following?
    a. spinous process
    b. lamina
    c. transverse process
    d. pedicle
95. Which number on the figure corresponds to the pedicle?
    a. 1
    b. 4
    c. 2
    d. 3
96. The intrathecal administration of an iodinated contrast agent in the patient in the figure would allow for greater visualization of the:
    1. spinal cord
    2. nerve roots
    3. anulus fibrosis
    a. 1 only
    b. 1 and 2 only
    c. 1 and 3 only
    d. 1, 2, and 3
97. Number 3 on the figure corresponds to which of the following?
    a. pedicle
    b. transverse process
    c. lamina
    d. spinous process

98. After initiation of rapid bolus administration of iodinated contrast material, the pancreatic phase of contrast enhancement occurs at approximately:
    a. 15-25 seconds
    b. 35-45 seconds
    c. 60-70 seconds
    d. 120-180 seconds
99. Following the IV administration of iodinated contrast media, a tumor that exhibits a greater density than the surrounding parenchyma is characterized as:
    a. hypervascular
    b. isovascular
    c. hypovascular
    d. cavernous
100. The retroperitoneum contains which of the following anatomic structures?
    a. spleen
    b. ovaries
    c. kidneys
    d. stomach
101. Which of the following is NOT a component of the "triple rule-out" MDCT protocol for patients complaining of chest pain?
    a. CTA of the pulmonary arteries
    b. prone HRCT of the lungs
    c. CTA of the aorta
    d. coronary CTA

FIGURE 6-10

102. During contrast-enhanced CT examinations of the chest, streaking artifact may obscure portions of the superior mediastinum because of dense concentrations of iodine in the:
    a. descending aorta
    b. superior vena cava
    c. ascending aorta
    d. pulmonary arteries

Use Fig. 6-10 to answer questions 103-106.

103. Number 3 on the figure corresponds to which of the following?
    a. esophagus
    b. left pulmonary vein
    c. trachea
    d. left primary bronchus

104. The image in the figure was most likely acquired during which of the following phases of contrast enhancement?
    a. pre-contrast
    b. arterial phase
    c. venous phase
    d. delayed phase

105. Number 2 on the figure corresponds to which of the following?
    a. left pulmonary artery
    b. descending aorta
    c. left brachiocephalic artery
    d. left subclavian artery

106. Number 6 on the figure corresponds to which of the following?
    a. right atrium
    b. pulmonary trunk
    c. ascending aorta
    d. descending aorta

107. The average density of a mass within the kidney measures −75 Hounsfield units (HU). The mass is most likely a:
    a. cyst
    b. lipoma
    c. stone
    d. hydrocele

PHYSICS AND INSTRUMENTATION

108. The component of the CT scanner responsible for the mathematical calculations of the image reconstruction process is the:
    a. DAS
    b. analog-to-digital converter (ADC)
    c. digital-to-analog converter (DAC)
    d. array processor

109. Filament sizes for modern CT x-ray tubes range between:
    a. 0.5 and 1.2 mm
    b. 2.0 and 3.0 mm
    c. 5.5 and 7.8 mm
    d. 25.0 and 31.5 mm

110. Which of the following is used to archive a hard copy of a CT image?
    a. laser film
    b. PACS
    c. CD-ROM
    d. LAN

111. Which of the following would serve to increase spatial resolution of a CT exam using a large focal spot size, 5-mm sections, and a 512^2 matrix?
    1. change to small focal spot size
    2. acquire 2.5-mm sections
    3. reconstruct images in a 320^2 matrix
    a. 1 only
    b. 1 and 2 only
    c. 1 and 3 only
    d. 1, 2, and 3

112. A CT image is formed in part by projecting back all of the attenuation values recorded during data acquisition onto a:
    a. pixel
    b. voxel
    c. matrix
    d. reformat

113. The mathematical process that allows MDCT images to be reconstructed at any point along the acquired volume is commonly referred to as:
    a. iteration
    b. filtered back-projection
    c. Fourier reconstruction
    d. z-filtering

114. Fourth-generation CT scanners use a _____ tube-detector configuration.
    a. rotate-translate
    b. electron beam–stationary
    c. rotate-stationary
    d. rotate-rotate

115. Which of the following is considered an equipment-induced CT image artifact?
    a. step artifact
    b. metallic artifact
    c. cupping artifact
    d. aliasing artifact

116. The measurement of CT system performance through quality testing procedures and evaluation of the test results is referred to as:
    a. calibration
    b. uniformity
    c. quality assurance
    d. linearity

117. During CT x-ray exposure, the product of the selected mA setting and the scan time is called the:
    a. effective mAs
    b. peak mAs
    c. absorbed mAs
    d. constant mAs

118. Which of the following mathematical reconstruction methods is used by most modern CT scanners?
    a. back-projection
    b. iterative methods
    c. Fourier transform
    d. filtered back-projection

119. What matrix size was used to reconstruct an image with the display characteristics DFOV 25 cm and pixel area 0.25 mm^2?
    a. 80 × 80 pixels
    b. 256 × 256 pixels
    c. 320 × 320 pixels
    d. 512 × 512 pixels

120. When one is viewing a minimum intensity projection (min-IP) image, each pixel represents:
    a. the maximum attentuation occurring within the voxel
    b. the average attenuation occurring within the voxel
    c. the minimum attenuation occurring within the voxel
    d. all attenuation occurring within the voxel above a set threshold value

121. Which of the following statements regarding pre-detector collimation of the CT x-ray beam is true?
    a. Pre-detector collimation reduces patient radiation dose.
    b. Pre-detector collimation reduces the production of scatter radiation.
    c. Pre-detector collimation determines the scan field of view (SFOV).
    d. Pre-detector collimation removes scatter radiation before it reaches the detectors.

122. Which of the following equations shows the Lambert-Beer law, which describes the relationship between matter and attenuation?
    a. $\text{Attenuation} = \dfrac{I_0}{I}$
    b. $\text{CT number} = \dfrac{\mu_t - \mu_w}{\mu_w \times K}$
    c. $I_0 = Ix^{-e\mu}$
    d. $I = I_0 e^{-\mu x}$

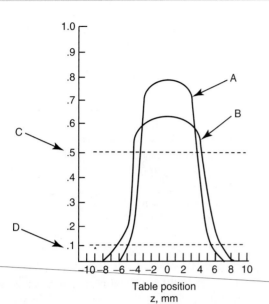

Table position
z, mm

FIGURE 6-11

Use Fig. 6-11 to answer questions 123 and 124.

123. The graph in the figure is used to evaluate which of the following components of CT image quality?
a. in-plane spatial resolution
b. longitudinal spatial resolution
c. temporal resolution
d. contrast resolution

124. On the basis of the information provided on the graph in the figure, which of the following statements is true?
a. The limiting resolution in section A is less than that in section B.
b. The signal-to-noise ratio (SNR) of section A is greater than that of section B.
c. The effective width of section B is greater than that of section A.
d. Section B is isotropic in dimension.

125. Which of the following would be considered the best method to reduce respiratory motion on the CT image?
a. good patient-technologist communication
b. reduced scan times
c. immobilization devices
d. glucagon administration

126. Which of the following types of gas is commonly used for gas ionization CT detectors?
a. xenon
b. cadmium tungstate
c. helium
d. nitrogen

127. Power output for a modern MDCT x-ray tube has an approximate range of:
a. 3-5 kilowatts (kW)
b. 15-20 kilowatts (kW)
c. 40-48 kilowatts (kW)
d. 60-100 kilowatts (kW)

128. The mathematical manipulations required during the reconstruction of a CT image are accomplished using a(n):
1. algorithm
2. kernel
3. mathematical filter function
a. 1 only
b. 1 and 2 only
c. 1 and 3 only
d. 1, 2, and 3

129. When an operator reduces the scan field of view for a particular body part, which of the following technical changes occurs?
a. The displayed image appears larger.
b. Spatial resolution increases.
c. A smaller number of detectors are activated.
d. The displayed image appears smaller.

130. An average CT number value for blood is:
a. −20 HU
b. +10 HU
c. +45 HU
d. +100 HU

131. The electronic combination of signals from adjacent detectors to form a CT image is called:
a. binning
b. interpolation
c. z-filtering
d. partial volume averaging

132. Which of the following technical adjustments may be employed to improve the temporal resolution of an MDCT system?
1. decrease in section width
2. image segmentation
3. physiologic gating
a. 1 only
b. 3 only
c. 1 and 2 only
d. 2 and 3 only

133. The streaking artifact that occurs in the area of the posterior fossa during a CT examination of the brain may be referred to as:
a. cupping
b. the "boiled egg" artifact
c. stairstep
d. the Hounsfield bar

134. The relative accuracy between calculated CT numbers and their respective linear attenuation coefficients is referred to as:
a. linearity
b. calibration
c. uniformity
d. contrast resolution

135. To maintain security and patient privacy when medical images are transmitted across a network, the images may be coded in a form decipherable only by software at the destination location. This process is referred to as:
    a. write-once, read-many (WORM)
    b. hypertext transfer protocol (HTTP)
    c. teleradiology
    d. encryption

136. Which of the following 3D imaging techniques is utilized to provide "fly-through" images during CT colonography?
    a. orthographic volume rendering
    b. shaded surface display (SSD)
    c. perspective volume rendering
    d. minimum intensity projection (min-IP)

137. Which of the following sets of technical factors would yield an isotropic data set when an MDCT image is reconstructed using a 512^2 matrix?
    a. 5.0-mm sections, 17-cm DFOV
    b. 3.0-mm sections, 25-cm DFOV
    c. 1.25-mm sections, 48-cm DFOV
    d. 0.625-mm sections, 32-cm DFOV

138. Which of the following is NOT commonly used as a CT scintillation detector material?
    a. ceramic rare earth
    b. silver halide
    c. bismuth germanate
    d. cadmium tungstate

139. The mathematical technique that involves the estimation of an unknown value from values on either side of it is known as:
    a. filtering
    b. interpolation
    c. convolution
    d. summation

140. During which of the following CT examinations is a misregistration artifact most likely to occur?
    a. brain
    b. pelvis
    c. neck
    d. abdomen

141. In a single-slice CT (SSCT) system, which of the following technical parameters may be adjusted retrospectively?
    1. section width
    2. section increment
    3. reconstruction algorithm
    a. 2 only
    b. 1 and 2 only
    c. 2 and 3 only
    d. 1, 2, and 3

142. Bow-tie filters are employed in a CT x-ray system to reduce:
    a. image noise
    b. low spatial frequency signal
    c. patient radiation dose
    d. high spatial frequency signal

143. Which of the following technical factors is/are involved in the determination of section width for MDCT images?
    1. scan field of view (SFOV)
    2. beam collimation
    3. detector configuration
    a. 2 only
    b. 1 and 2 only
    c. 1 and 3 only
    d. 2 and 3 only

144. The fluctuation of CT numbers in an image of uniform, homogeneous material may occur because of:
    a. linearity
    b. noise
    c. aliasing
    d. partial volume effect

145. A region of interest (ROI) measurement placed over a portion of a CT image provides which of the following?
    a. distance (mm)
    b. diameter (mm)
    c. linear attenuation coefficient (μ)
    d. average CT number (HU)

146. An MDCT image is reconstructed using a 512^2 matrix and a DFOV of 38 cm. If the detector collimation is set to a section width of 1.25 mm, what is the volume of each voxel?
    a. 0.69 mm^3
    b. 0.93 mm^3
    c. 1.26 mm^3
    d. 1.68 mm^3

W = 4000   L = 250

FIGURE 6-12

Use Fig. 6-12 to answer questions 147-149.

147. Which of the following is the common term for the artifact present on the image in the figure?
a. aliasing
b. streaking
c. edge gradient
d. tube arcing

148. Which of the following would be the most common cause of the artifact in the figure?
a. metallic dental fillings
b. partial volume averaging
c. beam hardening
d. detector malfunction

149. Reduction of the type of artifact seen in the figure on a coronal MDCT view of the sinuses may be accomplished through:
a. an increase in the mA
b. a decrease in the kVp
c. coronal MPR images built from an axial acquisition
d. a reduction in the scan field of view (SFOV)

150. First-generation CT scanners used a method of data acquisition based on a _____ principle.
a. multiplanar
b. rotation-only
c. translate-rotate
d. transaxial

151. The maximum beam collimation for an MDCT system with a detector array of 64 detectors, each 0.625 mm wide, is:
a. 1.25 mm
b. 5.00 mm
c. 10.00 mm
d. 40.00 mm

152. Compared with conventional radiography, computed tomography produces diagnostic images with better:
a. low-contrast resolution
b. spatial resolution
c. minute detail
d. patient radiation dose reduction

153. Writable CD and DVD media are optical disks that may be described as:
a. read-only
b. lossy
c. WORM
d. lossless

154. A CT system measures the average linear attenuation coefficient of a voxel of tissue to be 0.008. The linear attenuation coefficient of water for this scanner equals 0.181. The CT number assigned to the pixel representing this voxel of tissue equals:
a. −956 HU
b. −173 HU
c. +44 HU
d. +1044 HU

155. During data acquisition, a CT system may continuously adjust the mA relative to the measured image noise for a method of dose reduction referred to as:
a. iterative reconstruction
b. automatic tube current modulation
c. attenuation correction
d. Nyquist sampling

156. Which of the following statements comparing the efficiency of scintillation and gas ionization detectors is correct?
a. Both have approximately the same capture efficiency.
b. The scintillation detector has a higher capture efficiency.
c. Unlike the scintillation detector, the gas ionization detector has a problem with afterglow.
d. Gas ionization detectors have a higher conversion efficiency.

157. The data acquisition system (DAS) of a CT scanner is responsible for:
1. measuring transmitted intensity
2. conversion of the transmission data into a digital signal
3. sending the digital information to the computer for processing
a. 1 only
b. 2 only
c. 1 and 3 only
d. 1, 2, and 3

FIGURE 6-13

158. Which of the following is used to remove image blurring during the back-projection method of CT image reconstruction?
    1. z-filtering
    2. convolution kernel
    3. Feldkamp-Davis-Kress (FDK) algorithm
    a. 2 only
    b. 3 only
    c. 1 and 2 only
    d. 2 and 3 only

159. During CT x-ray production, the electromagnetic steering of the electron beam from the cathode to two alternating targets is referred to as:
    a. prospective gating
    b. ultrafast CT
    c. twin CAT
    d. flying focal spot

Use Fig. 6-13 *to answer questions 160-162.*

160. The region of interest (ROI) measurement in the figure provides an average density of +1.9 HU. This material is most likely:
    a. fat
    b. blood
    c. tumor
    d. water

161. The material within the ROI measurement in the figure has a linear attenuation coefficient of:
    a. 0.0007
    b. 0.185
    c. 0.206
    d. 0.530

162. The image in the figure was most likely displayed with the use of which of the following window widths?
    a. 70
    b. 400
    c. 1300
    d. 3800

163. Areas of a CT image that contain minimal changes in tissue density are electronically represented by:
    a. positive CT numbers
    b. high spatial frequencies
    c. negative CT numbers
    d. low spatial frequencies

164. A CT image is displayed in a window with a level of +200 and a width of 1000. Which of the following statements is correct?
    a. Pixels with values between +200 HU and −1000 HU will appear white.
    b. Pixels with values greater than +200 HU will appear black.
    c. Pixels with values between −300 HU and +700 HU will be assigned shades of gray.
    d. Pixels with values between −1200 HU and +1200 HU will be assigned shades of gray.

165. In the binary number system, a byte is a series of _____ bits of information.
    a. two
    b. four
    c. eight
    d. sixteen

Simulated Exam Three

PATIENT CARE

1. During CT examinations of the chest and abdomen, the highly radiosensitive breast tissue can be protected with minimal image artifact with the use of specialized shielding composed of:
   a. barium
   b. aluminum
   c. lead
   d. bismuth

2. The use of water as an oral contrast material for CT of the abdomen and/or pelvis has several potential advantages, including:
   1. increased palatability and improved patient comfort
   2. better demonstration of enhancing bowel wall
   3. no interference with 3D applications
   a. 1 only
   b. 1 and 2 only
   c. 1 and 3 only
   d. 1, 2, and 3

3. If all other technical factors remain constant, which of the following would serve to decrease patient radiation dose during a helical SSCT examination?
   a. decreased scan field of view (SFOV)
   b. decreased filtration
   c. increased pitch
   d. increased matrix size

4. A patient's blood pressure is measured as 140/70 mm Hg. The number 140 represents:
   a. the pressure within the arterial vessels during contraction of the heart
   b. the pressure exerted on the chambers of the heart while it is relaxed
   c. the pressure within the arterial vessels while the heart is relaxed
   d. the pressure exerted on the chambers of the heart during a contraction

5. A(n) _____ contrast material may be described as one that does not dissociate into charged particles in solution.
   a. neutral
   b. non-ionic
   c. osmolar
   d. ionic

6. Which of the following radiation dose indices is a measure of the total radiation exposure for an entire series of CT images?
   a. $CTDI_{100}$
   b. dose length product (DLP)
   c. $CTDI_{vol}$
   d. multiple scan average dose (MSAD)

7. Proper immobilization during a CT procedure may involve the use of:
   1. soft, hook-and-loop (e.g., Velcro) immobilization straps
   2. adhesive medical tape
   3. good patient communication
   a. 1 only
   b. 1 and 2 only
   c. 1 and 3 only
   d. 1, 2, and 3

8. The normal range of glomerular filtration rate (GFR) for men is:
   a. 50 ± 14 mL/min/m^2
   b. 60 ± 10 mL/min/m^2
   c. 70 ± 14 mL/min/m^2
   d. 80 ± 10 mL/min/m^2

9. *Effective dose* is a relative radiation dose measurement term that accounts for the:
   a. beam pitch
   b. tissue radiosensitivity
   c. detector pitch
   d. collimation

10. Risk factors for contrast-induced nephrotoxicity (CIN) include:
    1. diabetes
    2. advanced age
    3. hematuria
    a. 1 only
    b. 3 only
    c. 1 and 2 only
    d. 1, 2, and 3

11. The reduction in number of infectious organisms without a complete elimination is termed:
    a. medical asepsis
    b. sterilization
    c. surgical asepsis
    d. immunization

12. Which of the following is the preferred range for patient heart rate for optimal cardiac CT studies?
    a. 65-75 bpm
    b. 75-85 bpm
    c. 85-95 bpm
    d. > 100 bpm

13. Late effects of radiation, such as genetic mutations, may occur with even small doses of radiation and are termed:
    a. stochastic
    b. somatic
    c. nonstochastic
    d. chronic

14. *Urticaria* is which of the following?
    a. severe nausea with associated vomiting
    b. urinary tract infection
    c. hives
    d. bronchospasm

15. Which of the following type(s) of oral contrast material could cause peritonitis if leakage from the digestive tract occurs from perforation?
    a. iopamidol (Gastrografin)
    b. barium sulfate
    c. diatrizoate (Hypaque)
    d. effervescent granules

16. Which of the following is not an advantage of an automatic power injector over the manual bolus method of intravenous contrast agent administration?
    a. uniform contrast enhancement throughout the exam
    b. consistent contrast agent administration for all patients
    c. decreased risk of contrast-induced nephrotoxicity (CIN)
    d. shorter injection times

17. Which of the following is/are severe adverse reaction(s) to iodinated intravenous contrast media?
    1. anaphylaxis
    2. urticaria
    3. vomiting
    a. 1 only
    b. 1 and 2 only
    c. 1 and 3 only
    d. 1, 2, and 3

18. Which of the following laboratory values is the most dependable measure of renal function?
    a. BUN
    b. creatinine
    c. PT
    d. PTT

19. Which of the following angiocatheter sizes may be safely used for the automated power injection of iodinated contrast agents at flow rates higher than 3 mL/sec?
    1. 18-gauge
    2. 20-gauge
    3. 22-gauge
    a. 1 only
    b. 3 only
    c. 1 and 2 only
    d. 1, 2, and 3

20. Which of the following portions of the electrocardiogram (ECG) corresponds to the period of atrial systole?
    a. P wave
    b. QRS complex
    c. alpha wave
    d. T wave

21. Which of the following statements is true regarding the relationship between multiple scan average dose (MSAD) and image spacing during axial (step-and-shoot) scanning?
    a. MSAD decreases with overlapping scans.
    b. MSAD increases with overlapping scans.
    c. MSAD increases with noncontiguous scans.
    d. MSAD equals the product of image spacing and pitch.

22. Which of the following terms is used to describe the intravenous injection of medication or contrast agent in one complete dose over a short time?
    a. infusion
    b. bolus
    c. IV drip
    d. Infus-A-Port

23. Used in determining the biologic effect of iodinated contrast media, the term _____ refers to the number of ions formed when a substance dissociates in solution.
    a. solubility
    b. osmolality
    c. concentration
    d. iodination

24. The dosimetry index used to approximate the radiation dose for CT sections acquired during a helical scan is called the:
    a. $CTDI_W$
    b. effective dose
    c. $CTDI_{vol}$
    d. equivalent dose

25. The injection rate of an automatic injector is set at 1.5 mL/sec. What is the injection time for a contrast agent volume of 150 mL?
    a. 60 seconds
    b. 90 seconds
    c. 100 seconds
    d. 120 seconds
26. Which of the following must be included when one is obtaining informed consent for an invasive procedure?
    1. explanation of the examination techniques
    2. the possible risks and benefits of the exam
    3. alternatives to the procedure involved
    a. 1 only
    b. 1 and 2 only
    c. 1 and 3 only
    d. 1, 2 and 3
27. Which of the following techniques may be employed to reduce patient radiation dose during a cardiac CT examination?
    a. retrospective ECG gating
    b. z-axis interpolation
    c. prospective ECG gating
    d. multisegment reconstruction
28. Which of the following may be considered a low-osmolar contrast medium?
    1. iothalamate meglumine
    2. diatrizoate sodium
    3. iohexol
    a. 1 only
    b. 3 only
    c. 1 and 2 only
    d. 1, 2, and 3
29. Following the intrathecal injection of an iodinated contrast agent for a post-myelography CT study of the lumbar spine, the patient should be instructed to:
    a. take a cleansing enema
    b. resume normal activity
    c. rest for 8-24 hours with the head slightly elevated
    d. rest for 8-24 hours in the Trendelenburg position

30. Compared with single-slice CT (SSCT), patient radiation dose during a multidetector CT study may be higher because of:
    1. use of a cone beam of radiation
    2. acquisitions at thinner section widths
    3. higher-powered x-ray tubes
    a. 1 only
    b. 1 and 2 only
    c. 1 and 3 only
    d. 1, 2, and 3
31. Which of the following pharmaceuticals may be administered prior to a cardiac CT procedure in an effort to improve visualization of the coronary vessels?
    1. β-blocker
    2. nitroglycerin
    3. metformin
    a. 1 only
    b. 2 only
    c. 1 and 2 only
    d. 1, 2, and 3

IMAGING PROCEDURES

32. A _____ is a benign, highly vascular mass commonly found in the liver.
    a. hematoid
    b. vasculoma
    c. hemogenic carcinoma
    d. hemangioma
33. Which of the following is the preferred contrast enhancement phase for CT acquisition of the spleen?
    a. pre-contrast phase
    b. equilibrium phase
    c. arterial phase
    d. portal venous phase

FIGURE 7-1

Use Fig. 7-1 to answer questions 34-37.

34. Number 2 on the figure corresponds to which of the following?
   a. capitate
   b. lunate
   c. hamate
   d. scaphoid

35. The anatomic plane of the image in the figure can be best described as the:
   a. coronal plane
   b. sagittal plane
   c. axial plane
   d. oblique axial plane

36. Number 1 on the figure corresponds to which of the following?
   a. capitate
   b. lunate
   c. hamate
   d. scaphoid

37. Number 5 on the figure corresponds to which of the following?
   a. capitate
   b. lunate
   c. hamate
   d. scaphoid

38. Which of the following terms describes the appearance of an acute subdural hematoma on a CT image of the brain?
   a. radiolucent
   b. hyperdense
   c. hypodense
   d. isodense

39. The angiographic assessment known as a "CT run-off" evaluates the peripheral arterial tree from the renal arteries through the:
   a. aortic arch
   b. superior mesenteric artery
   c. aortic bifurcation
   d. distal lower extremity

40. During a PET-CT examination, the amount of FDG uptake in an anatomic region is directly proportional to the area's:
   a. size
   b. central vs. peripheral location
   c. radiosensitivity
   d. metabolic activity

Use Fig. 7-2 to answer questions 41-43.

41. Number 2 on the figure corresponds to which of the following?
   a. left ovary
   b. bladder
   c. sigmoid colon
   d. uterus

42. Number 4 on the figure corresponds to which of the following?
   a. left ovary
   b. bladder
   c. sigmoid colon
   d. uterus

43. Number 5 on the figure corresponds to which of the following?
   a. left ovary
   b. bladder
   c. sigmoid colon
   d. uterus

FIGURE 7-2

44. Accurate demonstration of _____ would most likely require the intravenous injection of an iodinated contrast agent during a CT study of the chest.
    a. pneumonia
    b. asbestosis
    c. a dissecting aortic aneurysm
    d. a solitary pulmonary nodule

45. Vascular components of the brain's blood supply known as the circle of Willis include the:
    1. internal carotid arteries
    2. basilar artery
    3. anterior communicating artery
    a. 2 only
    b. 1 and 2 only
    c. 1 and 3 only
    d. 1, 2, and 3

46. The benign mass of the eighth cranial nerve known as a *vestibular schwannoma* may also be termed a(n):
    a. acoustic neuroma
    b. hypoglossal adenoma
    c. olfactory neuroblastoma
    d. optic nerve glioma

Use Fig. 7-3 to answer questions 47-50.

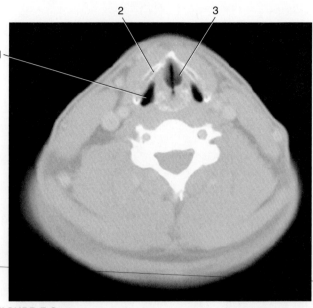

FIGURE 7-3

47. Number 3 on the figure corresponds to which of the following?
    a. cricoid cartilage
    b. piriform sinus
    c. aryepiglottic fold
    d. vocal cord

48. Number 1 on the figure corresponds to which of the following?
    a. trachea
    b. piriform sinus
    c. aryepiglottic fold
    d. vocal cord

49. Which of the following window settings was most likely used to display the image in the figure?
    a. WL −300, WW 1000
    b. WL −50, WW 50
    c. WL +50, WW 150
    d. WL +400, WW 3000

50. Number 2 on the figure corresponds to which of the following?
    a. hyoid bone
    b. cricoid cartilage
    c. thyroid cartilage
    d. mandible

51. The thick, layered portion of the peritoneum responsible for attaching portions of the intestines to the bowel wall is called the:
    a. Gerota fascia
    b. falciform ligament
    c. mesentery
    d. ligamentum teres

52. After initiation of rapid bolus administration of an iodinated contrast agent, the nephrographic phase of renal contrast enhancement occurs at approximately:
    a. 20-25 seconds
    b. 30-40 seconds
    c. 70-90 seconds
    d. 3-5 minutes

53. Retrospective ECG gating utilizes which of the following portions of the cardiac cycle for image reconstruction?
    1. atrial systole
    2. ventricular systole
    3. cardiac diastole
    a. 2 only
    b. 3 only
    c. 1 and 2 only
    d. 2 and 3 only

Use Fig. 7-4 to answer questions 54-57.

54. Number 9 on the figure corresponds to which of the following?
    a. ethmoid sinus
    b. nasal concha
    c. maxillary sinus
    d. sphenoid sinus
55. Number 5 on the figure corresponds to which of the following?
    a. optic nerve
    b. superior ophthalmic vein
    c. oculomotor nerve
    d. superior oblique muscle
56. Number 4 on the figure corresponds to which of the following?
    a. superior rectus muscle
    b. superior ophthalmic vein
    c. levator palpebrae superioris muscle
    d. superior oblique muscle
57. Number 6 on the figure corresponds to which of the following?
    a. optic nerve
    b. medial rectus muscle
    c. lateral rectus muscle
    d. oculomotor nerve

58. Which of the following is a common complication of CT-guided biopsy of the lung?
    a. pulmonary embolism
    b. aspiration
    c. pneumoconiosis
    d. pneumothorax
59. An enema is indicated prior to a CT examination of the pelvis to administer positive contrast material into the large bowel. Which of the following dosages would be sufficient to opacify the rectosigmoid region?
    a. 150-250 mL
    b. 300-500 mL
    c. 500-750 mL
    d. 900-1100 mL
60. A CT examination of the lumbar spine reveals a herniated disc at the level of L2-L3. Which of the following reformation planes would best demonstrate posterior compression of the disc material onto the spinal cord?
    a. coronal
    b. sagittal
    c. axial
    d. oblique

FIGURE 7-4

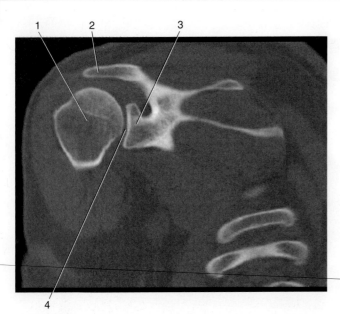

FIGURE 6-5

Use Fig. 6-5 to answer questions 65-67.

65. Number 3 on the figure corresponds to which of the following?
    a. coracoid process
    b. acromion
    c. glenoid process
    d. clavicle
66. The anatomic plane of the image in the figure can be best described as the:
    a. coronal plane
    b. sagittal plane
    c. axial plane
    d. oblique axial plane
67. Number 2 in the figure corresponds to which of the following?
    a. coracoid process
    b. acromion
    c. glenoid process
    d. clavicle
68. Which of the following contrast agent administration techniques should be used for a general CT survey of the abdomen?
    1. 400-600 mL oral contrast agent 45-90 minutes prior to the exam
    2. 250 mL oral contrast agent immediately before the exam
    3. 700-900 mL contrast agent administered as an enema immediately before the exam
    a. 1 only
    b. 1 and 2 only
    c. 1 and 3 only
    d. 1, 2, and 3

69. During CT perfusion studies, the quantity of blood (in mL) that moves through 100 g of tissue each minute is termed the:
    a. mean transit time (MTT)
    b. cerebral blood flow (CBF)
    c. cerebral blood volume (CBV)
    d. percentage washout value (PWV)

Use Fig. 6-6 to answer questions 70-73.

70. Which number in the figure corresponds to the trapezius muscle?
    a. 4
    b. 3
    c. 6
    d. 5
71. An adequate volume of intravenous contrast agent for the SSCT examination of the neck in this figure would be:
    a. 25 mL
    b. 50 mL
    c. 125 mL
    d. 225 mL
72. Number 1 on the figure corresponds to which of the following?
    a. common carotid artery
    b. external jugular vein
    c. internal jugular vein
    d. brachiocephalic artery
73. Number 4 on the figure corresponds to which of the following?
    a. erector spinae muscle
    b. rhomboid major muscle
    c. deltoid muscle
    d. levator scapulae muscle

FIGURE 6-6

FIGURE 7-5

Use Fig. 7-5 to answer questions 61-63.

61. Number 6 on the figure corresponds to which of the following?
    a. renal cortex
    b. renal pelvis
    c. renal calyx
    d. renal pyramid
62. Which of the following reformation techniques best describes the image in the figure?
    a. volume-rendered 3D
    b. multiplanar reformation (MPR)
    c. minimum intensity projection (min-IP)
    d. maximum intensity projection (MIP)
63. Number 1 on the figure corresponds to which of the following?
    a. ureteropelvic junction
    b. ureterovesical junction
    c. ureterocalyceal junction
    d. ureteropyramidal junction
64. A common formula used to calculate the maximum dosage of intravenous iodinated contrast material used in any CT examination is:
    a. 5 mg per kg of body weight
    b. 5 mL per lb of body weight
    c. 2 mL per kg of body weight
    d. 1 mL per lb of body weight
65. Which of the following MDCT examinations may include endobrachial views?
    a. virtual colonoscopy
    b. HRCT of the lungs
    c. virtual bronchoscopy
    d. CTA of the aorta

66. The Stanford type A dissecting aneurysm affects which portion of the aorta?
    a. ascending thoracic
    b. descending thoracic
    c. abdominal
    d. bifurcation
67. During HRCT of the lungs, edematous changes in the posterior lungs may be differentiated by positioning of the patient in the _____ position.
    a. supine
    b. right lateral decubitus
    c. left lateral decubitus
    d. prone
68. The firm, outer portion of each intervertebral disc is called the:
    a. nucleus pulposus
    b. nucleus prepositus
    c. anulus fibrosus
    d. anulus stapedius

Use Fig. 7-6 to answer questions 69-71.

69. Number 2 on the figure corresponds to which of the following?
    a. superior facet
    b. pedicle
    c. transverse process
    d. lamina
70. Number 1 on the figure corresponds to which of the following?
    a. spinal root
    b. superior articular recess
    c. anterior arch
    d. transverse foramen
71. Number 4 on the figure corresponds to which of the following?
    a. superior facet
    b. pedicle
    c. transverse process
    d. lamina

FIGURE 7-6

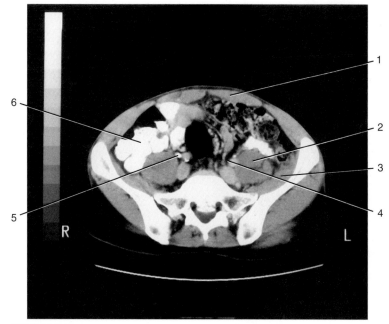

FIGURE 7-7

72. Which of the following refers to the surgical resection of the pancreas and duodenum for treatment of pancreatic carcinoma?
    a. endoscopic retrograde cholangiopancreatography (ERCP)
    b. cholecystectomy
    c. Roux-en-Y anastomosis
    d. Whipple procedure

73. During which of the following IV contrast phases does the bladder wall enhance?
    a. early arterial
    b. corticomedullary
    c. nephrographic
    d. excretory

74. Coronary artery calcium (CAC) quantitation by MDCT exam is used primarily to assess:
    a. aortic aneurysm
    b. atherosclerotic disease
    c. coronary artery stenosis
    d. ejection fraction

Use Fig. 7-7 to answer questions 75-78.

75. Number 4 on the figure corresponds to which of the following?
    a. left common iliac artery
    b. right common iliac artery
    c. left common iliac vein
    d. right common iliac artery

76. The best method for targeting the sacrum in the figure for detailed examination would be to:
    a. magnify the image 2×
    b. re-scan the patient using a small SFOV
    c. retrospectively reconstruct the image using a small DFOV
    d. decrease the matrix dimension

77. Number 5 on the figure corresponds to which of the following?
    a. right common iliac vein
    b. ureter
    c. right common iliac vein
    d. inferior mesenteric vein

78. Number 1 on the figure corresponds to which of the following?
    a. psoas muscle
    b. gluteus medius muscle
    c. iliacus muscle
    d. rectus abdominis muscle

79. A specialized CT examination involving the administration of an enteral contrast agent directly into the small bowel via nasogastric tube is called:
    a. CT enteroclysis
    b. CT colonography
    c. CT enterography
    d. CT colonoscopy

80. The epithelial lining of the urinary tract is called the:
    a. omentum
    b. haustrum
    c. urothelium
    d. pyelocalyx

81. A common area for inflammation, the primary drainage opening within the sinus cavities is referred to as the:
    a. mucosal fossa
    b. adenovestibular complex
    c. external olfactory canal
    d. ostiomeatal complex

FIGURE 7-8

Use Fig. 7-8 to answer questions 82-86.

82. Number 1 on the figure corresponds to which of the following?
    a. right brachiocephalic artery
    b. right pulmonary artery
    c. right pericardiacophrenic artery
    d. right subclavian artery

83. Which of the following best describes the type of image displayed in the figure?
    a. coronal maximum intensity projection (MIP)
    b. direct coronal acquisition
    c. coronal multiplanar reformation (MPR)
    d. coronal minimum intensity projection (min-IP)

84. Number 4 on the figure corresponds to which of the following?
    a. gastric artery
    b. inferior vena cava (IVC)
    c. superior mesenteric artery (SMA)
    d. descending aorta

85. The areas of image quality degradation indicated by number 3 on the figure are an example of:
    a. aliasing artifact
    b. windmill artifact
    c. pulsation artifact
    d. beam-hardening artifact

86. Number 2 on the figure corresponds to which of the following?
    a. aortic arch
    b. pulmonary trunk
    c. superior vena cava
    d. left anterior descending artery

87. During CT examination of the chest, the administration of a saline flush following the bolus injection of iodinated IV contrast media helps alleviate artifact from dense contrast in the:
    a. ascending aorta
    b. superior vena cava
    c. descending aorta
    d. inferior vena cava

88. Delayed post-contrast acquisition of the lower extremities following a CTA of the pulmonary arteries is termed:
    a. CT venography
    b. CT perfusion
    c. femoral CTA
    d. iliac CTA

FIGURE 7-9

Use Fig. 7-9 to answer questions 89-92.

89. Number 4 on the figure corresponds to which of the following?
    a. third ventricle
    b. quadrigeminal cistern
    c. fourth ventricle
    d. sagittal sinus

90. Number 2 on the figure corresponds to which of the following?
    a. left posterior cerebral artery
    b. left middle cerebral artery
    c. left anterior cerebral artery
    d. left posterior communicating artery

91. Number 5 on the figure corresponds to which of the following?
    a. posterior communicating artery
    b. anterior communicating artery
    c. internal carotid artery
    d. basilar artery

92. Number 3 on the figure corresponds to which of the following?
    a. left posterior cerebral artery
    b. left middle cerebral artery
    c. left anterior cerebral artery
    d. left posterior communicating artery

93. The overall quality of MPR and volume-rendered 3D images for a carotid artery CTA may be improved by:
    1. reducing the kVp for an increase in displayed vessel opacification and contrast
    2. retrospective reconstructions with a 50% overlap in section increment
    3. bolus-tracking software to maximize contrast enhancement
    a. 2 only
    b. 1 and 2 only
    c. 2 and 3 only
    d. 1, 2, and 3

94. Which of the following is the most common sign of GI pathology on CT images?
    a. fluid collection
    b. wall thickening
    c. air distention
    d. dense fecal matter

95. Often evaluated during body CTA examinations, the branches of the celiac axis are the:
    1. left gastric artery
    2. common hepatic artery
    3. splenic artery
    a. 1 only
    b. 3 only
    c. 2 and 3 only
    d. 1, 2, and 3

FIGURE 7-10

Use Fig. 7-10 to answer questions 96-99.

96. Number 2 on the figure corresponds to which of the following?
    a. right brachiocephalic vein
    b. left subclavian artery
    c. left brachiocephalic vein
    d. brachiocephalic artery
97. Number 5 on the figure corresponds to which of the following?
    a. right brachiocephalic vein
    b. left subclavian artery
    c. left brachiocephalic vein
    d. brachiocephalic artery
98. Number 1 on the figure corresponds to which of the following?
    a. right brachiocephalic vein
    b. left subclavian artery
    c. left brachiocephalic vein
    d. brachiocephalic artery
99. Which number on the figure corresponds to the left common carotid artery?
    a. 1
    b. 6
    c. 4
    d. 3

100. Vital components of a CT urogram (CT-IVP) protocol include:
    1. administration of 1200 to 1500 mL of a positive oral contrast agent 90 minutes prior to examination
    2. thin-section excretory phase imaging of the entire urinary tract
    3. volume-rendered 3D and maximum intensity projection (MIP) imaging of the urinary tract
    a. 2 only
    b. 1 and 2 only
    c. 2 and 3 only
    d. 1, 2, and 3
101. Arterial phase CT imaging of the liver is used to optimally demonstrate which of the following?
    a. fatty infiltration
    b. hepatic cysts
    c. portal vein thrombosis
    d. hepatocellular carcinoma (HCC)
102. Non-contrast CT of the urinary tract is a valuable tool in the investigation of:
    a. transitional cell carcinoma (TCC)
    b. urinary tract lithiasis
    c. renal artery stenosis
    d. ureteral duplication
103. Which of the following techniques may be used to improve visualization of the vocal cords during a CT examination of the neck?
    1. oral administration of thick barium paste
    2. CT acquisition with the mouth open as widely as tolerable
    3. scanning while the patient phonates the letter "E"
    a. 2 only
    b. 3 only
    c. 1 and 3 only
    d. 1, 2, and 3

6
1
2
3
4
5

R   L

W = 400   L = 39

FIGURE 7-11

Use Fig. 7-11 to answer questions 104-106.

104. Which number on the figure corresponds to the superior mesenteric vein?
    a. 3
    b. 5
    c. 1
    d. 2
105. Number 4 on the figure corresponds to which of the following?
    a. descending colon
    b. spleen
    c. adrenal gland
    d. renal vein
106. Number 6 on the figure corresponds to which of the following?
    a. duodenum
    b. terminal ileum
    c. appendix
    d. pancreas
107. Percutaneous drainage under CT guidance may be used for the aspiration of which of the following pathologic processes?
    a. chronic subdural hematoma
    b. hydrocephalus
    c. abdominal abscess
    d. dissecting aortic aneurysm

PHYSICS AND INSTRUMENTATION

108. The device constructed to house the x-ray tube and data acquisition system (DAS) for a CT scanner is called the:
    a. CPU
    b. generator
    c. array processor
    d. gantry

109. Third-generation CT scanners use which of the following scan geometries?
    a. translate-rotate
    b. rotate-stationary
    c. transaxial
    d. rotate-rotate
110. A quality control procedure determines that the low-contrast resolution of a CT scanner is extremely poor. Likely causes are:
    1. tube arcing
    2. increased electronic noise
    3. decreased tube output
    a. 1 only
    b. 1 and 3 only
    c. 2 and 3 only
    d. 1, 2, and 3
111. When one is viewing a maximum intensity projection (MIP) image, each pixel represents:
    a. the maximum attentuation occurring within the voxel
    b. the average attenuation occurring within the voxel
    c. the minimum attenuation occurring within the voxel
    d. all attenuation occurring within the voxel above a set threshold value
112. A CT image is reconstructed using a 512^2 matrix and a display field of view of 40 cm. What is the linear dimension of each pixel?
    a. 0.0015 mm
    b. 0.08 mm
    c. 0.78 mm
    d. 1.28 mm
113. Which of the following statements about collimation of the CT x-ray beam is false?
    a. Collimation of the x-ray beam occurs both before and after the patient.
    b. Collimation of the beam occurs in the z-axis, thus affecting slice thickness.
    c. Increases in collimation increase the intensity of the primary beam.
    d. Collimation of the CT x-ray beam is used to limit the detection of scatter radiation.
114. Which of the following terms may be used to describe the quantity of radiation emitted from the CT x-ray tube toward the patient?
    a. effective mAs
    b. photon flux
    c. constant mAs
    d. photon fluence
115. Which of the following mathematical techniques is used exclusively for image reconstruction with helical CT scanners?
    a. back-projection
    b. convolution
    c. interpolation
    d. iterative techniques

R   L

FIGURE 7-12

116. Which of the following is the most common type of noise found in the CT image?
    a. quantum noise
    b. electronic noise
    c. artifactual noise
    d. filter noise

117. A picture archival and communications system (PACS) is connected with imaging modalities and other peripheral devices on a computerized communications system called a:
    a. network
    b. web
    c. radiology information system (RIS)
    d. hospital information system (HIS)

Use Fig. 7-12 to answer questions 118-120.

118. Which of the following artifacts is evident on the image in the figure?
    a. blooming
    b. aliasing
    c. edge gradient effect
    d. ring artifact

119. Which of the following would serve to reduce the image artifact present in the figure?
    (1) increase in filtration
    (2) increase in kVp
    (3) increase in section width
    a. 1 only
    b. 1 and 2 only
    c. 1 and 3 only
    d. 1, 2, and 3

120. The image in the figure was most likely displayed in a window with a level of:
    a. −150
    b. 0
    c. +50
    d. +400

121. The major disadvantage of the back-projection method of image reconstruction is the appearance of the:
    a. partial volume effect
    b. ring artifact
    c. Gibb phenomenon
    d. star artifact

122. The most effective method of reducing involuntary motion on a CT image is:
    a. immobilization
    b. thorough explanation of the exam to the patient
    c. reduced scan times
    d. physical restraint

123. Soft copies of CT images are stored on which of the following media?
    1. hard drives
    2. magnetic optical disk
    3. laser film
    a. 3 only
    b. 1 and 2 only
    c. 1 and 3 only
    d. 2 and 3 only

124. The process of displaying CT images in a different orientation from the one used in the original reconstruction process is called:
    a. retrospective reconstruction
    b. prospective reconstruction
    c. multiplanar reformation
    d. multisegment reconstruction

125. The process of gray-scale mapping of the CT image may be referred to as:
    a. analog-to-digital conversion
    b. retrospective reconstruction
    c. prospective reconstruction
    d. windowing

126. In the formula used to calculate the linear attenuation coefficient, $I = I_0 e^{-\mu x}$, the symbol I_0 identifies:
    a. Euler constant
    b. incident intensity
    c. absorber thickness
    d. transmitted intensity

127. First-generation CT scanners possess which of the following characteristics?
    a. pencil-thin x-ray beam
    b. silver halide detectors
    c. rotate-rotate geometry
    d. nutating detector array

FIGURE 7-13

128. The intensity of the x-ray beam after it passes through an object to a detector is called the:
    a. incident intensity
    b. ray
    c. transmitted intensity
    d. primary beam

129. An accurate, modern CT scanner possesses a spatial resolution up to:
    a. 10 lp/mm
    b. 25 lp/mm
    c. 10 lp/cm
    d. 25 lp/cm

130. A high-resolution comb is utilized by an MSCT detector array in an effort to reduce:
    a. scatter radiation
    b. patient radiation dose
    c. low spatial frequency signal
    d. high spatial frequency signal

131. The distance between the centers of two adjacent reconstructed CT images is termed the:
    a. section width
    b. interpolation degree
    c. section interval
    d. sampling rate

132. The maximum number of simultaneous sections an MSCT system can acquire per gantry rotation is controlled by the number of:
    a. detector rows
    b. data channels
    c. focal spots
    d. x-ray tubes

133. *Matrix size* describes which of the following?
    a. aperture size used during data acquisition
    b. number of pixels used to display image
    c. relationship between the field of view and the algorithm
    d. the number of data channels available

Use Fig. 7-13 to answer questions 134-135.

134. The circle shown on the image in the figure is used to:
    a. magnify a portion of the image
    b. localize an area for percutaneous biopsy
    c. perform an ROI measurement
    d. produce an MPR image

135. The density measurement performed in the figure yielded an average CT number of zero. This area consists of:
    a. fat
    b. blood
    c. water
    d. air

136. The implementation of corrective actions to improve any identified performance inadequacies of the CT system is referred to as:
    a. quality control
    b. uniformity
    c. quality assurance
    d. linearity

137. The major disadvantage of the fan- or cone-shaped x-ray beams used in modern CT units in comparison with the "pencil-thin" beams of older units is:
    a. increased transmission measurements
    b. greater patient radiation dose
    c. decreased transmission measurements
    d. excess tube wear

138. When choosing a scan field of view (SFOV), the CT technologist is controlling the:
    1. diameter of data acquisition
    2. number of activated detectors within the array
    3. correction factors for the specific area of anatomic interest
    a. 2 only
    b. 1 and 2 only
    c. 1 and 3 only
    d. 1, 2, and 3

139. As the attenuation of a volume of tissue decreases, the transmitted intensity of a CT x-ray beam:
    a. increases
    b. remains unchanged
    c. decreases
    d. increases to a peak value and then rapidly decreases

140. Which of the following parameters or factors is improved by the selection of a smaller x-ray tube filament?
    a. scan time
    b. spatial resolution
    c. heat rating
    d. signal-to-noise ratio (SNR)

141. The geometric efficiency of a CT detector is influenced primarily by the:
    a. atomic number of the detector material
    b. size of the detector element
    c. size of the tube filament
    d. amount of interspace material between detectors

142. Which of the following factors may affect the attenuation of an object during CT data acquisition?
    a. beam pitch
    b. mA
    c. kVp
    d. algorithm

143. An image that is reconstructed a second time with some change in technical factor is said to be:
    a. reiterated
    b. post-processed
    c. retrospective
    d. reformatted

144. The Feldkamp-Davis-Kress (FDK) algorithm may be applied to MSCT acquisition data to overcome image artifacts from:
    a. patient motion
    b. beam hardening
    c. partial volume averaging
    d. beam divergence

145. MSCT systems are typically capable of differentiating adjacent objects with attenuation differences as small as:
    a. 3 HU
    b. 10 HU
    c. 25 HU
    d. 60 HU

146. The ability of an MSCT system to freeze motion and provide an image free of blurring is called:
    a. in-plane spatial resolution
    b. longitudinal spatial resolution
    c. temporal resolution
    d. contrast resolution

147. Ring artifacts on the CT image are associated with which of the following tube-detector geometries?
    a. rotate-nutate
    b. rotate-stationary
    c. rotate-rotate
    d. translate-rotate

148. What is the maximum beam collimation for an MSCT system with 16 rows of 1.25-mm detectors?
    a. 2.5 mm
    b. 5.0 mm
    c. 20.0 mm
    d. 40.0 mm

149. The polyenergetic x-ray beam emitted from a CT x-ray tube is susceptible to artifacts due to the phenomenon known as:
    a. beam hardening
    b. density bloom
    c. kerma
    d. partial volume

150. In an MSCT system, which of the following technical parameters determines the reconstructed section width?
    a. detector collimation
    b. number of data channels
    c. beam collimation
    d. detector pitch

151. Daily air or water calibration of the CT system is performed to evaluate which of the following components of image quality?
    a. contrast resolution
    b. temporal resolution
    c. uniformity
    d. linearity

152. The reduction in intensity of an x-ray beam as it interacts with matter is called:
    a. scatter
    b. attenuation
    c. transmission
    d. luminescence

153. Pixels whose average attenuation coefficients are less than the coefficient of water have which of the following types of CT number values?
    a. extremely large
    b. high positive
    c. negative
    d. high contrast

154. Which of the following actions would serve to magnify the CT image on the display monitor?
    a. decrease matrix size
    b. increase scan field of view
    c. decrease display field of view
    d. increase display field of view

155. The bit depth of a digital imaging system defines the number of information bits contained within each:
    a. pixel
    b. matrix
    c. axial image
    d. multiplanar reformation (MPR)
156. The technical factor(s) necessary for the acquisition of an isotropic data set is/are:
    1. thin detector collimation
    2. high mA setting
    3. small DFOV
    a. 1 only
    b. 1 and 3 only
    c. 2 and 3 only
    d. 1, 2, and 3

Use Fig. 7-14 to answer questions 157-159.

157. The limiting resolution of the bone algorithm in the figure is:
    a. 6.1 lp/cm
    b. 9.5 lp/cm
    c. 14.6 lp/cm
    d. 15.5 lp/cm
158. At an MTF of 20%, which reconstruction algorithm will demonstrate the greatest number of line pairs per centimeter (lp/cm)?
    a. bone
    b. standard
    c. smooth
    d. impossible to determine from the information provided
159. When one is assessing an MTF graph such as the figure, the limiting resolution is determined at a point where the signal frequency corresponding to a particular object has reached:
    a. 10%
    b. 20%
    c. 50%
    d. 100%
160. In multislice CT (MSCT), the combined thicknesses of all of the sections simultaneously acquired with each gantry rotation are called the:
    a. detector configuration
    b. beam pitch
    c. detector pitch
    d. total collimation
161. MSCT systems typically employ which of the following types of detectors?
    a. tungsten ring
    b. solid-state scintillation
    c. charged-coupled device (CCD)
    d. gas ionization

FIGURE 7-14

162. Which of the following technical adjustments may be employed to reduce step artifact in a multiplanar reformation CT image?
    1. acquisition of an isotropic data set
    2. overlapping section increment
    3. increase in effective mAs
    a. 1 only
    b. 1 and 2 only
    c. 2 and 3 only
    d. 1, 2, and 3
163. Which of the following is a manifestation of the partial volume artifact?
    a. cupping
    b. Hounsfield bar
    c. aliasing
    d. streaking
164. During volumetric CT acquisition, the slice sensitivity profile (SSP) graphically represents the:
    a. effective section width
    b. dose profile
    c. beam width
    d. detector collimation
165. An increase in the sampling rate during CT data acquisition corresponds to an increase in:
    a. views per rotation
    b. patient radiation dose
    c. image noise
    d. matrix size

Answer Key—Exam One

1. C

The partial thromboplastin time (PTT) is a laboratory measure of blood coagulation. This value is used for screening of patients for invasive procedures. Because of individual laboratory practices, the average range may fluctuate slightly.

2. B

A butterfly needle should be inserted at an angle of 15 degrees for the intravenous administration of contrast material. It is also important that the vein be properly stabilized and that the needle be inserted gently with the bevel facing upward.

3. D

The flow rate may be calculated by dividing the total contrast volume by the time of the injection. In this example, the total contrast volume is 125 mL and the time for the injection is 50 seconds. The flow rate programmed for this injection would be 125 ÷ 50, or 2.5 mL per second.

4. C

The CT dose index (CTDI) is used to quantify the radiation dose received by the patient during a CT scan. It involves the use of an ionization chamber to accurately measure radiation exposure for a given set of technical factors.

5. C

Prior reactions to contrast media and a history of asthma are factors that increase the incidence of adverse reaction to iodinated contrast media. It is therefore vital to question the patient regarding these factors prior to contrast agent administration. The presence of the human immunodeficiency virus (HIV) or hepatitis does not increase the incidence of adverse reaction to iodinated contrast media. Because universal precautions govern the protection of all patients and health care professionals, there is no need to question the patient regarding these factors.

6. D

GFR is calculated using the patient's measured serum creatinine level and takes into account the patient's age, sex, and race.

7. B

A bolus administration of contrast agent requires the entire volume of material to be injected over the shortest possible time. Accomplished by hand or with the use of an automatic injector, bolus administration provides the maximum plasma iodine concentration and subsequent tissue enhancement.

8. D

General signs and symptoms that a patient is going into shock include: rapid breathing, tachycardia, hypotension, weak pulse, pallor, cyanosis and cold, clammy skin.

9. D

SOLU-CORTEF is a brand name for hydrocortisone, which is a type of corticosteroid. This drug, or other types of corticosteroids, may be used during the treatment of anaphylactoid reactions to iodinated contrast materials.

10. C

With no consideration of image quality, reductions in mA and/or scan time (seconds) are direct methods of decreasing patient dose during a CT exam.

11. C

Non-ionic contrast media include iopamidol (Isovue), iohexol (Omnipaque), and iopromide (Ultravist).

12. B

The term dyspnea may be defined as the condition of difficult breathing.

13. C

An ionization chamber is a device used to accurately measure radiation exposure. Radiation causes ionization within the chamber, which is measured by an electrode. The amount of charged particles is proportional to the radiation exposure. The ionization chamber is an extremely accurate device that is used to quantify radiation exposure from a CT scan.

14. D

Implied consent occurs when a patient is in need of immediate medical services but is unconscious or physically unable to consent to treatment. The assumption is made that the patient would consent if able.

15. D

Complete cardiac diastole is the period of atrial and ventricular relaxation after heart contraction. The T wave of an ECG corresponds to cardiac diastole.

16. A

Iodinated water-soluble radiopaque contrast media (RCM) are injected directly into the joint space of interest during CT arthrography.

17. A

Iodixanol (Visipaque) is an example of a non-ionic iso-osmolar contrast agent. Iohexol (Omnipaque), iopamidol (Isovue), and ioversol (Optiray) are all non-ionic low-osmolar contrast media (LOCM).

18. D

Antecubital space refers to the anterior recess of the elbow. It contains the basilic vein medially and the cephalic vein laterally. Both veins are common sites for the IV administration of iodinated contrast media.

19. C

Contrast-induced nephrotoxicity (CIN) is a potentially serious delayed effect of contrast agent administration. It is a considerable decline in renal function that can occur after a patient receives an IV contrast agent. CIN is typically marked by an increase in serum creatinine concentration in comparison with a baseline measurement obtained prior to contrast agent administration.

20. C

Effective dose accounts for the type of tissue that the radiation is deposited in. Different tissues are assigned weighting factors on the basis of their individual radiosensitivities. Effective dose approximates the relative risk from exposure to low doses of ionizing radiation. The unit of measurement for effective dose is the sievert (Sv).

21. D

The use of a saline flush also improves the overall contrast agent utilization efficiency of the CT examination.

22. A

If not contraindicated, sublingual nitroglycerine may be administered just prior to the cardiac multislice CT (MSCT) study to cause dilation of the coronary vessels, improving their visualization. Please consult the referring physician and/or department protocol for further information regarding pharmaceutical administration for cardiac CT procedures.

23. B

The normal range for diastolic blood pressure in adults is 60-90 mm Hg. Diastolic pressure is the measurement of blood pressure at its lowest point, in between contractions of the heart.

24. B

Parenteral administration involves the injection of medication into the body. Common routes of parental medication administration include intramuscular, intravenous, intradermal, and subcutaneous.

25. D

The selected mA should be adapted to each patient according to size and/or weight. Eliminating unnecessary CT scans at the discretion of the physician is an additional way to reduce pediatric dose.

26. A

Certain harmful effects of exposure to diagnostic x-rays, such as cancer formation and genetic mutations, are said to be random, or stochastic, in nature. A *stochastic effect* is one that has no threshold dose but increases in probability with increasing dose.

27. C

Enteric precautions attempt to protect from the spread of infection through direct or indirect contact with fecal matter. Gowns and gloves are common protective devices used for enteric precautions. The use of a surgical mask is not warranted.

28. B

Ionic contrast media are salts consisting of sodium and/or meglumine.

29. A

CTDI$_w$ is calculated from measurements made with dosimeters positioned at the center and periphery of a phantom and accounts for the variance in dose distribution due to the effects of beam hardening.

30. A

Several factors may be regarded as contraindications to administration of iodinated contrast material, including known allergy to iodine, prior severe reaction, and renal insufficiency. Multiple myeloma and diabetes, although not absolute contraindications to IV administration of iodinated contrast agents, do require attention to the patient's hydration level to limit renal complications.

31. D

The dose length product (DLP) is the total patient dose over a given scan acquisition length (z) and can be illustrated as the product of CTDI$_{vol}$ and scan length. The DLP is expressed in units of milligrays per centimeter (mGy-cm).

32. D

Found typically in the emergency setting, a comprehensive acute stroke CT imaging protocol begins with a pre-contrast sequence to evaluate for hemorrhage. After the IV administration of an iodinated contrast agent, a

CTA acquisition is performed through the carotid vessels and brain. CTP is then performed to evaluate potential cerebral perfusion defects secondary to stroke.

33. A
Number 1 corresponds to the left pulmonary artery.

34. C
Number 4 corresponds to the superior vena cava.

35. D
Pleural effusions are commonly seen in the posterior portion of the lung field on images obtained with the patient in a supine position on the CT table. Differentiation between pleural effusion and pleural thickening is made when region of interest (ROI) measurements reveal fluid with density readings at or slightly above zero. Pleural effusion may be caused by multiple pathologic processes, including infection, neoplasm, and congestive heart failure.

36. B
Simple cysts contain primarily water and therefore exhibit CT numbers ranging from approximately 0 (or slightly below) to +20 Hounsfield units.

37. B
The arterial phase is the period of peak arterial enhancement typically occurring at 25 to 35 seconds after the initiation of contrast agent administration. During this phase, hypervascular tumors or tumors supplied by the hepatic artery undergo maximal enhancement.

38. C
Number 2 on the figure corresponds to the left internal carotid artery.

39. A
Number 5 on the figure corresponds to the right internal jugular vein.

40. D
Number 1 on the figure corresponds to the epiglottis.

41. D
The abdominal aorta descends to the level of the fourth lumbar vertebra (L4), where it bifurcates into the left and right common iliac arteries.

42. C
The least heart motion occurs at approximately 55% to 75% of the R-R interval, typically corresponding to the point of mid-diastole.

43. B
Small amounts of gas may appear in the areas of degenerated intervertebral discs. The accumulation of gases such as nitrogen occurs as a by-product of the physical breakdown of the disc material.

44. C
Spiral/helical CT examinations are obtained with the scanner continuously acquiring data as the patient travels through the gantry. The data acquired are volumetric, containing all of the attenuation information for a given area of anatomy.

45. C
Because of their increase in CT number, subdural hematomas may be well visualized without the IV administration of an iodinated contrast agent.

46. D
Excretory phase acquisitions after a delay of 3 to 15 minutes demonstrate the urinary tract while it is opacified with a contrast agent. Transitional cell lesions of the urothelium appear as filling defects within the bladder, ureters, and/or renal pelvis.

47. B
Number 1 on the figure corresponds to the stomach.

48. D
The location of the liver on the inferior portion of the image indicates that this patient is in the right lateral decubitus position.

49. B
The right lateral decubitus position is often used to differentiate the pancreatic head and the duodenum.

50. A
Number 2 on the figure corresponds to the right ureter.

51. C
A contiguous study with section widths ranging from 3 to 6 mm is sufficient for a general survey CT study of the neck.

52. C
Penumbra is the ischemic, yet still viable tissue immediately surrounding the infarct core. It can be described as the region of ischemic brain parenchyma where cerebral blood volume (CBV) is compromised but still higher than 2.5 mL per 100 g of tissue.

53. B
The wrist's scaphoid bone (navicular) is a common location for complex fracture.

54. D
Narrow sections (1-3 mm) are required in both the axial and coronal planes to properly demonstrate the orbits. Isotropic MDCT acquisition may provide multiplanar reformation images of sufficient quality to preclude the need for an additional scan in a second plane.

55. C

High-resolution CT is a specialized technique using narrow section widths and a high-resolution algorithm for image reconstruction. It is used to maximize detail of high spatial frequency tissue, such as the lungs and bony structures.

56. C

Electrocardiographic (ECG) gating can be utilized to eliminate pulsation artifacts due to cardiac motion during the study. Retrospective gating involves scanning throughout the entire cardiac cycle. Only data from specific user-determined portions of the ECG waveform are reconstructed into images.

57. B

The flow rate range 1.0 to 3.0 mL/sec should be sufficient to provide the enhancement necessary for proper evaluation of the abdomen. This is a general range that may be adjusted to meet the needs of the exam at the discretion of the physician and medical personnel involved for each patient.

58. B

Fatty liver disease, or hepatic steatosis, is a condition in which large quantities of fats (lipids) are retained within the liver. Whereas normal liver parenchyma exhibits attenuation values approximately 10 HU higher than those of the spleen, the liver with steatosis has attenuation values at least 10 HU below those of the spleen.

59. D

The renal pyramids are cone-shaped regions of the renal medulla. The wider bases of the renal pyramids border the renal cortex.

60. B

Beginning 30 to 40 seconds after the initiation of contrast agent administration, the corticomedullary phase demonstrates optimal enhancement of the renal cortex with maximum differentiation of the cortex from the renal medulla.

61. C

Number 2 on the figure corresponds to the right adrenal gland.

62. A

Number 6 on the figure corresponds to the psoas muscle.

63. A

Patient inspiration provides optimal chest expansion and allows for better demonstration of anatomic structures.

64. A

Routine CT scanning of the head should be performed with the gantry angled 15 degrees above the infraorbital-meatal line. This angle produces axial sections of the brain while limiting beam-hardening artifacts and direct orbital exposure.

65. D

The patient should be instructed to phonate the letter "E" during CT scanning of the larynx. As data are acquired during scanning, the patient's phonation requires vibration of the vocal cords, thus allowing for thorough evaluation of their mobility.

66. C

Number 2 on the figure corresponds to the cochlea.

67. D

Number 4 on the figure corresponds to the carotid canal.

68. A

Targeted reconstructions should be performed bilaterally utilizing a small display field of view (DFOV) or a higher zoom factor to maximize resolution of the small bony components of the inner ear.

69. A

Number 3 on the figure corresponds to the vestibule.

70. A

The *cul-de-sac* is the area posterior to the uterus and ovaries in the female patient. It is a common site for ascites in the patient with pelvic pathology.

71. A

Interstitial diseases of the lungs are usually diffuse pathologic processes involving the interstitium, or framework, of the lungs. Examples of interstitial diseases are bronchiectasis, emphysema, asbestosis, and sarcoidosis.

72. B

An enterovesical fistula is an abnormal communication between the bowel and the bladder. It typically results from inflammatory processes of the colon such as diverticulitis.

73. C

Catharsis describes the process of bowel cleansing that is required to improve the exam quality of CT colonography. A combination of restricted diet and bowel cleansing with polyethylene glycol (PEG) or magnesium citrate is used to achieve catharsis.

74. D

During a CT examination of the lumbar spine, a foam cushion should be placed under the patient's flexed knees. This maneuver reduces strain on the lower back, making the patient more comfortable and cooperative. It also reduces the lordotic curve of the lumbar spine, allowing for more accurate imaging of the intervertebral disc spaces.

75. C

The axial plane is parallel to the foot's plantar surface. The oblique axial plane is parallel to the metatarsals, approximately 20 to 30 degrees caudal from the direct axial plane.

76. B

Claudication refers to the condition of intermittent cramping pain in the legs due to poor circulation.

77. D

Ground-glass opacities are hazy areas of increased attenuation in the lungs and are often associated with the interstitial lung disease evaluated by HRCT.

78. C

Number 1 on the figure corresponds to the ascending aorta.

79. A

HRCT acquisitions of the chest should be performed with thin sections, within the range of 1 to 2 mm.

80. B

Number 2 on the figure corresponds to the anterior segment of the left upper lobe bronchus.

81. B

The pituitary and other structures involving the sella turcica are usually imaged in the coronal plane with CT. The coronal plane provides the best visualization of the pituitary gland with regard to its position within the sella turcica and involves less partial volume averaging of the pituitary with surrounding structures than scans obtained in the axial plane.

82. C

The spleen is the most common site of organ injury due to blunt abdominal trauma. Hematoma, hemorrhage, and laceration are typical signs of traumatic splenic injury.

83. B

Number 7 on the figure corresponds to the pancreatic head.

84. A

Number 2 on the figure corresponds to the superior mesenteric vein.

85. D

Number 8 on the figure corresponds to the ascending colon.

86. B

The spinal cord extends to the lower margin of the first or upper margin of the second lumbar vertebra. At this level it tapers to a point known as the *conus medullaris*.

87. C

Three-dimensional studies are best performed with the use of narrow sections acquired with no spacing or, preferably, an overlap. A detail (bone) algorithm is used for optimal demonstration of bony structures.

88. A

A *leiomyoma* is a benign mass of smooth muscle. It commonly occurs in the uterus and is readily identified on CT examination as a bulky, nonspecific uterine enlargement.

89. B

Number 4 on the figure corresponds to the ethmoid sinus.

90. A

The section thickness of a CT scan directly affects the detail and spatial resolution of the image. Narrow section widths result in greater detail for imaging of small anatomic parts such as the sinuses.

91. C

Number 2 on the figure corresponds to the zygomatic bone.

92. D

The peritoneal cavity is formed by the membranous sac called the *peritoneum*. It contains the stomach, liver, gallbladder, spleen, ovaries, transverse colon, and most of the small bowel.

93. C

Routine preparations for general studies of the abdomen and pelvis include the administration of an oral contrast agent for opacification of the GI tract. Patients are typically instructed to refrain from eating or drinking anything else for up to 6 hours prior to the exam. Polyethylene glycol (PEG) is used for bowel cleansing prior to a colonoscopy and may have certain applications for CT preparation limited to CT colonography.

94. A

Complete CT scans of the pelvis should include from the iliac crests to the pubic symphysis. This scan range may be extended if clinically warranted. Scan parameters (i.e., slice thickness, incrementation) can be adjusted to correlate with the patient's clinical history.

95. D

Acquisition of the cervical spine is performed with a large SFOV, 48 to 50 cm. Targeted reconstructions are made using a display field of view (DFOV) between 10 and 15 cm. Larger DFOV reconstructions may be used to retrospectively display a greater anatomic area as clinical indication dictates.

96. B

Number 4 on the figure corresponds to the cuboid.

97. C

The figure is a multiplanar reformation (MPR) in the sagittal plane.

98. A

Number 6 on the figure corresponds to the navicular.

99. D

Number 1 on the figure corresponds to the talus.

100. C

In comparison with the surrounding soft tissues, the thyroid gland is hyperdense on CT because it naturally contains iodine. This density increases further with administration of an iodinated contrast agent.

101. D

In the minimum intensity projection technique, displayed pixels represent the minimum attenuation value encountered along each sampled ray. Also referred to as min-IP, this type of multiplanar volume reconstruction (MPVR) can be applied to a volume of the thorax to demonstrate air trapping within the trachea and bronchial tree.

102. B

Number 5 on the figure corresponds to the anterior horn of the lateral ventricle.

103. B

Number 3 on the figure corresponds to the thalamus.

104. C

Number 4 on the figure corresponds to the septum pellucidum.

105. D

The small bowel consists of the duodenum, the jejunum, and the ileum. The cecum is the proximal portion of the large bowel; it is connected to the small bowel at the ileocecal valve.

106. C

Positron emission tomography (PET) is a functional nuclear medicine study utilizing fluorodeoxyglucose F 18 (FDG) as a radiopharmaceutical.

107. D

A CT cystogram involves the administration of an iodinated contrast agent directly into the bladder via a Foley catheter.

108. D

Multislice CT (MSCT) utilizes a cone-shaped beam that is incident upon an expanded array of detectors. The detector array consists of multiple rows along the z-axis and requires a cone-shaped beam to measure incident radiation.

109. C

Collimation of the x-ray beam in CT is accomplished by both pre-patient and pre-detector collimators, or detectors. The pre-patient detectors restrict the field size, directly influencing the reconstructed section thickness. The pre-detector or post-patient detectors absorb scatter radiation before it contributes to the signal produced by the detector array.

110. A

The *CT number* is a relative value based on the attenuation that occurs within a voxel of tissue. The Hounsfield unit is used for this value.

111. C

Interpolation is the mathematical process whereby data from tube rotations just above and just below a given slice position are used for image reconstruction. Interpolation allows for the reconstruction of a thin, motion-free image from a volumetric data set acquired from a moving patient.

112. A

The spatial resolution of a CT scanner can be measured by studying the amount of blurring that occurs around a point within the CT image. Known as the *point spread function* (PSF), this image unsharpness may be graphically represented. The spatial resolution can then be quantified by measuring the graph at half its maximum value. This measurement, called the *full width at half-maximum (FWHM)*, is used to illustrate the spatial resolution of a CT scanner.

113. C

First-generation CT scanners were based on a translate-rotate principle. The x-ray tube and detectors would translate across the patient's head and then rotate 1 degree. This process would repeat in a semicircular fashion, for 180 degrees around the patient's head.

114. B

Picture archival and communications systems (PACSs) are computerized networks charged with the responsibility of storing, retrieving, distributing, and displaying CT and other digital medical images.

115. C

The operator may control the contrast and brightness of the CT image by adjusting the "window" setting. As a form of gray-scale mapping, the window determines the pixels assigned shades of gray on the basis of their CT numbers.

116. B

Isotropic is used to describe voxels with equal dimensions along the x-, y- and z-axes. The ability to acquire an isotropic data set is a distinct advantage of MDCT.

117. D

Although the CT technologist must be able to readily identify them, ring artifacts are caused by detector malfunction and are beyond his/her control. Patient motion, partial volume averaging, and edge gradient artifacts can all be limited by the CT technologist through adequate preparation and careful scan procedures.

118. B

A standard MPR image is 1 voxel thick, with the pixels facing the viewer each representing the average attenuation occurring within the represented voxels.

119. D

Statistical noise is a term that may be used for quantum noise, or mottle. Caused by an insufficient number of photons being detected, this type of noise appears as graininess on the CT image.

120. C

The beam pitch for a given acquisition is equal to the table feed per rotation divided by the total collimation. The total collimation for this acquisition is equal to the total number of sections (detectors) multiplied by the detector dimension, or 64 × 0.625 mm. The table feed per rotation can be calculated as the product of the total collimation and the beam pitch, or 40 mm × 1.5, and equals 60 mm for the example provided.

121. B

The primary data processing component of the CT system is the array processor. It is responsible for receiving scan data from the host computer, performing all of the major processing of the CT image, and returning the reconstructed image to the storage memory of the host computer.

122. B

Retrospective reconstruction uses scan or "raw" data to change the matrix, DFOV, center, and/or algorithm used for a CT image. The slice thickness and SFOV are specifically used for data acquisition and cannot be altered retrospectively with a single-slice CT (SSCT) system. The advent of multislice CT (MSCT) technology has made retrospective adjustments in section width possible. The scan field of view (SFOV) remains an item that may not be altered retrospectively.

123. B

Misregistration is an artifact that occurs when a patient suspends respiration at different depths during consecutive scans. It results in the loss of anatomic information.

124. B

The analog-to-digital converter is responsible for transforming the analog signal from the detectors into a digital form that may be used by the computer. Analog information is based on a scale, whereas digital information is in numerical form.

125. C

The back-projection method of image reconstruction involves the acquisition of attenuation values, which are then projected back onto a matrix for subsequent display.

126. D

Magnetic optical disks vary in storage capacity, with some capable of storing several thousand 512^2 matrix CT images. This is considerably more than magnetic tape, which had previously been the standard choice for CT image archival.

127. B

The contrast of a CT image is controlled by the spatial frequencies of the tissue(s) within the section. Tissues of differing densities are represented electronically by different spatial frequencies. Adjacent tissues that greatly differ in density are represented by high spatial frequencies.

128. D

Noise is most commonly measured by scanning a water-filled phantom with a consistent set of technical factors. The image noise is equal to the standard deviation of pixel values within a region of interest (ROI) measurement of the image. Uniformity may also be evaluated by positioning several ROI measurements at different locations along the center and periphery of the image. The CT values should not differ by more than 2 HU from one location to another.

129. C

Beam hardening occurs as low-energy x-ray photons are absorbed while the beam passes through the patient. The average photon energy of the beam increases along the path and may result in a loss of system uniformity.

130. A

The image noise is equal to the standard deviation of pixel values within an ROI measurement of the image. ROI number 1 on the figure demonstrates the highest value for standard deviation (SD = 2.87).

131. B

An *algorithm* may be defined as a set of rules or steps used to solve a mathematical problem. The programs used by the CT computer to reconstruct the image are often referred to as algorithms.

132. C

The dimensions of a voxel are determined by multiplying the pixel dimensions by the slice thickness. The dimensions of a pixel are directly controlled by the matrix size and the field of view.

133. B

Increasing the display field of view (DFOV) for a reconstructed CT image decreases its displayed size.

Electronically magnifying the image on the display system results in a larger displayed image but has no effect on pixel or voxel dimension.

134. B
The average photon energy of the primary beam used in CT is approximately 70 keV. The average photon energy of any radiographic primary beam is typically 30% to 40% of the applied kilovoltage. The average photon energy of the CT beam is increased through beam filtration.

135. C
All MSCT systems utilize third-generation geometry and solid-state scintillation detectors.

136. B
Cine CT acquisition involves multiple axial scans obtained at a single anatomic level over a predetermined period. Clinical applications of cine CT acquisition include contrast bolus tracking, dynamic imaging of physiologic processes such as respiration, swallowing, and the cardiac cycle as well as for CT perfusion studies.

137. B
The rate at which a quantity of radiation (photon fluence) passes through a unit area over unit time is termed the *photon flux*. It may also be referred to as the *fluence rate*.

138. C
An average CT number value for bone is approximately +1000 HU. This may vary widely with the density of the particular bone in question and with the beam quality of the CT scanner.

139. A
Each CT image reconstructed on a 512^2 matrix is approximately 0.5 megabytes (MB) in digital size.

140. A
Linearity describes the relationship between the CT number and actual linear attenuation coefficients of an object. It is used to measure the accuracy of a CT scanner.

141. A
It is important that the calibration of a CT scanner be checked daily by the operator. CT units should be calibrated with their reference CT number for water at approximately zero. The CT number for air should be at approximately −1000.

142. D
Volume rendering adjusts the opacity of voxels included in the 3D model according to their tissue characteristics. Unlike the thresholding concept used for shaded-surface display (SSD), or surface rendering, volume rendering does not exclude voxels, but instead alters their appearance so that the 3D model contains the entire volume dataset.

143. A
The high-frequency generator used to produce the three-phase power used in modern CT scanners is located inside the gantry. It may be positioned in a corner of the gantry or fixed to the rotating tube assembly.

144. A
The *bit* is the smallest unit of information within the binary system. Its name is derived from the term "*binary digit*" and can appear as either a number 1 or 0. A sequence of eight bits constitutes a byte.

145. C
Eliminating the need for cables, slip-ring technology allows for continuous gantry rotation by utilizing a system of contact brushes that supply electricity to power the system, enabling the passage of transmission data to the computer system.

146. A
The process known as *convolution* is applied to reduce image unsharpness. An algorithm, or convolution kernel, acts as a mathematical filter, modifying the ray sum data and removing the unwanted blurring effect of the back-projection.

147. C
Contiguous images are those acquired with equal section thickness and interval. For example, 3.75-mm sections reconstructed every 3.75 mm completely cover a given volume of tissue with no unmeasured tissue.

148. B
When calculated by a formula comparing the attenuation coefficient of tissue with that of water, materials whose coefficients are greater than that of water are assigned positive CT numbers.

149. B
Pre-patient collimation influences the slice thickness by reducing the size of the primary beam. This is accomplished with the use of lead shutters that absorb the outer margins of the primary beam. Increases in pre-patient collimation diminish patient radiation dose by reducing the number of x-ray photons that reach the patient.

150. D
The Digital Imaging and Communications in Medicine (DICOM) standard confirms the process of recording, storing, printing, and transmitting medical image data.

151. A
The contrast resolution of a CT scanner depends on several factors, including section width, algorithm selection, detector sensitivity, and noise. The focal spot size is a geometric factor that influences the spatial resolution of a CT scanner.

152. B

The artifact present in the figure most likely represents an out-of-field artifact. This relatively large patient was incorrectly positioned, and a portion of the anatomy lies outside the scanned field of view. This improperly centered anatomy interferes with the reference detectors, thus causing a streak artifact near the unscanned area.

153. D

The out-of-field artifact present in this image could be easily reduced by properly centering the patient within the scan field of view.

154. B

Increases in filtration cause a greater amount of low-energy x-ray photons to be absorbed, thereby increasing the average photon energy of the beam. Higher mAs values increase the intensity of the beam but do not affect average photon energy.

155. C

Scintillation crystals are used in cooperation with photodiodes in a scintillation-type CT detector. The *photodiode* is a solid-state device that absorbs the light flashes given off by the crystal. The photodiode then emits an electrical signal in response to this light.

156. A

Automatic tube current modulation (ATCM) programs adjust the mA throughout an acquisition to reduce patient radiation dose to a minimum. ATCM automatically alters the applied mA on the basis of a predetermined noise index that is acceptable for appropriate image quality.

157. A

A uniform matrix array consists of multiple detectors in the longitudinal direction, each with the same dimensions.

158. B

The width of a window determines the range of pixel values that will be assigned shades of gray around a given level. In this example, all pixels within the range of −250 to +250 HU will be assigned shades of gray. Pixels below −250 HU will appear black, and pixels above +250 HU will appear white.

159. B

Orthogonal planes are at right angles to each other. Orthogonal reformations are perpendicular to the original plane of data acquisition.

160. A

The controlling factors of the temporal resolution of a CT system are the gantry rotation speed and reconstruction method. Temporal resolution can be improved by segmenting the data acquisition process into separate components of smaller rotation angles. Single-segment or half-scan acquisitions reconstruct data obtained from half of the rotation time. For example, this type of segmentation would yield a 250-msec temporal resolution from a 0.5-sec gantry rotation time.

161. D

Cone beam artifacts are unique to the cone beam geometry of MDCT systems and typically manifest much like partial volume artifacts.

162. C

The analytic methods of CT image reconstruction include the filtered back-projection and the Fourier transform method. These techniques are called *analytic* because they utilize precise formulas for image reconstruction.

163. B

The number of data channels controls the number of sections the scanner can simultaneously acquire with each gantry rotation. A 16-slice system possesses 16 data channels and is capable of acquiring 16 images per gantry rotation. The configuration of the detector array with regard to the size of individual detector elements controls the possible section widths for each reconstructed CT image.

164. D

The measurement of transmitted radiation made by an individual detector is called a *ray sum*. It equals the total attenuation occurring along a straight-line path from tube to detector.

165. C

The threshold setting is used to include and exclude information during the 3D reconstruction of a CT scan. For example, a high threshold (+150 HU) may be set to produce a 3D model of a bony structure. This threshold eliminates any density value below +150 HU from the data set. The reconstructed 3D model would include only bone tissue or any other substance with a Hounsfield value above +150.

Answer Key—Exam Two

1. A

Diastole refers to the relaxation of heart muscle. It is the period of the cardiac cycle that occurs between successive contractions of the heart muscle, which are known as systole.

2. C

High-osmolar contrast media (HOCM) are ionic agents that dissociate into charged particles (ions) in solution. Ionic contrast media are salts consisting of sodium and/or meglumine. Iothalamate meglumine and diatrizoate sodium are commonly known by the brand names Conray and HYPAQUE, respectively.

3. C

Many CT scanners allow the technologist to reduce the total rotation of the x-ray tube, thus reducing the scan time and subsequent patient radiation dose. This type of partial scan, commonly referred to as a "half-scan" or segmenting, is most often used to improve the temporal resolution of the acquisition.

4. C

Epinephrine (Adrenalin) is an adrenergic drug used as a bronchodilator. Diphenhydramine (Benadryl) may be used to block the physiologic effects of the body's release of histamine, thus reducing the allergic effect of the contrast material. Atropine should be used only to combat bradycardia during a vagal reaction to contrast material.

5. C

For all patients, regardless of age or sex indication, the CT protocol should be optimized according to size or weight.

6. D

The escape of contrast material from a needle or blood vessel into the subcutaneous tissues is called extravasation. It is also sometimes referred to as *infiltration*.

7. D

Good communication between the technologist and patient is an extremely important factor in the production of high-quality CT examinations. Patients can be made to feel more comfortable, and when they are given detailed instructions, their greater cooperation can improve the CT results.

8. A

MSAD (*multiple scan average dose*) accounts for the effects of image spacing, or bed index, on patient radiation dose during axial scanning. MSAD increases when slice thickness is greater than image spacing and decreases when slice thickness is less than the bed index.

9. B

Risk factors for contrast-induced nephrotoxicity (CIN) include pre-existing renal function compromise, dehydration, diabetes, myeloma, advanced age, and cardiovascular disease.

10. A

Because of the rotational nature of the x-ray tube, a patient receives exposure from all sides during a CT examination. Therefore, lead shielding should be placed above and below the patient.

11. D

Normal range of O_2 saturation as measured by a pulse oximeter is between 95% and 100%. Saturation levels below 95% may indicate respiratory insufficiency.

12. C

The laboratory measurements BUN (blood urea nitrogen) and serum creatinine (a component of urine) can be used to indicate the status of a patient's renal function.

13. D

Angiocatheters and higher-gauge needles are preferred for administration of a contrast agent with the use of a power injector. The stability of an angiocatheter maintains proper placement within the vein while withstanding the high pressure applied by the power injector.

14. D

The technologist and/or radiologist should always ask the patient about allergic history as well as current renal function status and history of cardiac illness (high blood pressure, congestive heart failure, and so on) prior to administration of any contrast material.

15. B

Nosocomial infections may be commonly referred to as health care–associated infections. They occur within the first 48 hours of a patient's stay in a health care facility.

16. A

As the beam traverses the patient, beam hardening alters the penetrability of the beam and affects the absorption across the field of view. The $CTDI_w$ is calculated by summing 2/3 of the exposure recorded at the periphery of the field with 1/3 of the centrally recorded radiation dose. This weighting yields a more accurate dose approximation.

17. B

The normal range for creatinine level is 0.5 to 1.5 mg/dL. The normal range for BUN levels is 7 to 25 mg/dL. Creatinine and BUN are laboratory measurements that may be used to evaluate the renal function of a patient scheduled to undergo a CT examination that involves intravenous administration of an iodinated contrast agent.

18. A

Larger-lumen (lower-gauge) needles allow for more rapid intravenous administration of contrast media. The lumen is considerably larger in a 19-gauge needle than in a 25-gauge needle. The viscosity of contrast material necessitates the use of a relatively large-bore needle.

19. A

The fetus is most susceptible to the harmful effects of ionizing radiation during the first trimester of the gestation period.

20. C

Patients may be assigned to a higher-risk group for an adverse reaction to iodinated contrast material on the basis of several factors, including previous allergic history and physical condition. Patients considered to be at high risk for adverse reactions should be administered non-ionic contrast material. Iso-osmolar contrast material is an alternative choice that may also reduce the risk of adverse reactions.

21. D

Examples of mild adverse reactions to iodinated contrast material are nausea, vomiting, mild urticaria, and a warm, flushed sensation. Dyspnea is a moderate reaction, whereas pulmonary edema and shock are severe reactions to contrast media.

22. D

The patient is required to provide informed consent prior to the start of any invasive procedure. The administration of intravascular contrast material is invasive in nature and requires the informed consent of the patient.

23. A

Because of the inherent differences in manufactured batches of tissue factor, the International Normalized Ratio (INR) is calculated to standardize PT results. The INR compares a patient's PT with a control sample for a more accurate result.

24. B

Insertion of any intravenous line requires the use of sterile technique to prevent microorganisms from entering the bloodstream.

25. B

All detectors of the MDCT array must be exposed to x-rays of equal intensity. The beam must be expanded even further to avoid exposing the detectors to undesirable "penumbra." This process is referred to as *overbeaming*.

26. D

Common sites for intravenous contrast injection are the antecubital, basilic, cephalic, and accessory cephalic veins.

27. A

Intrathecal injections of iodinated contrast material are used in the CT evaluation of the lumbar spine. This type of injection introduces contrast material directly into the subarachnoid space, which is located between the arachnoid and pia mater. The subarachnoid space contains the cerebrospinal fluid.

28. C

ATCM is a form of automatic exposure control for a CT system. It manages patient radiation dose on the basis of the size, density, and overall attenuation of the part being examined.

29. A

The serum iodine concentration is a measure of the amount of iodine within the bloodstream. The specific dose depends on the patient's age, weight, and renal function, as well as on the clinical indication for the CT procedure. The specific criteria of intravenous contrast administration must always be directed by a physician.

30. A

Additional components of the aseptic technique include cleaning the site of venipuncture in a circular motion with alcohol swab before injection, and applying pressure with an alcohol swab to the site after removal of the needle or catheter. It is *sterile* technique that involves establishing a sterile field around the area of an invasive procedure.

31. B

Kerma may be used to describe absorbed dose. *Air kerma* is the amount of radiation absorbed in a quantity of air.

32. D
Number 4 in the figure corresponds to the large colon (splenic flexure).

33. C
Number 2 in the figure corresponds to the portal vein.

34. A
Morison's pouch is the common name for the hepatorenal recess, which is indicated by number 7 in the figure. This space between the liver and right kidney is a common location for the abnormal collection of fluid known as ascites.

35. B
Number 6 in the figure corresponds to the superior mesenteric artery.

36. D
Number 3 in the figure corresponds to the pancreas.

37. A
Thin sections are required to properly assess abnormalities of the minute structures of the inner ear. The thinnest sections possible provide maximum detail.

38. A
The *Lisfranc joint* is the articulation between the tarsals and metatarsals; it can be the site of complex fractures and dislocations of the foot.

39. C
The Agatston scoring system quantifies the volume and density of calcium within the coronary arteries.

40. B
Adnexa is used to describe an appendage of an organ. The ovaries and fallopian tubes constitute the uterine adnexal region.

41. C
CTA of the neck is used primarily to evaluate the carotid arteries.

42. D
Opacification of the stomach and bowel loops is imperative during general CT examinations of the abdomen and pelvis. Effervescent agents may be used to ensure proper gastric distention. Intravenous contrast agents are used to opacify blood vessels and are helpful in anatomic differentiation and evaluation of mass vascularity.

43. C
The liver has a dual blood supply, receiving 75% of its supply from the portal vein and the remaining 25% from the hepatic artery.

44. A
Number 3 on the figure corresponds to the superior rectus muscle.

45. B
Number 2 on the figure corresponds to the optic nerve.

46. D
The image is a multiplanar reformation (MPR) image through the orbit in the oblique sagittal plane.

47. C
Number 1 on the figure corresponds to the inferior oblique muscle.

48. D
The acetabulum is a cup-shaped cavity that holds the head of the femur, forming the hip joint. It is composed of portions of the ilium, ischium, and pubis.

49. B
Number 6 on the figure corresponds to the azygos vein.

50. B
Number 4 on the figure corresponds to the pectoralis minor muscle.

51. C
With the lung fields black, the bony structures white, and the mediastinum and muscles gray, the image in the figure is displayed in a soft tissue window.

52. A
Number 1 on the figure corresponds to the superior vena cava.

53. C
It is widely recommended that volumetrically acquired CT sections be reconstructed with the use of at least a 50% overlap to improve the quality of 3D and MPR images.

54. A
Positron emission tomography (PET) provides a map of normal and abnormal tissue function. It offers excellent sensitivity for malignancy but suffers from an inability to accurately localize tumor activity. Fusion of PET with CT provides such precise anatomic localization.

55. A
Spondylolisthesis refers to the forward "slipping" of an upper vertebral body over the lower as a result of degenerative changes of the facet joints.

56. B
Number 2 on the figure corresponds to the sigmoid colon.

57. C
Number 3 on the figure corresponds to the seminal vesicles.

58. A
Number 1 on the figure corresponds to the rectus abdominis muscle.

59. C
Number 4 on the figure corresponds to the ureterovesical junction (UVJ).

60. C
Contrast enhancement greatly improves demonstration of lymphadenopathy within the chest in comparison with other mediastinal structures.

61. A
The frontal sinuses are absent at birth and do not usually fully develop until after puberty. The ethmoidal, maxillary, and sphenoidal sinuses begin to develop during gestation.

62. C
Thin-section (0.5-2.0 mm) helical acquisition specific to the larynx should extend from just above the hyoid bone inferiorly through the cricoid cartilage.

63. C
The most common indication for CT-guided percutaneous biopsy is to confirm the malignancy of a mass.

64. B
This technique allows for visualization of the relationship between the patella and the femur as the knee is increasingly flexed. The *patellofemoral congruence*, or the position of the patella within the patellar surface of the femur, may be measured at each point of flexion. Any medial or lateral displacement of the patella may indicate an abnormality of the patellofemoral joint.

65. C
Number 3 on the figure corresponds to the glenoid process.

66. A
The image is a multiplanar reformation (MPR) of the right shoulder in the coronal plane. This perspective demonstrates the relationship between the humeral head and the glenoid fossa (4).

67. B
Number 2 on the figure corresponds to the acromion.

68. B
The administration of an oral contrast agent is subject to specific departmental protocol considerations. Generally, 400 to 600 mL of oral contrast administered 45 to 90 minutes prior to the exam should opacify the small bowel. An additional dose of contrast agent (250 mL) immediately before the exam should ensure gastric opacification. Administration of contrast agents via enema is indicated for evaluation of the distal large bowel.

69. B
Cerebral blood flow (CBF) describes the quantity of blood (in mL) that moves through 100 g of brain tissue each minute. Normal CBF range in gray matter is 50 to 60 mL/100 g/min.

70. B
Number 3 in the figure corresponds to the trapezius muscle.

71. C
A total contrast agent volume between 100 and 150 mL is sufficient for imaging the neck. The precise volume and administration technique vary from one institution to another.

72. A
Number 1 on the figure corresponds to the common carotid artery.

73. D
Number 4 on the figure corresponds to the levator scapulae muscle.

74. B
Differentiation between a metastatic lesion and a benign adenoma of the adrenal can be accomplished by calculating the percentage of enhancement washout after a 10- to 15-minute delay. Pre-contrast, portal venous phase, and delayed acquisitions are obtained. On delayed post-contrast imaging, metastatic lesions of the adrenal gland remain enhanced longer than adrenal adenomas.

75. C
Ileus is used to describe an area of intestine that has lost normal contractile motion, resulting in obstruction.

76. B
Number 5 on the figure corresponds to the descending colon.

77. C
Number 3 on the figure corresponds to the abdominal aorta.

78. A
Demonstrating the same density and contrast as a conventional helically acquired axial image, the coronal display in the figure is a standard MPR image. *Multiplanar*

reformation (MPR) describes the process of displaying CT images in a different orientation from the one used in the original reconstruction process. The reformatted image is 1 voxel thick, with the pixels facing the viewer each representing the average attenuation occurring within the represented voxels.

79. C
Number 6 on the figure corresponds to the bladder.

80. A
The renal arteries are small structures that are optimally visualized with MDCT section widths of 1.25 mm or less.

81. C
The third and fourth ventricles communicate through the cerebral aqueduct, which is commonly referred to as the *aqueduct of Sylvius.*

82. C
Complete CT examination of the chest for bronchogenic carcinoma consists of an acquisition from the apices through the liver. The adrenal gland and liver are common sites for metastatic disease in patients with primary lung neoplasm. Scanning may be done in a caudocranial direction to ensure maximum contrast enhancement of the liver and adrenals when indicated.

83. C
The mediastinum is a potential space located between the two lungs. It contains the heart, great blood vessels, thymus, and portions of the trachea and esophagus.

84. D
The SFOV chosen must be larger than the width of the patient in order to eliminate out-of-field artifacts. Some CT scanners may have limited choices for SFOV values. Other common terminology includes full- or half-field, and body-cal and head-cal.

85. D
The kidneys are located in a portion of the retroperitoneum known as *Gerota's space.* They are held in place by fibrous connective tissue commonly referred to as *Gerota's fascia.*

86. C
The portal (or hepatic) venous phase is the period of peak hepatic parenchymal enhancement, when contrast material redistributes from the blood into the extravascular spaces. It occurs at approximately 60 to 70 seconds after the initiation of rapid bolus contrast agent administration.

87. D
Number 1 on the figure corresponds to the genu of the corpus callosum.

88. B
Number 6 on the figure corresponds to the falx cerebri.

89. B
Number 2 on the figure corresponds to the internal capsule.

90. A
Number 3 on the figure corresponds to the pineal gland.

91. C
The prone position during a post-myelogram CT study of the lumbar spine reduces pooling or layering of the intrathecal contrast material.

92. D
Bolus duration, or the time required to inject a specific volume of contrast agent, may be calculated as the product of injection flow rate and total contrast volume.

93. D
Low values for kVp and mA and short CT fluoroscopy time all reduce occupational radiation exposure. Greater distance from the source, as with the use of a needle holder to keep the operator's hands out of the CT fluoroscopy field, also greatly diminish exposure. Additional methods of exposure reduction are lead shielding, leaded patient drapes, and the utilization of a last-image-hold function to cut down on continuous CT fluoroscopy.

94. B
Number 4 on the figure corresponds to the lamina.

95. A
Number 1 on the figure corresponds to the pedicle.

96. B
Intrathecal administration of an iodinated contrast agent allows for greater visualization of the spinal cord and nerve roots after its introduction into the subarachnoid space.

97. D
Number 3 on the figure corresponds to the spinous process.

98. B
The pancreatic phase of contrast enhancement is a delayed arterial phase occurring approximately 35 to 45 seconds after the start of contrast agent administration, assuming an adequate volume injected at a rate of 3 mL/sec or greater.

99. A
Upon IV contrast enhancement, a tumor may be described as *hypovascular* if it is lower in density than the surrounding organ parenchyma or *hypervascular* if it is higher in density.

100. C

The *retroperitoneum* is the space located between the peritoneum and the posterior abdominal wall. It contains the duodenum, pancreas, adrenal glands, kidneys, ureters, and bladder.

101. B

The *"triple rule-out" MDCT procedure* is a comprehensive evaluation of the chest for cardiac and noncardiac pain. The single acquisition consists of a coronary CTA for coronary artery disease, a CTA of the aorta for aneurysm, and a CTA of the pulmonary arteries for embolism.

102. B

There is often significant artifact within the mediastinum from high concentrations of iodine in the superior vena cava. This artifact may be alleviated by administering a bolus of a contrast agent with reduced iodine concentration, which is achieved by diluting a full-strength contrast agent with saline.

103. D

Number 3 on the figure corresponds to the left primary bronchus.

104. B

Dense contrast opacification of the aorta and pulmonary arteries indicates that this image was obtained during the arterial phase, most likely within the first 20 to 30 seconds after bolus injection of contrast material.

105. A

Number 2 on the figure corresponds to the left pulmonary artery.

106. C

Number 6 on the figure corresponds to the ascending aorta.

107. B

The density of the mass in question indicates that it consists of fatty tissue. A *lipoma* is a benign mass consisting of fat cells. An *angiomyolipoma*, a common benign mass found in the kidney, consists of muscle cells, blood vessels, and fat. The average CT value range for fat is −50 to −100 Hounsfield units.

108. D

The *array processor* is a specialized component of the CT computer system. It is capable of performing the massive calculations required for CT image reconstruction.

109. A

Modern CT system x-ray tubes utilize dual-filament systems with focal spot sizes ranging between 0.5 and 1.2 mm in diameter.

110. A

Storage on film is considered to be a *hard copy*. The digital storage of CT images on PACS, CD-ROM, MOD, and so on, is referred to as *soft copy*.

111. B

The spatial resolution of a CT examination can be improved with the use of small focal spots, narrow sections, and large matrices.

112. C

The back-projection method of image reconstruction involves the acquisition of attenuation values, which are then projected back onto a matrix for subsequent display.

113. D

Multiple–detector row CT systems utilize the process called *z-filtering* during image reconstruction. Z-filtering allows for thin sections to be reconstructed at any point along the acquired z-axis volume. This interpolation technique utilizes multiple complimentary rays beyond those immediately above and below the particular slice plane.

114. C

Fourth-generation CT scanners operate with a rotating x-ray tube and a stationary ring of detectors. Some fourth-generation scanners also use a rotating x-ray tube with a nutating detector ring.

115. D

Aliasing is a type of streak artifact caused when an insufficient number of views (data samples) is obtained during data acquisition. It is typically due to a technical failure of the CT system.

116. C

Quality assurance refers to the measurement of the scanner's performance through quality testing procedures and evaluation of the test results. *Quality control* refers to the implementation of corrective actions to improve any identified performance inadequacies of the CT system found through quality assurance procedures.

117. D

The mA setting in coordination with the scan time (seconds) gives the constant mAs for a CT acquisition.

118. D

The filtered back-projection, or convolution, method of image reconstruction is used by most modern CT scanners.

119. D

The matrix size used to reconstruct an image can be calculated by dividing the display field of view (DFOV) by the pixel dimension. A pixel whose area is 0.25 mm² has a linear dimension of 0.5 mm. Dividing the DFOV of 250 mm by the pixel dimension 0.5 mm gives a matrix size of approximately 512 × 512 pixels.

120. C

Min-IP images display the minimum pixel value along each ray to the viewer. As the viewer faces a min-IP image, each pixel represents the minimum attenuation that occurs in the associated voxel. Min-IP reformations are used primarily during the evaluation of the biliary tree, colon, lungs, and trachea.

121. D

The purposes of pre-detector or post-patient collimation are to remove scatter radiation and to shape the portion of the beam that is incident on each detector.

122. D

The Lambert-Beer law or equation is properly written as $I = I_0 e^{-\mu x}$. This important exponential equation illustrates the mathematical relationship between the primary beam, the object thickness (density), and the radiation measured by each detector in the calculation of the linear attenuation coefficient (μ).

123. B

The longitudinal spatial resolution is usually qualified by the extent of broadening that occurs to the slice sensitivity profile (SSP) during volumetric acquisition. The section width (slice) for a volumetric acquisition may be graphically represented as a slice sensitivity profile (SSP).

124. C

The section width (slice) for a volumetric acquisition may be graphically displayed as a slice sensitivity profile (SSP). The effective section width is defined as the full-width at half-maximum (FWHM) of the SSP. The full-width at half-maximum is labeled in the figure as C. At this point of the graph, the section width of B is wider than that of A.

125. A

Thorough communication between the technologist and the patient is vital in ensuring superior exam quality. If the patient has been informed of the exam process, his/her anxiety may be reduced and cooperation improved. During all CT procedures, the patient must be instructed to hold still in an effort to reduce motion artifact on the CT images.

126. A

Because of its high atomic number and relative stability, xenon gas is commonly used in gas ionization CT detectors.

127. D

The power output of modern MDCT systems is vendor-specific, within a typical range of 60 to 100 kilowatts (kW).

128. D

The terms *algorithm*, *kernel*, and *mathematical filter function* may all be used interchangeably in describing the mathematical process used for the complex calculations required during CT image reconstruction.

129. C

The SFOV size is determined by the number of detectors activated along the in-plane (x-, y-) axes during data acquisition.

130. C

An average range of CT numbers for blood is +42 to +58. The CT number of any material is based on many factors, including the beam quality of a particular scanner.

131. A

Binning refers to the electronic combination of signal from adjacent detectors to form a reconstructed slice that is thicker than the individual detector width. For example, transmission data from four adjacent 1.25-mm detectors is combined to produce a CT section 5.0 mm thick.

132. D

Technical adjustments to improve the temporal resolution of the CT system may help reduce involuntary motion artifacts. Reductions in scan time (gantry rotation), image segmentation, and physiologic gating can be used to reduce the effects of involuntary motion.

133. D

The dense bony areas of the posterior fossa of the skull are especially prone to beam-hardening artifacts. *Hounsfield bar* is commonly used to describe this particular artifact.

134. A

The relative accuracy between calculated CT numbers and their respective linear attenuation coefficients is termed *linearity*. Calibration and routine vendor maintenance procedures work to establish and maintain CT system linearity.

135. D

Digital encryption is used to encode data that is transferred across a network into a form decipherable only by software at the destination location.

136. C

Perspective volume rendering provides one a viewpoint of being within the lumen of the object, similar to an endoscopic view. Also referred to as *immersive rendering*, this type of 3D reconstruction is commonly used during CT colonography and CT bronchography.

137. D

Thin-section reconstruction using the smallest display field of view (DFOV) possible results in the smallest pixel and voxel dimensions. Voxels with equal dimensions along the x-, y- and z-axes are described as *isotropic*.

138. B

CT does not employ silver halide crystal as a detector material.

139. B

Interpolation is a mathematical technique used in the reconstruction process of the spiral CT image. It involves the estimation of an unknown value from information above and below it.

140. D

Misregistration is the loss of anatomic information that occurs when a patient suspends respiration at different depths during consecutive scans. It occurs only during CT examinations in which suspended respiration of the patient is necessary. The ability of MDCT systems to volumetrically acquire entire anatomic areas in a single, short breath-hold has greatly reduced the occurrence of misregistration artifact.

141. C

Single-slice helical geometry allows for volumetric data acquisition. The reconstruction of CT sections at any point along the scanned volume is possible. The section width must be the same, however, and is controlled by the collimation (slice thickness) chosen prior to data acquisition. The advancement of multislice CT (MSCT) allows for retrospective reconstruction of sections at varying thicknesses.

142. C

Bow-tie filters, which are thicker at the ends than in the middle, help shape the beam to reduce patient radiation exposure. Because most body parts are circular or cylindrical, less radiation is necessary at the periphery than in the center. Bow-tie filters reduce beam intensity toward the outer margins, resulting in a reduction in patient radiation dose.

143. D

The thickness of the reconstructed section is controlled primarily by the detector configuration in an MDCT system. Beam collimation also exerts an indirect effect on section width by controlling the portion of the detector array exposed to transmitted radiation.

144. B

Noise appears on the CT image as an inaccuracy in CT number. The noise of a CT scanner may be measured by scanning a homogeneous object such as a water phantom. Fluctuations in CT number from pixel to pixel indicate the presence of noise.

145. D

The region of interest (ROI) measurement provides a quantitative analysis of the Hounsfield values of a specific anatomic area. System software calculates the average CT number in HUs within the defined ROI. The average ROI measurement provides information regarding tissue characteristics that may be helpful for clinical diagnosis.

146. A

The linear dimension of the pixel must first be calculated by dividing the DFOV, in mm, by the matrix (380 mm ÷ 512 = 0.74 mm) . This linear pixel dimension is squared to yield the pixel area in mm^2 (0.74 × 0.74 = 0.55 mm^2). The volume of the voxel may be calculated by multiplying the pixel area by the section width 0.55mm^2 × 1.25mm = 0.69 mm^3).

147. B

The presence of metal within the patient causes a streak artifact on the image. The artifact occurs when the dense metal absorbs a large amount of the radiation, interfering with the signal produced.

148. A

Metallic dental fillings often cause a streak artifact during CT examinations of the head.

149. C

An isotropic axial acquisition of the paranasal sinuses from the hard palate superiorly through the frontal sinus avoids artifact from dental fillings while providing excellent multiplanar reformations (MPRs) in any plane. Direct coronal acquisition may not be required because the detail provided by the reformatted images is usually sufficient. This technique also aids in reducing patient radiation dose.

150. C

The first-generation CT scanner acquired data through a process based on the principle of tube translation and rotation around the patient's head.

151. D

At a maximum, the MSCT cone beam may be collimated to a dimension equal to the entire multirow detector array. In the example, the total dimension of the detector array along the z-axis is 40.00 mm, or 64 × 0.625 mm.

152. A

Computed tomography has better low-contrast resolution over conventional radiography. The CT system is extremely sensitive to small changes in tissue density and also removes the problem of superimposition, both leading to greater contrast resolution.

153. C

Write-once, read-many (WORM) describes certain CD and DVD media capable of storing data only once.

The stored images can be read multiple times, but once recorded on, the media may not be reused.

154. A

The CT number of a pixel may be calculated by subtracting the linear attenuation coefficient of water from the linear attenuation coefficient of the tissue within the voxel ($0.008 - 0.181 = -0.173$). This number is divided by the linear attenuation coefficient of water ($-0.173 \div 1.81 = -0.956$). The quotient is multiplied by a contrast factor of 1000 to yield the value of the pixel in Hounsfield units.

155. B

Automatic tube current modulation (ATCM) programs adjust the mA throughout an acquisition to reduce patient radiation dose to a minimum. ATCM automatically alters the applied mA on the basis of a predetermined noise index that is acceptable for appropriate image quality.

156. B

Because of its solid nature, the scintillation detector interacts with a higher percentage of incident x-ray photons, giving it a better capture efficiency.

157. D

The DAS of a CT scanner consists of the detector array, the analog-to-digital convertor, and a transmission device used to send the converted digital information to the computer for image reconstruction.

158. A

During CT image reconstruction using the back-projection method, the data are manipulated with a convolution kernel or algorithm to remove image unsharpness (blurring). This method is called the filtered back-projection.

159. D

The oversampling technology known as *flying focal spot* involves the electromagnetic steering of the electron beam emitted from the cathode. The beam of electrons is directed toward two separate locations on the rotating anode, resulting in two sources of x-radiation. As the tube rotates around the patient, the number of data samples is essentially doubled because of the electronic switching between the two focal spots, improving the system's temporal and spatial resolution.

160. D

Water has a CT number at or near zero. This area in the ROI in the figure most likely represents a hepatic cyst.

161. C

At the range of photon energies employed during most CT examinations, water exhibits an approximate attenuation coefficient value of 0.206.

162. B

The width of a window used to display a CT image of the abdomen should be within the range of 350 to 600 HU. This range allows for excellent visualization of the soft tissue structures.

163. D

The contrast of a CT image is controlled by the spatial frequencies of the tissue(s) within the section. Tissues of differing densities are represented electronically by different spatial frequencies. Adjacent tissues with similar densities or areas of tissue with minimal differences in density are represented by low spatial frequencies.

164. C

The width of a window determines the range of pixel values that will be assigned a shade of gray around a given level. In this example, all pixels within the range of -300 to $+700$ HU will be assigned shades of gray. Pixels below -300 HU will appear black, and pixels above $+700$ HU will appear white. This calculation is performed by dividing the width in half ($1000/2 = 500$) and subtracting and adding this value to the level ($+200$ HU $+ 500 = +700$ HU, $+200$ HU $- 500 = -300$ HU).

165. C

A *byte* is a series of eight bits. Bits and bytes are part of the binary language used by computers to process information.

1. D

In-plane bismuth shielding of particularly radiosensitive areas such as the orbits, thyroid, and breast tissue can substantially reduce effective radiation dose.

2. D

The use of water as a negative contrast agent is becoming increasingly common for many CT applications for the abdomen and pelvis.

3. C

With an SSCT system, pitch equals the ratio of the table speed with the section thickness. As the detector pitch is increased, the patient translates through the gantry at a greater rate relative to each rotation of the x-ray tube, resulting in the acquisition of a given volume of anatomy with fewer tube-detector rotations and shorter scan times. Increases in pitch therefore allow for reduced patient radiation dose while covering the necessary anatomic area.

4. A

The top number of a blood pressure measurement is the *systolic* pressure. This is a measure of the pressure exerted on the arterial walls during a contraction of the heart.

5. B

Non-ionic contrast materials do not dissociate into charged particle (ions) when placed in solution. *Ionic* contrast materials are salts that form independent particles in aqueous solutions.

6. B

The $CTDI_{vol}$ is a measure of dose to each slice along a helically acquired volume. The dose length product (DLP) is calculated by multiplying the $CTDI_{vol}$ by the total scan length.

7. C

CT manufacturers routinely supply comfortable, nonadhesive straps and cushions to help maintain motion-free patient positioning. Adhesive tape should not be routinely used because of the abrasive effects of tape removal. Good patient communication is a key immobilization technique. Proper instructions for remaining still, suspending respiration, not swallowing, and so on, help ensure patient cooperation and yield higher-quality CT examinations.

8. C

Normal range of GFR is 70 ± 14 mL/min/m^2 for men and 60 ± 10 mL/min/m^2 for women.

9. B

Effective dose accounts for the type of tissue that the radiation is deposited in. Different tissues are assigned weighting factors on the basis of their individual radiosensitivities.

10. C

Risk factors for contrast-induced nephrotoxicity (CIN) include pre-existing compromise of renal function, dehydration, diabetes, myeloma, advanced age, and cardiovascular disease.

11. A

Medical asepsis is the reduction in number of infectious agents without the complete elimination of the organisms. It is accomplished through the use of soap, water, and many other types of disinfectant materials.

12. A

Patients with slower heart rates exhibit longer diastolic phases, which yield higher-quality cardiac CT exams. The preferred heart rate for optimal imaging on most MSCT systems is 65 beats per minute (bpm). Newer systems at the 64-slice level and beyond are capable of acquiring adequate cardiac CT images at higher heart rates.

13. A

A *stochastic,* or random, effect of radiation exposure is one having no threshold dose. Common examples of stochastic radiation effects are genetic mutations and cancer.

14. C

Urticaria is a common adverse reaction to iodinated intravenous contrast material. Characterized by the presence of wheals or localized skin eruptions, it is commonly referred to as "hives."

15. B

Barium sulfate is not water soluble and is not easily absorbed by the body. If it leaks out of the digestive tract because of perforation, this agent may cause peritonitis.

16. C

The use of automatic injectors does not decrease the risk of CIN in comparison with the manual bolus technique. Automatic injectors do offer shorter injection times, more consistent administration, and greater enhancement.

17. A

Severe reactions to iodinated contrast material include anaphylaxis, shock, cardiac arrest, and death. Urticaria and vomiting may be considered mild or moderate reactions, depending on their severity.

18. B

Serum creatinine levels are the most accurate and dependable laboratory measures of renal function. The blood urea nitrogen (BUN) level may be affected by many variables and is not a suitable test of renal function by itself. BUN levels are usually evaluated in conjunction with creatinine levels for a more accurate measurement of renal function.

19. C

22-gauge angiocatheters are sufficient for flow rates up to 3 mL/sec. 20-gauge or larger angiocatheters should be utilized whenever flow rates exceed 3 mL/sec.

20. A

Atrial systole refers to the contraction of the left and right atria. The onset of the P wave on an ECG corresponds to atrial systole.

21. B

During axial scanning, overlapping scans increase the patient radiation dose, whereas gaps between slices decrease the dose.

22. B

A *bolus injection* is one in which the entire volume of medication or contrast agent is administered at once over a short period.

23. B

Osmolality or *osmotic concentration* is the number of ions or particles formed when a substance (solute) dissociates in a given solution. It is described as the number of particles in solution per kg of water.

24. C

$CTDI_{vol}$ is used to approximate the dose from a helical scan. It corresponds to the axially acquired $CTDI_w$ divided by the helical pitch. Whereas $CTDI_w$ approximates dose along the x- and y-axes of the acquired CT image, $CTDI_{vol}$ also includes dose along the z-axis of the scan acquisition. As pitch increases, the dose per section, or $CTDI_{vol}$, decreases.

25. C

The total injection time may be calculated by dividing the contrast agent volume by the flow rate. In this example, the flow rate is 1.5 mL/sec, for a total of 150 mL. The time required for this injection would be 100 seconds.

26. D

Informed consent must be obtained from the patient prior to any invasive procedure. The components of informed consent are thorough explanations of the procedure, any possible risks in addition to the proposed benefits, and alternatives to the procedure.

27. C

During MSCT cardiac studies, prospective gating can be used to reduce patient radiation dose. In this technique, ECG-triggered tube current modulation allows for pulses of x-ray energy to be used rather than continuous exposure. Both retrospective ECG gating and multisegment reconstruction require constant radiation exposure throughout multiple heartbeats.

28. B

Low-osmolar contrast media (LOCM) are non-ionic agents that do not dissociate into charged particles (ions) in solution. Examples of LOCM are iohexol (Omnipaque), iopamidol (Isovue), and ioversol (Optiray).

29. C

In an effort to reduce the possibility of headaches after a CT examination involving an intrathecal injection of contrast material, the patient should rest for 8 to 24 hours with the head slightly elevated (35-45 degrees).

30. B

Dose can be considerably higher with MSCT owing to a decrease in the focal spot–detector distance, the use of a cone beam instead of a more z-axis–collimated fan beam, an increase in number of imaging phases enabled by shorter scan times, and the acquisition of thinner sections for improvement of 3D and MPR images.

31. C

β-Adrenergic receptor blocking agents (β-blockers) may be used to reduce a patient's heart rate, and sublingual nitroglycerin may be administered to cause dilation of the coronary vessels. The use of these pharmaceuticals may improve the overall visualization of the coronary vessels during a cardiac CT examination. Please consult the physician and/or department protocol for further information regarding pharmaceutical administration for cardiac CT procedures.

32. D
A *hemangioma* is a congenital, benign mass containing blood-filled spaces. It is commonly found in the liver and spleen.

33. D
The preferred timing for CT acquisition of the spleen is the portal venous phase (60-70 sec), when a more homogeneous pattern of enhancement is demonstrated.

34. D
Number 2 on the figure corresponds to the scaphoid.

35. A
The image in the figure is a multiplanar reformation (MPR) of the wrist in the coronal plane. MPR images are particularly helpful for trauma indications, such as fracture of the distal radius, labeled number 3 on the figure.

36. A
Number 1 on the figure corresponds to the capitate.

37. B
Number 5 on the figure corresponds to the lunate.

38. B
Subdural hematomas are collections of blood that occur throughout the subdural space after traumatic injury to the head. An acute subdural hematoma is one that has manifested clinically during the first 24 hours after the injury. During this stage, the hematoma appears hyperdense compared with normal brain tissue because of the initial clotting that has occurred and the concentration of hemoglobin in fresh blood.

39. D
The angiographic assessment of the peripheral arterial tree from the renal arteries through the feet is commonly referred to as a "CT runoff."

40. D
Malignant cells demonstrate an increase in metabolic activity and glucose utilization. Once administered, fludeoxyglucose F 18 (FDG) mimics glucose and is taken up by normal and abnormal tissue. The amount of FDG uptake is directly proportional to the area's metabolic activity. Malignant cells will take up a disproportionately larger amount of FDG than metabolically normal tissue.

41. A
Number 2 on the figure corresponds to the left ovary.

42. D
Number 4 on the figure corresponds to the uterus.

43. B
Number 5 on the figure corresponds to the bladder.

44. C
Intravenous administration of an iodinated contrast agent is vital to making an accurate diagnosis of a dissecting aortic aneurysm. The contrast agent helps outline the wall of the aorta and improves visualization of any division within it. Because of differences in blood flow, CT numbers within the actual lumen of the aorta are different from those in the dissected portion.

45. C
The circle of Willis is composed of the anterior cerebral, anterior communicating, internal carotid, posterior cerebral, and posterior communicating arteries. The basilar artery is an important vessel supplying blood to the brain, but it is not part of the circle of Willis

46. A
The eighth cranial nerve is the vestibulocochlear nerve responsible for both hearing and balance. Vestibular schwannoma may also be referred to as *acoustic neuroma*. This type of mass most often involves the vestibular portion of the nerve bundle, with deleterious effects on balance and equilibrium.

47. D
Number 3 on the figure corresponds to the vocal cord.

48. B
Number 1 on the figure corresponds to the piriform sinus.

49. A
A wide window setting (WL −300, WW 1000) may be used to properly demonstrate the small soft tissue vocal structures from the surrounding air-filled endolarynx.

50. C
Number 2 on the figure corresponds to the thyroid cartilage.

51. C
The *mesentery* is a double fold of the peritoneum that attaches the jejunum and ileum of the small bowel to the abdominal wall.

52. C
The nephrographic phase occurs between 70 and 90 seconds after the start of injection. Enhancement of the

renal cortex and medulla reaches equilibrium, providing optimal sensitivity for parenchymal lesions.

53. B
Complete cardiac diastole is the period of relaxation after heart contraction. *Diastole* is the portion of the cardiac cycle when coronary artery motion is the slowest and cardiac motion is at its lowest. For evaluation of the coronary arteries, the MDCT system utilizes only the diastolic portion of the acquisition in the reconstruction process.

54. C
Number 9 on the figure corresponds to the maxillary sinus.

55. B
Number 5 on the figure corresponds to the superior ophthalmic vein.

56. D
Number 4 on the figure corresponds to the superior oblique muscle.

57. C
Number 6 on the figure corresponds to the lateral rectus muscle.

58. D
Pneumothorax is one of the most common complications of CT-guided needle biopsy of the lung. The term *pneumothorax* describes a collection of air in the pleural space. A pneumothorax causes a portion of the lung to collapse, often resulting in the placement of a chest tube to re-inflate the lung.

59. A
Positive contrast material can be administered into the large bowel via enema to achieve thorough opacification. A dosage of 150 to 250 mL should be sufficient to opacify the rectosigmoid region. Doses of 300 to 500 mL may be necessary to opacify the large bowel in its entirety.

60. B
A sagittally reformatted image would demonstrate the relationship of the disc material as it protrudes posteriorly into the spinal cord.

61. C
Number 6 on the figure corresponds to the renal calyx.

62. D
Maximum intensity projection (MIP) images display only the maximum pixel value along a ray traced through the object to the viewer's assumed perspective in front of the viewing monitor. Tissue with lower attenuation values is not displayed, leaving high-attenuation structures such as bone and contrast-enhanced soft tissue structures free of superimposition.

63. A
Number 1 on the figure corresponds to the ureteropelvic junction (UPJ).

64. C
Dosage calculations for intravenous contrast agent administration should adhere to the general guiding principle of injecting the smallest quantity of contrast agent possible to meet the technical requirements of the examination. The maximum dose for any procedure should not exceed 2 mL per kg of body weight.

65. C
CT bronchography is a three-dimensional examination of the tracheobronchial tree. It may include detailed endobrachial views, on which the viewer has the perspective of flying through the trachea and bronchi, as in conventional bronchoscopy. These specialized 3D reconstructions are commonly referred to as *virtual bronchoscopy*.

66. A
Stanford type A dissecting aneurysms affect the ascending aorta. Stanford type B dissecting aneurysms affect the descending aorta.

67. D
HRCT images with the patient in the prone position can be acquired to differentiate the dependent edematous changes often seen in the lung bases.

68. C
The outer portion of an intervertebral disc is the anulus fibrosus.

69. C
Number 2 on the figure corresponds to the transverse process.

70. D
Number 1 on the figure corresponds to the transverse foramen.

71. D
Number 4 on the figure corresponds to the lamina.

72. D
Whipple procedure is the surgical resection of the pancreas and duodenum (pancreaticoduodenectomy) for the treatment of pancreatic carcinoma.

73. C
Nephrographic (70-90 sec) imaging provides enhancement of the bladder wall, which is used to evaluate the extent of tumor infiltration.

74. B

The primary clinical indication for MDCT coronary artery calcium (CAC) quantitation is the assessment of atherosclerotic disease. The presence of coronary artery calcium (CAC) is a specific indicator of atherosclerotic disease.

75. C

Number 4 on the figure corresponds to the left common iliac vein.

76. C

Portions of the CT image may be enlarged on the display screen by either of two methods. The image may be magnified to offer the viewer a closer, enlarged look at a specific area. A CT image may also be "targeted" through a decrease in the display field of view (DFOV) size. A targeted image places the area of interest over the entire display matrix, providing greater resolution and more detail than a magnified image.

77. B

Number 5 on the figure corresponds to the ureter.

78. D

Number 1 on the figure corresponds to the rectus abdominis muscle.

79. A

CT enteroclysis is a specialized evaluation of the small bowel whereby a nasogastric catheter is placed into the duodenum under fluoroscopic guidance. 1.5 to 2.0 L of enteral contrast agent is administered directly into the small intestine for maximal opacification. Non–IV contrast, thin-section (0.6-1.25 mm) CT images are acquired through the abdomen and pelvis.

80. C

The urothelium lines most of the urinary tract, including the renal pelvis, ureters, and bladder. The transitional portion of the urothelium can be the site of transitional cell carcinoma (TCC), a common malignancy of the bladder, ureters, and kidneys.

81. D

The *ostiomeatal complex* is an important sinus opening that allows for drainage of the frontal, ethmoid, and maxillary sinuses. It is a common area for sinusitis, or inflammation of the sinuses.

82. B

Number 1 on the figure corresponds to the right pulmonary artery.

83. A

Maximum intensity projection (MIP) images are a routine component of CTA examinations of the chest.

This CTA of the pulmonary arteries (CTPA) demonstrates the well-opacified pulmonary vasculature in coronal thick-slab format. From the perspective of the viewer, each pixel displays the maximum attenuation value contained within the thickness of the slab.

84. D

Number 4 on the figure corresponds to the descending aorta.

85. C

Pulsation artifacts are unique to cardiac imaging and CTA procedures of the mediastinum. They appear as a type of stair-step artifact and result from the diastolic heart motion occurring during relatively long exposure times. Improving the temporal resolution of the scan and ECG gating are methods employed to reduce pulsation artifact.

86. B

Number 2 on the figure corresponds to the pulmonary trunk.

87. B

The use of a saline flush reduces artifact from dense contrast in the superior vena cava. The streaking artifact can hamper visualization of the upper mediastinum and surrounding lung tissue.

88. A

Shortly after a CTPA study, CT venography (CTV) of the lower extremities for the identification of deep vein thrombosis (DVT) may also be performed. After the CTPA acquisition, a delay of 2 to 3 minutes is employed, and an acquisition is made from the iliac crest to the ankles.

89. C

Number 4 on the figure corresponds to the fourth ventricle.

90. B

Number 2 on the figure corresponds to the left middle cerebral artery.

91. D

Number 5 on the figure corresponds to the basilar artery.

92. A

Number 4 on the figure corresponds to the left posterior cerebral artery.

93. D

Reductions in kVp, overlapping axial sections, and precise bolus timing are all important factors in the production of high-quality CTA examinations.

94. B

The most important identifying sign of GI pathology on CT examination is wall thickening. The ability to evaluate the gastric and bowel walls is a crucial component of the successful CT evaluation of the GI system. Distention and opacification with oral media, coupled with contrast enhancement through IV administration, offer the best demonstration of the GI wall.

95. D

The branches of the celiac axis are the left gastric artery, common hepatic artery, and splenic artery.

96. B

Number 2 on the figure corresponds to the left subclavian artery.

97. A

Number 5 on the figure corresponds to the right brachiocephalic vein.

98. C

Number 1 on the figure corresponds to the left brachiocephalic vein.

99. C

Number 4 on the figure corresponds to the left common carotid artery.

100. C

Water is the preferred oral contrast material for CT urograms, because its use avoids the interference seen with denser materials when one is producing volume-rendered and MIP images. Additional protocol considerations include pre-contrast acquisition of the urinary tract and post-contrast nephrographic phase imaging. Excretory phase imaging occurs after a delay of 5 to 15 minutes and may be aided by the IV drip administration of approximately 250 mL of normal (0.9%) saline to improve urinary tract opacification.

101. D

Hepatocellular carcinomas (HCCs) are hypervascular lesions that appear hyperdense in comparison with surrounding normal hepatic parenchyma during the arterial phase of contrast enhancement.

102. B

Lithiasis refers to the presence of stones. Unenhanced helical CT of the urinary tract has become the standard for the investigation of urinary tract lithiasis.

103. B

Phonation during acquisition may be used to demonstrate abnormal mobility of the vocal cord(s). A thin-section (0.5-2 mm) sequence is obtained during which the patient is instructed to phonate a low, steady "E" sound during the entire scan duration.

104. C

Number 1 on the figure corresponds to the superior mesenteric vein.

105. B

Number 4 on the figure corresponds to the spleen.

106. D

Number 6 on the figure corresponds to the pancreas.

107. C

Computed tomography is commonly used during percutaneous aspiration and drainage procedures. CT images enable the radiologist to view the precise location of abnormal fluid collections and allow for accurate planning of a safe access route for the aspiration procedure. When performed properly, CT-guided aspiration of an abdominal abscess can be a valuable nonsurgical therapeutic technique. This type of procedure can also be used to reduce other types of abnormal fluid collections, including cysts, bilomas, urinomas, and lymphoceles.

108. D

The x-ray tube and data acquisition system (DAS) are housed within the gantry of a CT scanner. The gantry aperture is the circular opening through which the patient moves during scanning.

109. D

Both the x-ray tube and detector array rotate around the patient during scanning with a third-generation CT unit.

110. C

The scanner's reduced low-contrast resolution is most likely the cause of increased noise. When the noise level of a CT image increases, the low-contrast resolution decreases. Decreased patient radiation dose implies that the signal-to-noise ratio has decreased, thus raising the noise level of the image. The same situation would apply for an increase in electronic noise.

111. A

MIP images display only the maximum pixel value along a ray traced through the object to the viewer's assumed perspective in front of the viewing monitor. As the viewer faces an MIP image, each pixel represents the maximum attenuation that occurs in the associated voxel.

112. C

The dimension of a pixel may be calculated by dividing the field of view by the matrix size. The DFOV of 40 cm must first be converted into 400 mm. This is then divided by 512 mm, for a pixel dimension of 0.78 mm. Keep in mind that the pixel is a square, two-dimensional item and that the measurement of 0.78 mm corresponds to only one side.

113. C
Collimation occurs as lead shutters close down upon the beam, limiting its projected area. Constructed of lead, the collimator shutters absorb portions of the primary beam, thereby reducing its intensity.

114. D
Photon fluence may be described as the quantity of x-radiation passing through a unit area.

115. C
Interpolation is a mathematical technique used in helical CT. In interpolation, approximations of information above and below a section level are made to overcome the fact that a complete revolution of tube and detectors was not performed for each image.

116. A
The most common cause of CT image noise is the fluctuation in the number of x-ray photons measured by the detectors. When a CT scanner attempts to reconstruct an image from an insufficient amount of transmitted radiation measurements, *quantum noise* occurs.

117. A
A computer network is a communication system designed to facilitate the transfer of data between computers. A PACS works on a network, which connects each of the involved imaging modalities, viewing stations, printers, and so on.

118. C
The edge gradient effect occurs when the CT x-ray beam passes through areas of abrupt changes in density that are represented by high spatial frequencies. This type of streak artifact commonly occurs at the interface of dense bone and soft tissue in anatomic areas such as the brain.

119. B
Streaking edge gradient artifacts may be reduced with increases in the beam's average photon energy. Increases in kVp and filtration would accomplish this. This type of artifact may also be reduced with a decrease in reconstructed section width, which helps minimize the edge gradient effect. A decrease in partial volume averaging may lessen the streaking that is apparent from edge gradient inconsistencies.

120. C
The level chosen for a given window setting should correspond to the average density value of the tissue(s) of interest. Areas of soft tissue, such as the brain, are often displayed at window levels of approximately +50 HU.

121. D
The star artifact was an unwanted by-product of the back-projection method of image reconstruction used in older CT scanners. It is now removed by the process of convolution used in the modern reconstruction method known as filtered back-projection.

122. C
Involuntary motion is beyond control of the patient and includes peristalsis, cardiac contraction, and tremors. The most effective method of reducing involuntary motion on a CT scan is reduction of scan times. Many scanners offer segmenting or "half-scan" options whereby images may be reconstructed after a partial revolution of the tube-detector system. In the case of digestive involuntary motion, glucagon administration is an additional option.

123. B
Storage of CT images in digital file format is referred to as *soft copies*. Hard copies of CT images are those stored on laser film.

124. C
Multiplanar reformation (MPR) describes the process of displaying CT images in a different orientation from the one used in the original reconstruction process. Unlike retrospective reconstruction, reformation does not change the makeup of the image voxels. Reformation merely alters the viewing perspective of the images to a different anatomic plane.

125. D
Windowing is used to describe the process of gray-scale mapping the CT image, during which the display system assigns a shade of gray to an individual pixel on the basis of its CT number (HU).

126. B
The Lambert-Beer law, $I = I_0 e^{-\mu x}$ is used to calculate the attenuation coefficient of a volume of material. The symbol "I_0" represents the intensity of the radiation incident upon the tissue being imaged. It is compared with the intensity of the radiation passing through the tissue (I) during the calculation of the linear attenuation coefficient.

127. A
The x-ray beam of a first-generation CT scanner was highly collimated to the size of a single detector. It was often referred to as a "pencil beam."

128. C
The *transmitted intensity* is the amount of energy that passes through the patient onto a detector.

129. D
The limiting resolution of a modern CT scanner is approximately 25 lp/cm. This resolution varies greatly with scan factors and is considerably less than that of projection radiography.

130. A

Post-patient collimation occurs through a high-resolution comb placed over the detector array. Functioning like a grid, it removes unwanted scatter radiation and off-axis photons that result from the more divergent nature of the MSCT beam.

131. C

Section interval describes the spacing between two adjacent CT images. It is measured as the distance between the center of one section and the center of the adjacent section.

132. B

The number of data channels controls the number of sections the scanner can simultaneously acquire with each gantry rotation. For example, a four-slice MSCT system has 16 1.25-mm detectors in its array. However, with only four data channels, the maximum number of sections that may be reconstructed from each gantry rotation is four. The system combines transmission information from the individual detectors through its four data channels, resulting in the acquisition of four sections per gantry rotation.

133. B

Consisting of an arrangement of pixels in rows and columns, the *matrix* is used to organize the attenuation information from the anatomic section into a digital image. The size of the matrix is given as the number of pixels across multiplied by the number of pixels down.

134. C

Region of interest (ROI) measurements may be made by superimposing a cursor over an area and instructing the computer to average the CT numbers included within the region.

135. C

The CT number for water has an average value of zero.

136. A

Quality control refers to the implementation of corrective actions to improve any identified performance inadequacies of the CT system found through quality assurance procedures.

137. B

The use of a fan- or cone-shaped x-ray beam during CT increases the total volume of tissue irradiated, thereby increasing the amount of scatter radiation produced. This change results in a significantly higher patient radiation dose than the "pencil beam" radiation used in older CT scanners.

138. D

Each CT scanner has several choices for SFOV. The choice made by the technologist activates a certain percentage of the detector array so that information is acquired from a circular portion of the anatomic section. Built into the SFOV selection are additional correction factors used to process different types of tissue. For example, a CT scanner may have a specific selection for scans of the head, which attempts to limit the artifact occurring at the delineation of bone from brain tissue.

139. A

The transmitted intensity of a CT x-ray beam and the attenuation of the tissue imaged are inversely related. As the tissue begins to attenuate less radiation, the transmitted intensity of the beam increases. Areas of less dense tissue allow more radiation to pass onto the detectors, and vice versa.

140. B

Smaller focal spots improve the geometric efficiency of the x-ray beam, leading to greater spatial resolution.

141. D

The geometric efficiency of a CT detector is influenced primarily by the amount of interspace material necessary between adjacent detectors. Although valuable in limiting interference (cross talk) between adjacent detectors, the interspace material reduces geometric efficiency by absorbing transmitted x-ray energy.

142. C

The degree of attenuation depends on multiple factors, including the x-ray energy and the atomic structure and density of the exposed tissue.

143. C

Retrospective reconstruction occurs when an image is reconstructed a second time with an adjustment in a technical factor. The scan data or "raw" data are used to reconstruct the image with a different display matrix, display field of view, algorithm, and so on.

144. D

The beam divergence inherent to the cone beam geometry of MSCT can cause difficulty during the image reconstruction process. Specific cone beam algorithms such as the Feldkamp-Davis-Kress (FDK) and advanced single-slice rebinning (ASSR) algorithms attempt to overcome the issues resulting from the divergent path of the x-ray beam from tube to the widened detector array.

145. A

Each 1.0% difference in contrast between adjacent objects amounts to a difference in pixel value of approximately 10 HU. MSCT systems are typically capable of differentiating adjacent objects with attenuation differences as small as 3 HU.

146. C

The stop-motion capability of a CT system is referred to as *temporal resolution*. Temporal resolution quantifies the CT system's ability to freeze motion and provide an image free of blurring.

147. C

Ring artifacts are associated with the use of third-generation CT scanners. Both the x-ray tube and the detector array rotate around the patient with third-generation scanners. A malfunctioning detector or series of detectors in a third-generation CT scanner causes a ring artifact to appear on the image as a result of the rotational nature of the detector array.

148. C

At a maximum, the MSCT cone beam may be collimated to a dimension equal to the entire multirow detector array. In the example, the total dimension of the detector array along the z-axis is 16×1.25 mm, or 20.0 mm.

149. A

The polyenergetic CT x-ray beam consists of photons of varying energy. As the beam traverses the patient, low-energy photons are absorbed first, increasing the average intensity of the beam as it travels along its path. This change, referred to as *beam hardening,* can have an artifactual result on the CT image.

150. A

With MSCT, detector collimation determines the width of the reconstructed section. By electronically adjusting the detector dimension, the operator can control the width of the x-ray beam contributing to a reconstructed section. Beam collimation no longer directly controls section width.

151. D

The accuracy between calculated CT numbers and their respective linear attenuation coefficients is termed *linearity*. Daily system calibration and routine vendor maintenance procedures work to establish and maintain CT system linearity.

152. B

Attenuation is the reduction in intensity of an x-ray beam as it interacts with matter. Several interactions are responsible for the attenuation of primary radiation, including Compton scatter and photoelectric effect. Each of these interactions reduces the energy and/or number of the x-ray photons in a primary beam.

153. C

When a formula comparing the attenuation coefficient of tissue with that of water is used, materials whose coefficients are less than that of water are assigned negative CT numbers.

154. C

Referred to as *targeting,* decreasing the display field of view (DFOV) causes an increase in the image size on the monitor. The DFOV controls the amount of scanned information to be displayed on the matrix. If a small portion of information is to be displayed on the entire matrix, it will appear larger to the viewer.

155. A

The *bit depth* of a digital imaging system defines the number of information bits contained within each pixel. This parameter ultimately controls the total range of CT values that may be assigned to a given pixel. For example, a bit depth of 12 results in 4096 possible CT values ($2^{12} = 4096$).

156. B

Isotropic voxels have equal dimensions along the x-, y-, and z-axes. Use of a thin reconstructed section width and small DFOV minimizes each voxel dimension.

157. C

The limiting resolution of a particular CT scan is determined at a point on the graph where the signal frequency corresponding to a particular object has reached 10% (MTF = 0.1).

158. A

According to the MTF diagram, the bone algorithm has a resolution of approximately 12 lp/cm. The standard algorithm and smooth algorithm are approximately 10 and 7 lp/cm, respectively.

159. A

The limiting resolution of a particular CT scan is determined at a point on the graph where the signal frequency corresponding to a particular object has reached 10%. When the MTF is lower that 10% (0.1), the object is no longer resolved.

160. D

Total collimation equals the combined thicknesses of all the sections that are simultaneously acquired with each gantry rotation. For example, a given MSCT system has an array of 64 detectors, each 0.625 mm wide. If the beam is collimated to expose the entire array, the total collimation for the acquisition is equal to 0.625 mm $\times$ 64, or 40 mm.

161. B

All modern MSCT systems utilize solid-state detectors consisting primarily of a scintillating crystal material. Solid-state detectors are preferred for MSCT because of their ability to accurately record incident x-ray energy from any angle. This flexibility is important when one considers the widened cone beam geometry inherent to MSCT systems.

162. B

In modern MSCT systems, the highest-quality 3D and multiplanar reformation (MPR) images are obtained with the acquisition of an isotropic or near-isotropic data set. The other equally important piece is an overlapping data set, for which the reconstruction interval is less than the section width.

163. A

The cupping artifact that occurs at the superior portion of the skull is another form of partial volume artifact. The dense skull table averages with the low-attenuating brain tissue, causing an artifact by which the brain parenchyma may appear abnormally dense.

164. A

The *effective section width* corresponds to the SSP of the reconstructed section in consideration of the widening that occurs during helical data acquisition.

165. A

The sampling rate may be quantified as *views per rotation (VPR)*. As the sampling rate rises, the number of views per rotation (VPR) increases.

180-degree linear interpolation (180LI) Type of algorithm used for MSCT image reconstruction in which data acquired from a shorter distance (180 degrees) away from the reconstructed slice location are interpolated.

360-degree linear interpolation (360LI) Type of algorithm used for MSCT image reconstruction in which two sets of projection data acquired 360 degrees apart are used to form an image at a precise z-axis location.

absorbed dose The amount of x-ray energy absorbed in a unit of mass. It is measured in grays (Gy).

absorption efficiency The ability of an individual CT detector to absorb and measure the transmitted x-ray intensity incident upon it. Primarily controlled by the characteristics and physical makeup of the detector material.

adaptive array The type of MSCT detector array configured with the thinnest detectors at the center, surrounded by detectors of incrementally increasing widths along the z-axis.

advanced single-slice rebinning (ASSR) algorithm Cone beam correction algorithm utilized to overcome potential attenuation calculation errors from the divergent beam of MSCT systems.

afterglow The tendency of a scintillation-type CT detector to continue to glow in response to x-radiation after the exposure source has been terminated.

Agatston score Quantification of the volume and density of calcium within the coronary arteries. As calculated during a CT coronary artery calcification (CAC) examination, the Agatston score is used to indicate a patient's risk of suffering a cardiac event.

ALARA Acronym for *as low as reasonably achievable*, the cardinal principle of radiation dose reduction for all radiologic procedures, including CT.

algorithm Mathematical filter applied to raw data during CT image reconstruction to remove blurring artifact inherent to back-projection. May also be referred to as a *kernel*.

aliasing A form of streak artifact caused by an insufficient number of views (data samples) obtained during data acquisition.

analog-to-digital converter (ADC) Component of the data acquisition system (DAS) responsible for converting the electronic signal emitted by the CT detectors into digital form.

archival The storage of CT data in either hard (film) or soft (digital) form.

array processor (AP) Component of the CT computer system responsible for receiving raw scan data, performing all of the major processing of the CT image, and returning the reconstructed image to the storage memory of the host computer.

arterial phase Period of peak arterial enhancement following the bolus IV administration of iodinated contrast material. For example, the hepatic arterial phase occurs approximately 25 to 35 seconds after the initiation of contrast agent administration.

artifact A form of noise on the CT image resulting from errors during the measurement of transmitted radiation by the detectors.

attenuation The reduction in intensity of a radiation beam as it passes through a substance.

attenuation coefficient The value assigned to an object quantifying its ability to attenuate an x-ray beam.

automatic tube current modulation (ATCM) CT system software used to adjust the mA throughout an acquisition to reduce patient radiation dose to a minimum.

back-projection The mathematical process of CT image reconstruction whereby ray sum data are projected back onto a matrix.

beam hardening The phenomenon whereby low-energy photons are absorbed as the x-ray beam passes through an object, resulting in an increase in the average photon energy of the beam.

beam pitch The ratio of table feed per gantry rotation to the total collimation used during acquisition with a multislice CT (MSCT) system.

beam width The dimension of the primary beam in the longitudinal or z-axis as controlled by the pre-patient collimator.

binning The process of electronically combining signal from adjacent detector elements to produce a reconstructed CT image that is thicker than the individual detector width.

bit depth The number of information bits contained within each pixel.

blood urea nitrogen (BUN) A measurement of renal function, determined as the amount of nitrogen in the blood in the form of the waste product urea. The normal range of BUN in adults is 7 to 25 mg/dL.

bow-tie filter A type of filter added to the CT x-ray tube to compensate for the cylindrical shape of most body parts. The filter is thicker at the ends and helps shape the beam to reduce patient radiation exposure.

cardiac cycle The series of blood flow–related events that occur from the beginning of one heartbeat to that of the next.

cerebral blood flow (CBF) A common measurement during CT perfusion studies of the brain. CBF is the quantity of blood (mL) that moves through 100 g of brain tissue each minute. Normal range in gray matter is 50 to 60 mL/100 g/min.

cerebral blood volume (CBV) A common measurement during CT perfusion studies of the brain. CBV is the quantity of blood (mL) contained within a 100-g volume of brain tissue. Normal range is 4 to 5 mL/100 g.

cerebral perfusion The level of blood flow throughout brain tissue.

constant mAs The product of milliamperage (mA) and scan time (seconds) utilized for a CT acquisition.

contiguous images CT images acquired with equal section thicknesses and reconstruction intervals.

contrast resolution The ability of a CT system to detect an object with a small difference in linear attenuation coefficient from the surrounding tissue. May also be referred to as *low-contrast detectability* or *sensitivity*.

contrast-induced nephrotoxicity (CIN) A substantial decline in renal function that can occur after a patient receives IV contrast material. It is usually signified by a marked increase in serum creatinine over a baseline measurement obtained prior to contrast agent administration.

convolution Mathematical filtration used by the CT system to remove blurring artifact during the back-projection method of image reconstruction.

corticomedullary phase A late arterial phase of renal enhancement beginning 30 to 40 seconds after the initiation of contrast agent administration. Optimal enhancement of the renal cortex and renal veins occurs during this period.

creatinine A waste product of metabolism found in the bloodstream and measured as an indicator of renal function. Normal range of creatinine is 0.5 to 1.5 mg/dL.

CT arthrography CT evaluation of a joint after the intra-articular injection of iodinated contrast material.

CT bronchography Specialized MSCT examination of the tracheobronchial tree consisting of MPR and volume-rendered 3D images reconstructed from thin, overlapping MDCT axial images through the airways.

CT colonography Specialized CT evaluation of the large intestine used primarily for colon cancer screening. The large intestine is extended and scanned with thin-section CT. 2D and 3D models are constructed, including virtual endoscopic fly-through views.

CT cystography Specialized CT examination of the bladder whereby iodinated contrast material is administered directly under gravity into the bladder via Foley catheter.

CT dose index (CTDI) An approximate measure of the radiation dose received in a single CT section or slice.

CT enteroclysis Specialized CT evaluation of the small bowel whereby enteral contrast material is administered directly into the duodenum through a nasogastric catheter placed under fluoroscopic guidance.

CT enterography Specialized CT evaluation of the small bowel after the oral administration of low-density (0.1%) barium.

CT fluoroscopy Continuous, real-time CT imaging used predominantly for CT-guided interventional procedures.

CT myelography CT evaluation of the spinal cord and nerve roots after the intrathecal administration of iodinated contrast material.

CT number Relative value assigned to each pixel to quantify the attenuation occurring in each voxel in comparison with the attenuation of water. The calculated CT number for a given pixel is given in Hounsfield units (HU). May also be referred to as *pixel value*.

CT runoff The CT angiographic assessment of the peripheral arterial tree from the renal arteries through the lower extremities.

CT simulation The process of obtaining anatomic information with CT imaging that is used to calculate the beam arrangement for radiotherapy.

CT urogram A comprehensive, multiphasic CT evaluation of the urinary tract. Consists primarily of pre-contrast, post-contrast, and delayed CT acquisitions

through the kidneys, ureters, and bladder. It may also be commonly referred to as a *CT-IVP*.

cupping artifact An error occurring in the superior portion of the skull, where dense bone averages with the low-attenuating brain tissue. This partial volume artifact may result in abnormally dense-appearing brain parenchyma.

data acquisition system (DAS) The electronic components of a CT system responsible for measuring the transmitted x-radiation absorbed by the detectors.

data channel Pathway of data transmission from the detectors to the computerized components of the system's data acquisition system. The number of data channels of a CT system determines the maximum number of sections that may be acquired with each gantry rotation.

data transfer rate The speed at which a computerized storage drive is able to transfer data.

deconvolution Mathematical image processing technique used to generate blood perfusion maps during CT perfusion studies of the brain.

detector Device responsible for measuring transmitted radiation and converting it into a proportionate electronic signal to be used for image reconstruction.

detector array The CT image receptor, consisting of a series of detectors arranged in varying configurations.

detector collimation The process of determining section width in the MSCT system as determined by the defined beam width and the number and thickness of detectors utilized for image reconstruction.

detector configuration The number, length, and organization of the individual detector elements in an MSCT system.

detector pitch The ratio of table feed per gantry rotation to the acquired section width. This definition of pitch is used for helical single-slice CT (SSCT).

diastole Portion of the cardiac cycle when the heart muscle is relaxed. Diastolic blood pressure reflects the force exhibited on the arterial walls during relaxation of the heart muscle. It is the bottom or second number provided during the assessment of blood pressure.

DICOM Acronym for the Digital Imaging and Communications in Medicine standard for the process of recording, storing, printing, and transmitting medical image data.

display field of view (DFOV) The diameter of the acquired attenuation data displayed across the image matrix. May also be referred to as the *zoom factor* or *target view*.

dose length product (DLP) The measurement of dose for an entire series of CT images. DLP is equal to the calculated dose per section multiplied by the length of a CT acquisition along the z-axis.

dose profile The section of the patient exposed to radiation at the gantry isocenter.

dual-energy CT Simultaneous acquisition, by an MSCT system, of attenuation data for a single anatomic section with two x-ray beams, each having a different energy spectrum. Dual-energy CT systems rapidly switch between or alternate kVp settings during data acquisition, allowing for improved contrast between substances of differing densities.

dual-source CT   CT system that consists of two separate x-ray tubes and detector arrays mounted 90 degrees from each other within the gantry, allowing for dual-energy CT acquisition.

edge gradient   Streak artifact that occurs at the interface between a high-density object and the lower-attenuation material surrounding it.

effective dose   Approximation of the relative risk from exposure to ionizing radiation; is calculated by assigning weighting factors to different tissues on the basis of their individual radiosensitivities. It is measured in Sieverts (Sv).

effective mAs   The calculated mAs per acquired slice with a multislice CT (MSCT) system.

effective section width   The slice sensitivity profile (SSP) of the reconstructed CT section. It is measured at the full width at half maximum (FWHM) of the SSP for a given CT acquisition.

electrocardiogram (ECG)   A graphical representation of the electrical activity of the heart recorded over time through electrodes placed on the patient's skin.

electron beam CT (EBCT)   Specialized CT design devoid of moving parts. Utilizes a beam of electrons bombarding a tungsten target to produce x-radiation. EBCT systems are capable of extremely short exposure times and have their greatest application in cardiac imaging.

equilibrium phase   Contrast phase of the liver when hepatic parenchymal enhancement dissipates and there is minimal attenuation difference between the intravascular and extravascular spaces. Usually occurs at 2 to 3 minutes after the initiation of contrast agent administration.

excretory phase   A delayed imaging renal enhancement phase that begins approximately 3 minutes after the initiation of contrast agent administration. Contrast material has been excreted into the renal calyces, opacifying the renal pelvis and the remainder of the urinary collecting system (ureters, bladder).

exposure   The ability of x-rays to ionize a volume of air. It is measured in roentgens (R).

extravasation   The escape of contrast material outside the blood vessel into the surrounding soft tissue.

fan angle   Angle of coverage by the x-ray beam as it emerges from the tube housing and exposes the detector array within the scan plane (x-y axis).

Feldkamp-Davis-Kress (FDK) algorithm   Cone beam correction algorithm utilized to overcome potential attenuation calculation errors from the divergent beam of MSCT systems.

filtered back-projection   The mathematical process of CT image reconstruction that involves convolution of the raw data prior to their projection back onto a matrix.

filtration   Removal of the low-energy x-ray photons emitted from the x-ray tube to improve beam quality and reduce patient radiation dose.

flat-panel detector   Large-area detector consisting of a film of scintillating crystals bonded to a matrix of silicon photosensors. May be used in place of the segmented detector rows found in MDCT systems.

flying focal spot   Electronic switching technique whereby the electron beam is electromagnetically steered toward two separate locations on the rotating anode. Results in the emission of two sources of x-radiation from the CT x-ray tube and a doubling of the data samples acquired from each gantry rotation.

full width at half maximum (FWHM)   The midpoint of a slice sensitivity profile (SSP), where the effective section width for a CT acquisition is determined.

gantry   The assembly that houses the x-ray tube, detectors, and additional data acquisition components of a CT system. The patient is positioned within the gantry during CT data acquisition.

geometric efficiency   The ability of a detector array to absorb and measure the transmitted x-ray intensity incident upon it. Primarily controlled by the physical arrangement of detectors within the array and the amount of interspace material required between adjacent detectors.

glomerular filtration rate (GFR)   An approximation of creatinine clearance or the rate by which creatinine is filtered from the bloodstream. GFR is utilized as a measure of renal function with normal ranges of 70 ± 14 mL/min/m^2 for men and 60 ± 10 mL/min/m^2 for women.

helical   The type of CT acquisition whereby the x-ray tube and patient continuously move during scanning, yielding a data set in the form of a helix. May also be commonly referred to as *spiral*.

Hounsfield bar   Specific type of streaking beam-hardening artifact that occurs in the posterior fossa of the brain.

Hounsfield unit   The unit of the CT number scale assigned to each pixel to quantify relative attenuation.

hybrid-array   The type of MSCT detector array with narrower detectors positioned midline, flanked by the wider detectors.

hyperdense   Possessing CT attenuation values greater than the values of the surrounding tissue.

hypodense   Possessing CT attenuation values less than the values of the surrounding tissue.

image compression   Complex computer technique that reduces the size of digital CT image data.

image data   The reconstructed data that have been projected back onto a matrix after convolution by an algorithm and displayed on a monitor as a gray-scale CT image.

immersive rendering   *See* perspective volume rendering.

insufflation   The introduction of air into an organ or cavity for distention and improved visualization.

interpolation   The mathematical process used for helical CT image reconstruction whereby data from tube rotations just above and just below a given slice position are used for image reconstruction.

isocenter   The center point of gantry rotation.

isodense   Possessing CT attenuation values equal to the values of the surrounding tissue.

isotropic   Having equal dimensions along the x-, y-, and z-axes; in CT, describes voxels with this property.

kerma   Quantity of energy deposited in a unit of mass. *Kerma* is used to describe the absorbed dose of x-radiation.

kernel   Mathematical filter applied to raw data during CT image reconstruction to remove the blurring artifact inherent to back-projection. May also be referred to as an *algorithm*.

linear attenuation coefficient (μ) The value assigned to an object to quantify the extent to which it attenuates x-ray.

linearity The relative accuracy between calculated CT numbers and their respective linear attenuation coefficients.

lossless compression The reversible process whereby the CT image is digitally compressed in size without loss of data and is identical to the original.

lossy compression The irreversible process whereby data are lost during the compression process and the CT image does not exactly match the original.

matrix Two-dimensional grid of numbers arranged in rows and columns.

maximum intensity projection (MIP) Multiplanar reformation technique that displays only the maximum pixel value along a ray traced through the object to the viewer's assumed perspective in front of the viewing monitor.

mean transit time (MTT) A common measurement during CT perfusion studies of the brain. MTT refers to the average transit time, in seconds, needed for blood to pass through a given region of brain tissue.

minimum intensity projection (min-IP) Multiplanar reformation technique that displays the minimum pixel value along each ray to the viewer.

misregistration Artifact that occurs when patient motion between consecutive acquisitions causes misalignment of data and the potential loss of anatomic information.

modulation transfer function (MTF) A graphical representation of a CT system's response to a spatial frequency that serves as a measurement of the system's in-plane spatial resolution.

monoenergetic Consisting of a uniform photon energy; used in CT to describe a beam of x-radiation.

multi-slice CT (MSCT) A CT system with a detector array capable of acquiring more than one section for each gantry rotation. May also be referred to as *multidetector CT (MDCT)*.

multiphase CT data acquisition during multiple timed phases of contrast enhancement.

multiplanar reformation (MPR) The process of displaying CT images in a different orientation from the one used in the original reconstruction.

multiple scan average dose (MSAD) A calculation of the average cumulative radiation dose to each anatomic slice within the center of a CT scan consisting of multiple slices.

multisegment reconstruction A method of improving the temporal resolution of a CT system whereby the data acquisition process is subdivided into separate components of smaller rotation angles.

nephrographic phase Renal enhancement phase occurring between 70 and 90 seconds after the start of injection of a contrast agent. Enhancement between renal cortex and medulla reaches equilibrium, providing optimal sensitivity for parenchymal lesions.

noise Grainy appearance on the CT image due primarily to an insufficient x-ray photon flux per voxel. May also be described as any portion of the signal that contains no useful information, as evident in certain CT image artifacts.

Nyquist theorem A sampling law dictating that the data sampling frequency must be at least twice the object's spatial frequency in order for the object to be resolved by the CT system.

O-arm Portable CT-fluoroscopy unit with a telescoping gantry used to acquire 3D CT images and standard fluoroscopy during invasive or surgical procedures.

opacification The increase in CT density of a structure due to filling with positive contrast material.

operating system (OS) The main software of the CT computer, controlling the utilization of the hardware resources including the available memory, CPU time, disk space, and so on.

orthogonal Imaging planes that are perpendicular to each other.

orthographic volume rendering Technique yielding a 3D model with the perspective of externally viewing the reconstructed object.

osmolality The propensity of an iodinated contrast medium to cause fluid from outside the blood vessel to move into the bloodstream.

out-of-field artifact Hyperdense streaking that occurs when a portion of the patient has been positioned outside the scan field of view (SFOV).

overbeaming Expansion of the primary beam in an MSCT system to ensure that all detectors of the array are exposed to x-rays of equal intensity.

overlapping images CT images produced with a reconstruction interval that is less than the section width.

overranging The process of applying radiation dose before and after the acquisition volume to ensure sufficient data collection for the interpolation algorithms of helical CT reconstruction.

PACS Acronym for a picture archival and communications system. Responsible for storing, retrieving, distributing, and displaying CT and other digital medical images.

pancreatic phase A delayed arterial enhancement phase occurring approximately 35 to 45 seconds after the start of contrast agent administration, if an adequate volume has been injected at a rate of 3 mL/sec or greater.

parallel processing The ability of a computer to perform multiple functions simultaneously.

partial volume artifact An error that occurs when a structure is only partly positioned within a voxel and the attenuation for the object is not accurately represented by a pixel value.

partial volume averaging Inaccuracy in pixel values that occurs when the associated voxels contain attenuation coefficients for multiple tissue types. The values are averaged together to yield a single pixel value that attempts to represent an assortment of different materials.

perspective volume rendering Technique yielding a 3D model with the perspective of being within the lumen of the object, similar to an endoscopic view. May also be referred to as *immersive rendering*.

phantom A quality control device typically composed of a radiolucent plastic material containing specialized inserts that is used to measure specific image quality criteria.

photodiode   Device used by a solid-state CT detector to convert the light emitted by a scintillation crystal into a proportional electronic signal.

photon fluence   Quantity of x-ray photons passing through a specified area.

photon flux   The rate at which a quantity of x-ray photons (fluence) passes through a unit area over a unit time.

pipelining   A form of parallel processing used by a computer to improve computation speed.

pitch   The relationship between collimation and table movement per gantry rotation.

pixel   Abbreviation of *picture element*. Refers to the individual boxes arranged in the matrix used to display the CT image.

pixel value   *See* CT number.

point spread function (PSF)   A measure of a CT system's in-plane spatial resolution that evaluates the amount of spread inherent in an orthogonal image of a thin wire.

polyenergetic   Consisting of a spectrum of differing energies; used in CT to describe the beam of x-radiation.

portal venous phase   Period of peak hepatic parenchymal enhancement when contrast material redistributes from the blood into the extravascular spaces. Typically occurs 60 to 70 seconds after the initiation of contrast agent administration.

prospective ECG gating   Method of improving the temporal resolution of an MSCT system during examinations of the heart and mediastinum. Data are acquired in an axial "step-and-shoot" mode and only during the diastolic portion of the R-R interval.

prospective reconstruction   The initial construction of the acquired raw data into CT image data with selected display field-of-view, algorithm, image center, and so on.

pseudoenhancement   Minimal increase in attenuation demonstrated by a structure that typically does not enhance following intravenous contrast administration. Most common during MSCT evaluation of cysts.

pulse oximeter   An electronic device placed on a patient's finger, toe, or earlobe to measure pulse and blood oxygen levels.

quality assurance   The measurement of the scanner's performance through quality testing procedures and evaluation of the test results.

quality control   The implementation of corrective actions to improve any identified performance inadequacies of the CT system.

raw data   The transmission measurements obtained by the detectors used to mathematically reconstruct the CT image.

ray   The portion of the x-ray beam transmitted through the patient and incident upon a single detector.

ray sum   The measurement of transmitted radiation made by an individual detector used to determine the attenuation occurring along a ray.

region of interest (ROI)   A user-defined graphic outline that calculates the average CT number of a given anatomic area.

rendering   Use of three-dimensional (3D) algorithms to provide a specific perspective to the construction of a 3D model.

response time   The ability of a CT detector to quickly measure x-ray and then recover before the next measurement.

retrospective ECG gating   Method of improving the temporal resolution of an MSCT system during CT examinations of the heart and mediastinum. Only data acquired during diastole are used for image reconstruction, allowing for a reduction of motion artifact in the CT image.

retrospective reconstruction   Reconstruction performed after the initial prospective reconstruction. Multiple retrospective reconstructions of raw data are possible, with changes to display field of view, algorithm, image center, and so on.

ring artifact   An incorrect ring of density on the reconstructed CT image resulting from detector malfunction.

saline flush   Injection of a volume of normal saline solution immediately following the bolus administration of an iodinated contrast agent. The saline flushes any remaining contrast agent through the automated injector tubing, improving the efficiency of contrast agent utilization.

scan delay   The time between the initiation of contrast agent administration and CT data acquisition. The chosen scan delay determines the phase of contrast enhancement for a given CT acquisition.

scan field of view (SFOV)   A parameter that controls the diameter of the circular data acquisition field within the CT gantry as determined by the number of activated detectors along the x-y axes. May also be referred to as the *calibration field*.

scintillation   The production of light energy by a CT detector material in response to absorbed x-ray energy.

scout image   Digital survey radiograph acquired by the CT system for the purpose of prescribing the cross-sectional acquisition. Similar to a conventional radiograph, the scout view is produced by translating the patient through the gantry without tube and detector rotation. May also be referred to as a *topogram, scanogram,* or *survey radiograph*.

section interval   The distance between the center of one CT section and the center of the next adjacent section.

section width   The dimension of a reconstructed CT slice along the longitudinal direction of acquisition (z-axis). Commonly referred to as *slice thickness*.

shaded surface display (SSD)   *See* surface rendering.

signal   Electronic current emitted by the CT detector in response to the absorption and measurement of transmitted radiation.

signal-to-noise ratio (SNR)   Quantification of the amount of noise in a displayed CT image. SNR is calculated as the standard deviation in the ROI measurement of a water phantom image.

single-slice CT (SSCT)   A CT system with a single row of detectors capable of acquiring only one image section for each gantry rotation.

slice sensitivity profile (SSP)   Graph demonstrating the broadening of the section width that is inherent to volumetric (helical) CT acquisition.

slice thickness   *See* section width.

slip-ring   The rotating assembly used to enable the passage of electrical signal during continuous rotation of the helical CT system.

spatial frequency   The waveform of signal that represents the varied objects imaged by a CT system.

spatial resolution   The ability of a CT imaging system to display fine details separately. Given in units of line pairs per centimeter (lp/cm).

spiral   *See* helical.

step artifact   The unwanted appearance of individual sections on a multiplanar or 3D reformation image resulting in a loss of sharpness and detail.

stranding   Hazy increase in density of the fat surrounding an organ on CT examination that usually indicates an inflammatory process.

surface rendering   Construction of a three-dimensional (3D) model of a specific tissue type by limiting the displayed volumetric data on the basis of an attenuation threshold. May also be referred to as *shaded surface display (SSD)*.

systole   Portion of the cardiac cycle when the heart muscle is in contraction. Systolic blood pressure reflects the force exhibited on the arterial walls during ventricular contraction. It is the top or first number provided during the assessment of blood pressure.

teleradiology   The transmission of image data across networks from the imaging facility to an off-site location for review and interpretation.

temporal resolution   The ability of a CT system to freeze motion and provide an image free of blurring.

total collimation   The combined thickness of all of the sections that are simultaneously acquired with each gantry rotation during MSCT acquisition.

triple rule-out   Comprehensive MSCT examination of the chest for cardiac and noncardiac pain. The single acquisition evaluates for coronary artery disease, aortic aneurysm, and pulmonary embolism.

tube arcing   Short circuiting within the x-ray tube during data acquisition that results in severe streak artifacts in the CT image.

uniform matrix array   The type of MSCT detector array that utilizes multiple detectors in the longitudinal direction, each of the same length.

uniformity   Maintenance of relatively consistent CT values across the entire image of an object of equal density.

urticaria   Itchy, red rash commonly referred to as *hives.*

view   Each data sample made by the DAS during CT data acquisition.

views per rotation (VPR)   The sampling rate of transmission measurements acquired during each gantry rotation.

virtual bronchography   Three-dimensional (3D) fly-through endobrachial views included in a CT bronchography examination.

volume rendering   A three-dimensional (3D) modeling technique that utilizes the entire acquired data set but adjusts the opacity of voxels included in the 3D image according to their tissue characteristics.

voxel   Abbreviation of *volume element.* Refers to the volume of tissue represented by a pixel in the matrix used to display the CT image.

window   The user-defined range of pixel values that will be assigned a particular shade of gray.

window level (WL)   The pixel value, given in Hounsfield units (HU), at the center of the window width. Window level controls the brightness (density) of the CT image.

window width (WW)   The range of pixel values assigned a shade of gray in the displayed CT image. Window width controls the contrast of the CT image.

windowing   The process of gray-scale mapping of the CT image on the basis of the CT number (Hounsfield value) assigned to each pixel.

x-y axis   The plane perpendicular (orthogonal) to the axis of data acquisition (z-axis). The x-y axis is parallel to the plane of the CT gantry.

z-axis   Longitudinal direction of the coordinate system used to spatially describe the location of acquired CT sections. The z-axis corresponds to the axis of data acquisition.

z-filtering   Mathematical process utilized by MSCT systems to reconstruct thin sections at any point along the acquired z-axis volume.

Abbara S, Soni AV, Cury RC: Evaluation of cardiac function and valves by multidetector row computed tomography, *Semin Roentgenol* 43:145-153, 2008.

American College of Radiology: *ACR practice guideline for the performance of high-resolution computed tomography (HRCT) of the lungs in adults*, Reston, VA, 2005, American College of Radiology.

American College of Radiology: *Manual on contrast media, version 6*, Reston, VA, 2008, American College of Radiology.

Adler AM, Carlton RR: *Introduction to radiologic sciences and patient care*, ed 4, Philadelphia, 2007, Elsevier.

Agarwal PP, Chughtai A, Matzinger FRK, Kazerooni EA: Multidetector CT of thoracic aortic aneurysms, *Radiographics* 29:537-552, 2009.

Aird EGA, Conway J: CT simulation for radiotherapy treatment planning, *Br J Radiol* 75:937-949, 2002.

Akbar SA, Mortele KJ, Baeyens K, et al: Multidetector CT urography: techniques, clinical applications, and pitfalls, *Semin Ultrasound CT MRI* 25:41-54, 2004.

Bae KT, Heiken JP, Siegel GL, Bennett HF: Renal cysts: is attenuation artifactually increased on contrast-enhanced CT images? *Radiology* 216:792-796, 2000.

Barrett CP, Anderson LD, Holder L, Poliakoff S: *Primer of sectional anatomy with MRI and CT correlation*, ed 2, Baltimore, 1994, Williams & Wilkins.

Barrett JF, Keat N: Artifacts in CT: recognition and avoidance, *Radiographics* 24:1679-1691, 2004.

Bauhs JA, Vrieze TJ, Primak AN, et al: CT dosimetry: comparison of measurement techniques and devices, *Radiographics* 28:245-253, 2008.

Becker CR, Wintersperger B, Jakobs TF: Multi-detector-row CT angiography of peripheral arteries, *Semin Ultrasound CT MR* 24:268-279, 2003.

Belden CJ, Zinreich SJ: Orbital imaging techniques, *Semin Ultrasound CT MR* 18:413-422, 1997.

Belfiore G, Tedeschi E, Ronza FM, et al: CT-guided radiofrequency ablation in the treatment of recurrent rectal cancer, *AJR Am J Roentgenol* 192:137-141, 2009.

Berland LL: *Practical CT: technology and techniques*, New York, 1987, Raven Press.

Bettmann MA: Frequently asked questions: iodinated contrast agents, *Radiographics* 4:S3-S10, 2004.

Bhalla S, West OC: CT of nontraumatic thoracic aortic emergencies, *Semin Ultrasound CT MR* 26:281-304, 2005.

Blake MA, Kalra MK, Sweeney AT, et al: Distinguishing benign from malignant adrenal masses: multi-detector row CT protocol with 10-minute delay, *Radiology* 238:578-585, 2006.

Blebea JS, Meilstrup JW, Wise SW: Appendiceal imaging: which test is best? *Semin Ultrasound CT MR* 24:91-95, 2003.

Blodgett T: Best practices in PET/CT: consensus on performance of positron emission tomography-computed tomography, *Semin Ultrasound CT MR* 29:236-241, 2008.

Blodgett TM, Meltzer CC, Townsend DW: PET/CT: form and function, *Radiology* 242:360-385, 2007.

Bluemke DA, Urban B, Fishman EK: Spiral CT of the liver: current applications, *Semin Ultrasound CT MR* 15:107-121, 1994.

Bo WJ, Wolfman NT, Krueger WA, Meschan I: *Basic atlas of sectional anatomy with correlated imaging*, ed 2, Philadelphia, 1990, Saunders.

Boone JM: Multidetector CT: opportunities, challenges, and concerns associated with scanners with 64 or more detector rows, *Radiology* 241:334-337, 2006.

Boonn WW, Litt HI, Charagundla SR: Optimizing contrast injection for coronary CT angiography and functional cardiac CT: applications in cardiac imaging, *Appl Radiol* (Suppl), January 2007.

Brink M, deLange F, Oostveen LJ, et al: Arm raising at exposure-controlled multidetector trauma CT of thoracoabdominal region: higher image quality, lower radiation dose, *Radiology* 249:661-670, 2008.

Brown MA: Imaging acute appendicitis, *Semin Ultrasound CT MR* 29:293-307, 2008.

Budoff MJ, Gul K: Computed tomographic cardiovascular imaging, *Semin Ultrasound CT MR* 27:32-41, 2006.

Bushberg JT, Seibert JA, Leidholdt EM, Boone JM: *The essential physics of medical imaging*, Baltimore, 2001, Williams & Wilkins.

Bushong SC: *Computed tomography*, New York, 2000, McGraw-Hill.

Bushong SC: *Radiologic science for technologists*, ed 9, St. Louis, 2008, Elsevier.

Buzug TM: *Computed tomography: from photon statistics to modern cone-beam CT*, Berlin, 2008, Springer-Verlag.

Cademartini F, Luccichenti G, van Der Lugt A, et al: Sixteen-row multislice computed tomography: basic concepts, protocols, and enhanced clinical applications, *Semin Ultrasound CT MR* 25:2-16, 2004.

Carr DH: *Contrast media*, London, 1988, Churchill Livingstone.

Chen JS: Noninvasive coronary plaque evaluation by cardiac CT: applications in cardiac imaging, *Appl Radiol* (Suppl), January 2007.

Chen MY: Coronary artery disease assessment with cardiac CT: applications in cardiac imaging, *Appl Radiol* (Suppl), January 2007.

Chiu LC, Lipcamon JD, Yiu-Chiu VS: *Clinical computed tomography for the technologist*, New York, 1995, Raven Press.

Christian PE, Waterstram-Rich KM: *Nuclear medicine and PET/CT*, ed 6, St. Louis, 2007, Mosby.

Cody DD, Mahadevappa M: Technologic advances in multidetector CT with a focus on cardiac imaging, *Radiographics* 27:1829-1837, 2007.

Cody DD: AAPM/RSNA physics tutorial for residents: topics in CT: image processing in CT, *Radiographics* 22:1255-1268, 2002.

Copstead LEC, Banasik JL: *Pathophysiology*, ed 3, St. Louis, 2005, Elsevier.

Costello P: Spiral CT of the thorax, *Semin Ultrasound CT MR* 15:90-106, 1994.

Crim JR, Moore K, Brodke D: Clearance of the cervical spine in multitrauma patients: the role of advanced imaging, *Semin Ultrasound CT MR* 22:283-305, 2001.

Crim JR, Ripp D: Multidetector CT of the spine, *Semin Ultrasound CT MR* 25:55-66, 2004.

Curry TS, Dowdey JE, Murry RE: *Christensen's physics of diagnostic radiology*, ed 4, Philadelphia, 1990, Lea & Febiger.

Dalrymple NC, Prasad SR, El-Merhi FM, Chintapalli KN: Price of isotropy in multidetector CT, *Radiographics* 27:49-62, 2007.

Dalrymple NC, Srinivasa RP, Freckleton MW, Kedar NC: Informatics in radiology (infoRAD): introduction to the language of three-dimensional imaging with multidetector CT, *Radiographics* 25:1409-1428, 2005.

DeMaio D: *Registry review in computed tomography*, Philadelphia, 1996, Saunders.

Desser TS, Gross M: Multidetector row computed tomography of small bowel obstruction, *Semin Ultrasound CT MR* 29:308-321, 2008.

DeWever W, Bogaert J, Verschakelen JA: Virtual bronchoscopy: accuracy and usefulness—an overview, *Semin Ultrasound CT MR* 26:364-373, 2005.

Ehrlich RA, McCloskey ED, Daly JA: *Patient care in radiography*, ed 6, St. Louis, 2004, Mosby.

Einstein AJ, Moser KW, Thompson RC, et al: Radiation dose to patients from cardiac diagnostic imaging, *Circulation* 116:1290-1305, 2007.

El-Khoury GY, Montgomery WJ, Bergman RA: *Sectional anatomy by MRI and CT*, ed 3, Philadelphia, 2007, Churchill Livingstone.

Fefferman NR, Roche KJ, Oinkney LP, et al: Suspected appendicitis in children: focused CT technique for evaluation, *Radiology* 220:691-695, 2001.

Filipek MS, Gosselin MV: Multidetector pulmonary CT angiography: advances in the evaluation of pulmonary arterial diseases, *Semin Ultrasound CT MR* 25:83-98, 2004.

Firooznia H, Golimbu CN, Rafii M, et al: *MRI and CT of the musculoskeletal system*, St. Louis, 1992, Mosby-Year Book.

Fishman EK, Jeffrey RB: *Spiral CT: principles, techniques and clinical applications*, New York, 1995, Raven Press.

Fiss DM: Normal coronary anatomy and anatomic variations: applications in cardiac imaging, *Appl Radiol* (Suppl), January 2007.

Fleischmann D: A practical approach to contrast delivery for peripheral CTA, *Appl Radiol* (Suppl), December 2004.

Flohr TG, Schaller S, Stierstorfer K, et al: Multi-detector row CT systems and image-reconstruction techniques, *Radiology* 235:756-773, 2005.

Flukinger T, White CS: Multidetector computed tomography in the evaluation of chest pain in the emergency department, *Semin Roentgenol* 43:136-144, 2008.

Foley WD, Kerimoglu U: Abdominal MDCT: liver, pancreas, and biliary tract, *Semin Ultrasound CT MR* 25:122-144, 2004.

Frank ED, Long BW, Smith BJ: *Merrill's atlas of radiographic positioning and procedures*, ed 11, St. Louis, 2007, Mosby.

Frush DP, Soden B, Frush KS, Lowry C: Improved pediatric multidetector body CT using a size-based color-coded format, *AJR Am J Roentgenol* 178:721-726, 2002.

Frush DP: Review of radiation issues for computed tomography, *Semin Ultrasound CT MR* 25:17-24, 2004.

Furlow B: *Computed tomography and magnetic resonance angiography*, 1999, American Society of Radiologic Technologists (ASRT).

Gedgaudas-McClees RK, Torres WE: *Essentials of body computed tomography*, Philadelphia, 1990, Saunders.

Gerber TC, Breen JF, Kuzo RS, et al: Computed tomographic angiography of the coronary arteries: techniques and applications, *Semin Ultrasound CT MR* 27:42-55, 2006.

Goldman LW: Principles of CT and CT technology, *J Nucl Med Technol* 35:115-128, 2007.

Goldman LW: Principles of CT: multislice CT, *J Nucl Med Technol* 36:57-68, 2008.

Goldman LW: Principles of CT: radiation dose and image quality, *J Nucl Med Technol* 35:213-225, 2007.

Gonzalez-Beicos A, Nunez DB: Role of multidetector computed tomography in the assessment of cervical spine trauma, *Semin Ultrasound CT MR* 30:159-167, 2009.

Green D, Parker D: CTA and MRA: visualization without catheterization, *Semin Ultrasound CT MR* 24:185-191, 2003.

Grenier PA, Beigelman-Aubry C, Fetita C, Martin-Bouyer Y: Multidetector-row CT of the airways, *Semin Roentgenol* 38:146-157, 2003.

Gruden JF, Tigges S, Baron MG, Pearlman H: MDCT pulmonary angiography: image processing tools, *Semin Roentgenol* 40:48-63, 2005.

Gupta R, Cheung AC, Bartling SH, et al: Flat-panel volume CT, fundamental principles, technology, and applications, *Radiographics* 28:2009-2022, 2008.

Guyton AC, Hall JE: *Textbook of medical physiology*, ed 11, Philadelphia, 2006, Saunders.

Haaga JR, Lanzieri CF, Gilkeson RC: *CT and MR imaging of the whole body*, ed 4, St. Louis, 2003, Mosby.

Haage P, Schmitz-Rode T, Hübner D, et al: Reduction of contrast material dose and artifacts by a saline flush using a double power injector in helical CT of the thorax, *AJR Am J Roentgenol* 174:1049-1053, 2000.

Herts BR, O'Malley CM, Wirth SL, et al: Power injection of contrast media using central venous catheters: feasibility, safety, and efficacy, *AJR Am J Roentgenol* 176:447-453, 2001.

Hoeffner EG, Case I, Jain R, et al: Cerebral perfusion CT: technique and clinical applications, *Radiology* 231:632-644, 2004.

Hofer M: *CT teaching manual*, ed 3, New York, 2007, Thieme.

Hofmann LK, Becker CR, Flohr T, Schoepf UJ: Multidetector-row CT of the heart, *Semin Roentgenol* 38:135-145, 2003.

Hollingsworth C, Frush DP, Cross M, Lucaya J: Helical CT of the body: a survey of techniques used for pediatric patients, *AJR Am J Roentgenol* 180:401-406, 2003.

Hopper KD: CT bronchoscopy, *Semin Ultrasound CT MR* 20:10-15, 1999.

Hopper KD: Orbital, thyroid, and breast superficial radiation shielding for patients undergoing diagnostic CT, *Semin Ultrasound CT MR* 23:423-427, 2002.

Huda W, Ogden KM, Khorasani MR: Converting dose-length product to effective dose at CT, *Radiology* 248:995-1003, 2008.

Huda W, Ravenel JG, Scalzetti EM: How do radiographic techniques affect image quality and patient doses in CT? *Semin Ultrasound CT MR* 23:411-422, 2002.

Hunsaker AR: Multidetector-row CT and interstitial lung disease, *Semin Roentgenol* 38:176-185, 2003.

Hurwitz LM, Yoshizumi TT, Goodman PC, et al: Radiation dose savings for adult pulmonary embolus 64-MDCT using bismuth breast shields, lower peak kilovoltage, and automatic tube current modulation, *AJR Am J Roentgenol* 192:244-253, 2009.

Israel GM, Bosniak MA: How I do it: evaluating renal masses, *Radiology* 236:441-450, 2005.

Jacobs JE, Birnbaum BA: CT imaging in acute appendicitis: techniques and controversies, *Semin Ultrasound CT MR* 24:96-100, 2003.

Jakobs TF, Wintersperger BJ, Becker CR: MDCT-imaging of peripheral arterial disease, *Semin Ultrasound CT MR* 25:145-155, 2004.

Jeffrey RB: CT angiography of the abdominal and thoracic aorta, *Semin Ultrasound CT MR* 19:405-412, 1998.

Jensen SC, Peppers MP: *Pharmacology and drug administration for imaging technologists*, ed 2, St. Louis, 2006, Elsevier.

Judy PF: Multidetector-Row CT image quality and radiation dose: imaging the lung, *Semin Roentgenol* 38:186-192, 2003.

Kalender WA: *Computed tomography*, ed 2, Erlangen, 2005, Germany, Publicis Corporate Publishing.

Kalender WA: Technical foundations of spiral CT, *Semin Ultrasound CT MR* 15:81-89, 1994.

Kalender WA: Thin-section three-dimensional spiral CT: is isotropic imaging possible? *Radiology* 197:578-580, 1995.

Kalra MK, Maher MM, Toth TL, et al: Strategies for CT radiation dose optimization, *Radiology* 230:619-628, 2004.

Kalra MK, Maher MM, Toth TL, et al: Techniques and applications of automatic tube current modulation for CT, *Radiology* 233:649-657, 2004.

Kanada D, Catanzano TM: The role of cardiac CT for function: evaluation of perfusion, volumetric analysis, and regional wall motion assessment: applications in cardiac imaging, *Appl Radiol* (Suppl), January 2007.

Kapoor V, McCook BM, Torok FS: An introduction to PET-CT imaging, *Radiographics* 24:523-543, 2004.

Katz DS, Loud PA, Hurewitz AN, et al: CT venography in suspected pulmonary thromboembolism, *Semin Ultrasound CT MR* 25:67-80, 2004.

Katzberg RW: *The contrast media manual*, Baltimore, 1992, Williams & Wilkins.

Kawamoto S, Johnson PT, Fishman EK: Three-dimensional CT angiography of the thorax: clinical applications, *Semin Ultrasound CT MR* 19:425-438, 1998.

Kawashima A, Vrtiska TJ, LeRoy AJ, et al: CT urography, *Radiographics* 24:S35-S58, 2004.

Kelley LL, Petersen CM: *Sectional anatomy for imaging professionals*, ed 2, St. Louis, 2007, Mosby.

Knollman F, Coakley FV: *Multislice CT: principles and protocols*, Philadelphia, 2006, Elsevier.

Kuszyk BS, Beauchamp NJ, Fishman EK: Neurovascular applications of CT angiography, *Semin Ultrasound CT MR* 19:394-404, 1998.

Kuszyk BS, Fishman EK: Technical aspects of CT angiography, *Semin Ultrasound CT MR* 19:383-393, 1998.

Lake DR, Kavanagh JJ, Ravenel JG, et al: Computed tomography and pulmonary embolus: a review, *Semin Ultrasound CT MR* 26:270-280, 2005.

Lane A, Sharfaei H: *Modern sectional anatomy*, Philadelphia, 1992, Saunders.

Lane JI, Lindell EP, Witte RJ, et al: Middle and inner ear: improved depiction with multiplanar reconstruction of volumetric CT data, *Radiographics* 26:115-124, 2006.

Laudicina P, Wean D: *Applied angiography for radiographers*, Philadelphia, 1994, Saunders.

Lawler LP, Pannu HK, Fishman EK: MDCT evaluation of the coronary arteries, 2004: how we do it—data acquisition, postprocessing, display, and interpretation, *AJR Am J Roentgenol* 184:1402-1412, 2005.

Lee CH, Goo JM, Lee HJ, et al: Radiation dose modulation techniques in the multidetector CT era: from basics to practice, *Radiographics* 28:1451-1459, 2008.

Lee JKT, Sagel SS, Stanley RJ, Heiken JP: *Computed body tomography with MRI correlation*, ed 4, Philadelphia, 2006, Lippincott Williams & Wilkins.

Lee MJ, Kim S, Lee SA, et al: Overcoming artifacts from metallic orthopedic implants at high-field-strength MR imaging and multidetector CT, *Radiographics* 27:791-803, 2007.

Lell MM, Anders K, Uder M, et al: New techniques in CT angiography, *Radiographics* 26:S45-S62, 2006.

Lewis MA: Patient dose reduction in CT, *Br J Radiol* 78:880-883, 2005.

Loud PA, Katz DS, Belfi L, Grossman ZD: Imaging of deep venous thrombosis in suspected pulmonary embolism, *Semin Roentgenol* 40:33-40, 2005.

Luetmer PH, Mokri B: Dynamic CT myelography: a technique for localizing-high-flow spinal cerebrospinal fluid leaks, *Am J Neuroradiol* 24:1711-1714, 2003.

MacDonald SLS, Mayo JR: Computed tomography of acute pulmonary embolism, *Semin Ultrasound CT MR* 24:217-231, 2003.

Maglinte DDT, Sandrasegaran K, Lappas JC, Chlorean M: CT enteroclysis, *Radiology* 245:661-671, 2007.

Mahesh M: The AAPM/RSNA physics tutorial for residents: search for isotropic resolution in CT from conventional through multiple-row detector, *Radiographics* 22:949-962, 2002.

Mahesh M, Scatarige JC, Cooper J, Fishman EK: Dose and pitch relationship for a particular multislice CT scanner, *AJR Am J Roentgenol* 177:1273-1275, 2001.

Mayo JR, Leipsic JA: Radiation dose in cardiac CT, *AJR Am J Roentgenol* 192:646-653, 2009.

McCollough CH: Standardization in CT terminology: a physicist's perspective, *Radiology* 241:661-662, 2006.

McCollough CH, Bruesewitz MR, Kofler JM: CT dose reduction and dose management tools: overview of available options, *Radiographics* 26:503-512, 2006.

McNitt-Gray MF: AAPM/RSNA physics tutorial for residents: topics in CT: radiation dose in CT, *Radiographics* 22:1541-1553, 2002.

Menke J: Comparison of different body size parameters for individual dose adaptation in body CT of adults, *Radiology* 236:565-571, 2005.

Mochizuki T, Hosoi S, Higashino H, et al: Assessment of coronary artery and cardiac function using multidetector CT, *Semin Ultrasound CT MR* 25:99-112, 2004.

Moloo J, Shapiro MD, Abbara S: Cardiac computed tomography: technique and optimization of protocols, *Semin Roentgenol* 43:90-99, 2008.

Mosby's Dictionary of Medicine: *Nursing & health professions*, ed 8, St. Louis, 2009, Mosby.

Moser T, Dosch JC, Moissoui A, et al: Multidetector CT arthrography of the wrist joint: how to do it, *Radiographics* 28:787-800, 2008.

Moss AA, Gamsu GG, Genant HK: *Computed tomography of the body with magnetic resonance imaging*, ed 2, Philadelphia, 1992, Saunders.

Mullins ME, Kircher MF, Ryan DP, et al: Evaluation of suspected appendicitis in children using limited helical CT and colonic contrast material, *AJR Am J Roentgenol* 176:37-41, 2001.

Murray JG, Gean AD, Evans SJJ: Imaging of acute head injury, *Semin Ultrasound CT MR* 17:185-205, 1996.

Naidich DP, Webb WR, Müller NL, et al: *Computed tomography and magnetic resonance of the thorax*, ed 4, Philadelphia, 2007, Lippincott Williams & Wilkins.

Newbold K, Partridge M, Cook G, et al: Advanced imaging applied to radiotherapy planning in head and neck cancer: a clinical review, *Br J Radiol* 79:554-561, 2006.

Newman J, Hladik WB: Pharmacology for the radiologic technologist. Part 2: intravascular radiopaque contrast media, *ASRT Homestudy Series* 2(2), 1997.

Nghiem HV, Jeffrey RB: CT Angiography of the visceral vasculature, *Semin Ultrasound CT MR* 19:439-446, 1998.

Nguyen BT, Mulins ME: Computed tomography follow-up imaging of stroke, *Semin Ultrasound CT MR* 27:168-176, 2006.

Nickoloff EL, Lu ZF, Dutta AK, So JC: Radiation dose descriptors: bERT, COD, DAP, and other strange creatures, *Radiographics* 28:1439-1450, 2008.

Parry RA, Glaze SA, Archer BR: The AAPM/RSNA physics tutorial for residents: typical patient radiation doses in diagnostic radiology, *Radiographics* 19:1289-1302, 1999.

Patel S, Lieberman S: Computed tomography of coronary artery disease, *Semin Roentgenol* 43:122-135, 2008.

Paulsen SR, Huprich JE, Fletcher JG, et al: CT enterography as a diagnostic tool in evaluating small bowel disorders: review of clinical experience with over 700 cases, *Radiographics* 26:641-662, 2006.

Pickhardt PJ: Screening CT colonography: how I do it, *AJR Am J Roentgenol* 189:290-298, 2007.

Pomerantz SR, Harris GJ, et al: Computed tomography angiography and computed tomography perfusion in ischemic stroke: a step-by-step approach to image acquisition and three-dimensional postprocessing, *Semin Ultrasound CT MR* 27:243-270, 2006.

Prat-Gonzalez S, Sanz J, Garcia MJ: Cardiac CT: indications and limitations, *J Nucl Med Technol* 36:18-24, 2008.

Primak AN, McCollough CH, Bruesewitz MR, et al: Relationship between noise, dose, and pitch in cardiac multidetector row CT, *Radiographics* 26:1785-1794, 2006.

Putman CE, Ravin CE: *Textbook of diagnostic imaging*, ed 2, Philadelphia, 1994, Saunders.

Ravenel JG, Kipfmueller F, Schoepf UJ: CT angiography with multidetector-row CT for detection of acute pulmonary embolus, *Semin Roentgenol* 40:11-19, 2005.

Rivitz SM, Drucker EA: Power injection of peripherally inserted central catheters, *J Vasc Interv Radiol* 8:857-863, 1997.

Rubin GD, Rofsky NM: *CT and MR angiography: comprehensive vascular assessment*, Philadelphia, 2008, Lippincott Williams & Wilkins.

Rubin GD: CT angiography of the thoracic aorta, *Semin Roentgenol* 38:115-134, 2003.

Rumberger JA: Coronary artery calcium scanning using computed tomography: clinical recommendations for cardiac risk assessment and treatment, *Semin Ultrasound CT MR* 29:223-229, 2008.

Saini S, Rubin GD, Kalra MK: *MDCT: a practical approach*, Milan, 2006, Springer-Verlag.

Saini S: Multi-detector row CT: principles and practice for abdominal applications, *Radiology* 233:323-327, 2004.

Schnapauff D, Zimmermann E, Dewey M: Technical and clinical aspects of coronary computed tomography angiography, *Semin Ultrasound CT MR* 29:167-175, 2008.

Schoepf UJ, Costello P: CT angiography for diagnosis of pulmonary embolism: state of the art, *Radiology* 230:329-337, 2004.

Schoepf UJ, Costello P: Multidetector-row CT imaging of pulmonary embolism, *Semin Roentgenol* 38:106-114, 2003.

Schwartz RB: Neuroradiological applications of spiral CT, *Semin Ultrasound CT MR* 15:139-147, 1994.

Seeram E: *Computed tomography*, ed 3, St. Louis, 2009, Saunders.

Seeram E: *Computed tomography: a study guide and review*, Philadelphia, 1997, Saunders.

Semba CP, Rubin GD, Dake MD: Three-dimensional spiral CT angiography of the abdomen, *Semin Ultrasound CT MR* 15:133-138, 1994.

Shanmuganathan K: Multi-detector row CT imaging of blunt abdominal trauma, *Semin Ultrasound CT MR* 25:180-204, 2004.

Sheth S, Fishman EK: Multi-detector row CT of the kidneys and urinary tract: techniques and applications in the diagnosis of benign disease, *Radiographics* 24:e20, 2004.

Shetty SK, Lev MH: CT perfusion in acute stroke, *Semin Ultrasound CT MR* 26:404-421, 2005.

Shreve P: PET/CT: changing the practice of medical imaging—PET-CT protocols and techniques. In *Program and abstracts of the society of nuclear medicine mid-winter educational symposium*, January 29–30, 2005, Tampa, FL.

Silverman PM: *Multislice computed tomography*, Philadelphia, 2002, Lippincott Williams & Wilkins.

Silverman SG, Leyendecker JR, Amis ES: What is the current role of CT urography and MR urography in the evaluation of the urinary tract? *Radiology* 250:309-323, 2009.

Singh J, Daftary A: Iodinated contrast media and their adverse reactions, *J Nucl Med Technol* 36:69-74, 2008.

Sistrom CL, Gay SB, Peffley L: Extravasation of iopamidol and iohexol during contrast-enhanced CT: report of 28 cases, *Radiology* 180:707-710, 1991.

Smith AB, Dillon WP, Lau BC, et al: Radiation dose reduction strategy for CT protocols: successful implementation in neuroradiology section, *Radiology* 247:499-506, 2008.

Smith PA, Fishman EK: Three-dimensional CT angiography: renal applications, *Semin Ultrasound CT MR* 19:413-424, 1998.

Snopek AM: *Fundamentals of special radiographic procedures*, ed 5, St. Louis, 2006, Elsevier.

Srinivasan A, Goyal M, Al Azri F, Lum C: State-of-the-art imaging of acute stroke, *Radiographics* 26:S75-S95, 2006.

Staffey KS, van Beek EJR, Jagasia D: Clinical performance and considerations in coronary CTA: applications in cardiac imaging, *Appl Radiol* (Suppl).

Standring S: *Gray's anatomy*, ed 40, St. Louis, 2008, Elsevier.

Strauss KJ, Goske MJ, Frush DP, et al: Image gently vendor summit: working together for better estimates of pediatric radiation dose from CT, *AJR Am J Roentgenol* 192:1169-1175, 2009.

Taber's cyclopedic medical dictionary, ed 20, Philadelphia, 2005, FA Davis.

Tack D, Gevenois PA: Efforts for lowering radiation dose delivered with CT: raising arms, or is there more? *Radiology* 249:413-415, 2008.

Takakuwa KM, Halpern EJ: Evaluation of a "triple rule-out" coronary CT angiography protocol: use of 64-Section CT in low-to-moderate risk emergency department patients suspected of having acute coronary syndrome, *Radiology* 248:438-446, 2008.

Taourel P, Thuret R, Devaux-Hoquet M, et al: Computed tomography in the nontraumatic renal causes of acute flank pain, *Semin Ultrasound CT MR* 29:341-352, 2008.

Tepel M, Aspelin P, Lameire N: Contrast-induced nephropathy: a clinical and evidence-based approach, *Circulation* 113:1799-1806, 2006.

The merck manual, ed 18, Whitehouse Station, NJ, 2006, Merck Research Laboratories.

Thomas BP, Strother MK, Donnelly EF, Worrell JA: CT virtual endoscopy in the evaluation of large airway disease: review, *AJR Am J Roentgenol* 192:S20-S30, 2009.

Torres LS: *Basic medical techniques and patient care*, ed 4, Philadelphia, 1993, JB Lippincott.

Tortorici MR, Apfel PJ: *Advanced radiographic and angiographic procedures*, Philadelphia, 1995, FA Davis.

Trotman-Dickenson B, Baumert B: Multidetector-row CT of the solitary pulmonary nodule, *Semin Roentgenol* 38:158-167, 2003.

Valentin J: International commission on radiation protection: managing patient dose in multi-detector computed tomography (MDCT): ICRP publication 102, *Ann ICRP* 37:1-79, 2007.

Vining DJ: Virtual colonoscopy, *Semin Ultrasound CT MR* 20:56-60, 1999.

von Schulthess GK, Steinert HC, Hany TF: Integrated PET/CT: current applications and future directions, *Radiology* 238:405-422, 2006.

Vu D, Lev MH: Noncontrast CT in acute stroke, *Semin Ultrasound CT MR* 26:380-386, 2005.

Wang CL, Cohan RH, Ellis JH, et al: Frequency, management, and outcome of extravasation of nonionic iodinated contrast medium in 69,657 intravenous injections, *Radiology* 180:707-710, 1991.

Wang ZJ, Coakley FV, Fu Y, et al: Renal cyst pseudoenhancement at multidetector CT: what are the effects of number of detectors and peak tube voltage, *Radiology* 248:910-916, 2008.

Webb WR, Brant WE, Major NM: *Fundamentals of body CT*, ed 3, Philadelphia, 2006, Elsevier.

Webb WR, Müller NL, Naidich DP: *High-resolution of the lung*, ed 4, Philadelphia, 2009, Lippincott Williams & Wilkins.

Wesolowski JR, Lev MH: CT: history, technology, and clinical aspects, *Semin Ultrasound CT MR* 26:376-379, 2005.

Wicke L: *Atlas of radiologic anatomy*, ed 5, Philadelphia, 1994, Lea & Febiger.

Wiest PW, Locken JA, Heintz PH, Mettler FA: CT scanning: a major source of radiation exposure, *Semin Ultrasound CT MR* 23:402-410, 2002.

Wijetunga R, Doust B, Bigg-Wither G: The CT diagnosis of acute appendicitis, *Semin Ultrasound CT MR* 24:101-106, 2003.

Williamson EE, McKinney JM: Assessing the adequacy of peripherally inserted central catheters for power injection of intravenous contrast agents for CT, *J Comput Assist Tomogr* 25:932-937, 2001.

Wintersperger BJ, Nikolaou K, Becker CR: Multidetector-row CT angiography of the aorta and visceral arteries, *Semin Ultrasound CT MR* 25:25-40, 2004.

Wolbarst AB: *Physics of radiology*, Norwalk, CT, 1993, Appleton & Lange.

Wyatt SH, Fishman EK: Spiral CT of the pancreas, *Semin Ultrasound CT MR* 15:122-132, 1994.

Zimmermann E, Schnapauff D, Dewey M: Cardiac and coronary anatomy in computed tomography, *Semin Ultrasound CT MR* 29:176-181, 2008.

Zompatori M, Sverzellati N, Poletti V, et al: High-resolution CT in diagnosis of diffuse infiltrative lung disease, *Semin Ultrasound CT MR* 26:332-347, 2005.

Note: Page numbers followed by *b* indicates boxes, *f* indicates figures and *t* indicates tables.